SPORT FIRST AID

Fifth Edition

Melinda J. Flegel, MS, ATC, LAT, CSCS

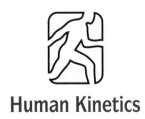

Human Kinetics

Library of Congress Cataloging-in-Publication Data

Flegel, Melinda J., 1958-
  Sport first aid / Melinda J. Flegel, MS, ATC, LAT, CSCS. -- Fifth edition.
      pages cm
  Includes bibliographical references and index.
  1. Sports injuries--Treatment. 2. First aid in illness and injury. I. Title.
  RD97.F525 2013
  617.1'027--dc23

                              2013022686

ISBN: 978-1-4504-6890-9 (print)

Developmental Editor: Christine M. Drews; **Managing Editor:** Julie Marx Goodreau; **Copyeditors:** Patrick Connolly and Jan Feeney; **Indexers:** Marie Rizzo and Alisha Jeddeloh; **Permissions Manager:** Martha Gullo; **Graphic Designer:** Fred Starbird; **Graphic Artist:** Tara Welsch; **Cover Designer:** Keith Blomberg; **Photograph (cover):** David Allio/Icon SMI; **Photographs (interior):** © Human Kinetics, unless otherwise noted; **Photo Asset Manager:** Laura Fitch; **Visual Production Assistant:** Joyce Brumfield; **Photo Production Manager:** Jason Allen; **Art Manager:** Kelly Hendren; **Associate Art Manager:** Alan L. Wilborn; **Illustrations:** © Human Kinetics, unless otherwise noted; **Printer:** Versa Press

Human Kinetics books are available at special discounts for bulk purchase. Special editions or book excerpts can also be created to specification. For details, contact the Special Sales Manager at Human Kinetics.

Printed in the United States of America   20 19 18 17 16

The paper in this book is certified under a sustainable forestry program.

Human Kinetics
1607 N. Market Street
Champaign, IL 61820
USA

United States and International
Website: **US.HumanKinetics.com**
Email: info@hkusa.com
Phone: 1-800-747-4457

Canada
Website: **Canada.HumanKinetics.com**
Email: info@hkcanada.com

Tell us what you think!
Human Kinetics would love to hear what we
can do to improve the customer experience.
Use this QR code to take our brief survey.

E6157

Contents

Preface

Being a successful coach requires knowing more than just the skills and strategies of a sport. It includes being able to teach techniques and tactics, motivate athletes, and manage a myriad of details. *And* it involves fulfilling the role of being a competent first responder to athletes' injuries and illnesses.

The National Federation of State High School Associations (NFHS) reported that 7,692,520 high school youth participated in sports programs in 2011-2012. In a study of nine sports (football, boys' and girls' basketball, boys' and girls' soccer, baseball, softball, volleyball, and wrestling) from a randomly selected sample of 100 U.S. high schools in 2011-2012, researchers estimated that approximately 1,392,262 injuries occurred among athletes participating in those sports (Comstock et al., 2012). The researchers estimated that approximately 740,493 of the injuries occurred during competition, while 651,769 occurred during practice.

Ideally you would have medical professionals such as certified athletic trainers (ATs) or emergency medical technicians (EMTs) available for every competition and practice. Unfortunately less than 42% of U.S. high schools have access to certified athletic trainers who are specially trained to evaluate, treat, and prevent athletic injuries. If athletic trainers are available at your school, they won't be able to attend every practice and competition for every sport. EMTs or physicians may attend some competitions, but they aren't at every competition or any practices. So as a coach, you will often be the one responsible for administering first aid to your injured athletes.

To help you meet the challenge of administering first aid to your injured athletes, the American Sport Education Program (ASEP) has developed the Sport First Aid course. This fifth edition of *Sport First Aid* serves as the text for that course.

Sport First Aid and the accompanying Sport First Aid course cover protocols for these tasks:

1. Conducting emergency action steps
2. Conducting the physical assessment and administering first aid for bleeding, tissue damage, and unstable injuries
3. Moving injured athletes and returning athletes to play

In addition to the Sport First Aid course, ASEP also offers the widely used Coaching Principles course and the Coaching [Sport] Technical and Tactical Skills courses. Together, these courses compose ASEP's Bronze Level curriculum (see appendix B). ASEP delivers these courses to interscholastic coaches throughout the nation through the ASEP Professional Coaches Education Program, adopted in whole or in part by 30 state high school associations.

Throughout its development and revision *Sport First Aid* was reviewed by experts representing key areas of sports medicine specialization. Their close scrutiny and invaluable feedback ensure that this is a scientifically sound, relevant, and current text for coaches. The protocols described here also have been revised to reflect the 2010 American Heart Association Guidelines for Cardiopulmonary Resuscitation and Emergency Cardiovascular Care.

However, ASEP wants to emphasize that this is a *sport first aid* book, not a general guide to medical procedures. The contents of this text are tailored to the athletic context, with the perspective that the coach is the initial responder to most athletes' injuries and is not medically trained to provide care beyond the initial first aid response.

Sport First Aid focuses on the recognition and emergency treatment of sports injuries on the playing field. Most basically, this book explains what you should do and what you should not do when an athlete suffers an injury.

Part I of this text introduces you to the teamwork and preparation needed for effective sport first aid. Chapter 1 covers your role on the athletic health care team, including your responsibilities and limitations. You will learn what others, including parents and the legal system, expect from you as a sport first aider. You'll learn about other members of the athletic health care team and how to interact with them to make your efforts successful. Chapter 2 includes guidelines on how to prepare for your duties on the athletic health care team. This includes using preseason conditioning programs, creating safe playing environments, planning for weather emergencies, ensuring proper fitting and use of protective equipment, enforcing proper sports skills and safety rules, and developing a medical emergency plan. Using these strategies, you can greatly reduce your athletes' risk of injury or illness.

In part II you will learn the fundamentals of sport first aid. Chapter 3 covers anatomy and sport first aid terminology. Chapter 4 explains how to conduct the emergency action steps and provide first aid for life-threatening conditions such as choking. It includes updated guidelines for performing cardiopulmonary resuscitation (CPR), performing the Heimlich maneuver, and using an automated external defibrillator (AED). Evaluating and caring for the more common conditions of bleeding, shock, unstable injuries, and local tissue damage are outlined in chapter 5, which focuses on the physical assessment. Chapter 6 shows you how to safely move an injured athlete.

Part III covers over 110 different injuries and illnesses, and includes evaluation, first aid, prevention, and return to play strategies for each of these injuries and illnesses. Chapters 7 through 11 cover potential life-threatening problems such as respiratory conditions, head, spine, and nerve injuries, internal organ injuries, sudden illnesses, and temperature-related illnesses. Though these problems occur infrequently, when they do, you'll need to be prepared to provide quick and appropriate first aid, because it may help you save an athlete's life. In chapters 12 through 15, you'll learn how to recognize and provide first aid for more common sport-related upper body and lower body musculoskeletal injuries, face and scalp injuries, and skin conditions.

ASEP originally developed this book as the text for its Sport First Aid course. It was designed to provide interscholastic and club sport coaches with first aid skills and a basic understanding of sports injuries. In its fifth edition, this text continues to be a primary resource for the Sport First Aid course, which now is delivered two ways—in the classroom and online. For more information on either version of the Sport First Aid course, including when the next classroom course will be offered near you, contact ASEP by phone (800-747-5698) or e-mail (asep@hkusa. com), or visit ASEP's website (www.asep.com).

Armed with this information and skills from this *Sport First Aid* text and the accompanying course, ASEP believes you'll be able to administer first aid to your athletes confidently and competently. The health and success of your athletes depend on it.

REFERENCES

Comstock, R.D., Collins, C.L., Corlette, J.D. and Fletcher, E.N. 2013. National High School Sports-Related Injury Surveillance Study: 2011-2012. Retrieved on June 6, 2013, from http://www.nationwidechildrens.org/cirp-rio-study-reports.

Field, J.M. et al. 2010. Part 1: Executive summary: 2010 American Heart Association Guidelines for Cardiopulmonary Resuscitation and Emergency Cardiovascular Care. *Circulation* 122 (suppl 3): S640 –S656.

National Federation of State High School Associations. 2011-12 High School Athletics Participation Survey Results. Downloaded on June 6, 2013 from http://www.nfhs.org/content. aspx?id=3282.

Travers, A.H., et al. 2010. Part 4: CPR overview: 2010 American Heart Association Guidelines for Cardiopulmonary Resuscitation and Emergency Cardiovascular Care. *Circulation* 122 (suppl 3): S676 –S684.

Acknowledgments

Lord . . . all that we have accomplished you have done for us.

Isaiah 26:12

A project of this magnitude would not be possible without the help of many people. So, I would like to extend my heartfelt gratitude to everyone who assisted in any way with this fifth edition. Chris Drews, Julie Marx Goodreau, Martha Gullo, Fred Starbird, and many other dedicated employees at Human Kinetics helped me shape the revisions for this new edition and assisted with the book's development, production, and distribution. I would also like to thank my family, friends, and coworkers for providing their never-ending support and encouragement. Last, but not least, I want to thank you, the reader, for your commitment to providing a safe sport environment for your athletes.

PART I

Introduction to Sport First Aid

"Individual commitment to a group effort—that is what makes a team work . . ."

Vince Lombardi

Being a successful athletic health care team requires teamwork and a will to prepare. No athlete who is out of shape or unfamiliar with the team can walk onto a playing field and expect to contribute toward a victory. The same is true of being an effective sport first aider.

Chapter 1 introduces you to your role on the athletic health care team, including your responsibilities and limitations. You'll learn what parents and the legal authorities expect from you as a sport first aider. And you will become familiar with other members of the athletic health care team and how to interact with them to make your efforts successful.

Just as an athlete needs preseason preparation or conditioning to achieve success, you also need to be prepared for your duties on the athletic health care team. Part of the preparation involves developing strategies for injury prevention. Chapter 2 will get you started by offering tips on utilizing preseason conditioning programs, creating safe playing environments, planning for weather emergencies, and enforcing proper sport skills and safety rules. This chapter also helps you prepare for sport first aid situations by giving you guidelines for formulating a medical emergency plan. Using these strategies, you can greatly reduce your athletes' risk of injury or illness.

Your Role on the Athletic Health Care Team

IN THIS CHAPTER, YOU WILL LEARN:

▸ What the athletic health care team is and who is part of it.

▸ What your role is on the athletic health care team.

▸ What first aid knowledge parents expect you to have.

▸ What types of physicians you might work with and what your role is in working with them.

▸ What emergency medical personnel, athletic trainers, and physical therapists do and what your role is in working with them.

▸ Why treatment and rehabilitation are important parts of first aid followup.

From the starter's gun to the finish line, a winning relay team runs like a well-oiled machine. Each team member has a special role—the leadoff is expected to get a fast start, the second leg executes a quick and smooth transition, the third leg helps establish a lead, and the final leg confidently and coolly competes under pressure. One person makes a mistake and the whole team could lose. The same is true for the athletic health care team. Each member has a specific role in ensuring proper emergency evaluation and care of injured or ill athletes. If one team member is slow to start, drops the baton, or oversteps the bounds of that member's role, the athlete will ultimately suffer. It can cause further injury, delay the athlete's recovery, or have catastrophic consequences.

There are four legs in the race to keep athletes healthy (figure 1.1). The first leg is injury and illness prevention. The second is injury and illness recognition and first aid care. The third leg is assessment or diagnosis and treatment, and the fourth leg is rehabilitation.

Many different team members can participate:

- Athlete
- Parents
- Coach
- Emergency medical technician or paramedic
- Doctors
- Athletic trainer
- Physical therapist
- Dentist or oral surgeon
- Optometrist

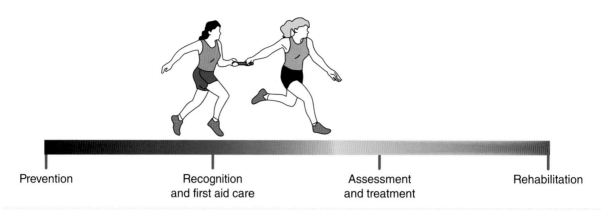

Figure 1.1 Athletic health care relay legs.

- Strength and conditioning coach
- Equipment manager

This relay race is unique in that the various members may participate in more than one leg. For example, as athletic health specialists, athletic trainers may participate in three or four legs of the race. Athletes themselves are in each leg of the race.

Before further discussing each of the team members and each member's role, let's explore some of your roles on the athletic health care team.

COACH'S ROLE ON THE ATHLETIC HEALTH CARE TEAM

As a coach you are likely to be involved in each portion of the athletic health care relay—prevention, recognition and first aid care, assessment and treatment, and rehabilitation.

Your roles are defined by

- certain rules of the legal system and rules of your school administration,
- expectations of parents, and
- interactions with other athletic health care team members.

Legal Definitions of Your Role

Basically, the legal system supports the theory that a coach's primary role is to minimize the risk of injury to the athletes under the coach's supervision. This encompasses a variety of duties.

1. Properly plan the activity.
   - Teach the skills of the sport in the correct progression.
   - Consider each athlete's developmental level and current physical condition. Evaluate your athletes' physical capacity and skill level with preseason fitness tests, and develop practice plans accordingly.
   - Keep written records of fitness test results and practice plans. Don't deviate from your plans without good cause.

2. Provide proper instruction.
   - Make sure that athletes are in proper condition to participate.
   - Teach athletes the rules and the correct skills and strategies of the sport. For example, in football teach athletes that tackling with the head (spearing) is illegal and also a potentially dangerous technique.
   - Teach athletes the sport skills and conditioning exercises in a progression so that the athletes are adequately prepared to handle more difficult skills or exercises.
   - Keep up-to-date on better and safer ways of performing the techniques used in the sport.
   - Provide competent and responsible assistants. If you have coaching assistants, make sure that they are knowl-

edgeable in the skills and strategies of the sport and act in a mature and responsible manner.

3. Warn of inherent risks.
- Provide parents and athletes with both oral and written statements of the inherent health risks of their particular sport.
- Also warn athletes about potentially harmful conditions, such as playing conditions, dangerous or faulty equipment, and the like.

4. Provide a safe physical environment.
- Monitor current environmental conditions (i.e., windchill, temperature, humidity, and severe weather warnings).
- Periodically inspect the playing areas, the locker room, the weight room, and the dugout for hazards.
- Remove all hazards.
- Prevent improper or unsupervised use of facilities.

5. Provide adequate and proper equipment.
- Make sure athletes are using equipment that provides the maximum amount of protection against injury.
- Inspect equipment regularly.
- Teach athletes how to fit, use, and inspect their equipment.

6. Match your athletes appropriately.
- Match the athletes according to size, physical maturity, skill level, and experience.
- Do not pit physically immature or novice athletes against those who are in top condition and are highly skilled.

7. Evaluate athletes for injury or incapacity.
- Require all athletes to submit to preseason physicals and screenings to detect potential health problems.
- Withhold an athlete from practice and competition if the athlete is unable to compete without pain or loss of function (e.g., inability to walk, run, jump, throw, and so on without restriction).

→ Playing It Safe...
With Return to Play

Under no circumstances should athletes be allowed to return to activity if they exhibit any of the following conditions:

- Loss of function. This means not being able to walk, run, sprint, jump, or hop without limping. For the arms, it may mean not being able to throw, catch, hit a ball, or grip with the hand.
- Fever.
- Headaches, memory loss, dizziness, ringing in the ears, or unresponsiveness from a head injury.
- Heat- or cold-related illnesses.
- Pain with activity.

An athlete with any of these problems must be examined and released by a physician before returning to full activity.

8. Supervise the activity closely.
- Do not allow athletes to practice difficult or potentially dangerous skills without proper supervision.
- Forbid horseplay, such as "wrestling around."
- Do not allow athletes to use sports facilities without supervision.

9. Provide appropriate emergency assistance.
- Learn sport first aid and cardiopulmonary resuscitation (CPR). (Take a course through the American Red Cross, American Heart Association, or the National Safety Council.)
- Take action when needed. The law assumes that you, as a coach, are responsible for providing first aid care for any injury or illness suffered by an athlete under your supervision. So, if no medical personnel are present when an injury occurs, you are responsible for providing emergency care.

- Use only the skills that you are qualified to administer and provide the specific standard of care that you are trained to provide through sport first aid, CPR, and other sports medicine courses.
- If athlete is a minor, obtain a signed written consent form from their parents before the season. For injured adult athletes, specifically ask if they want help. If they are unresponsive, consent is usually implied. If they refuse help, you are not required to provide it. In fact, if you still attempt to give care, they can sue you for assault.

Some states expect coaches to meet additional standards of care. Check with your athletic director to find out if your state has specific guidelines for the quality of care to be provided by coaches.

You should become familiar with each of these 9 legal duties. The first 8 duties deal mainly with preventive measures, which are explained more thoroughly in chapter 2. This book is primarily designed to help you handle duty number 9.

Parental Expectations

Parents will look to you for direction when their child is injured. They may ask questions such as these:

What do you think is wrong with my child's knee?

Will it get worse if my child continues playing?

Should my child see a doctor?

Does my child need to wear protective knee braces for football?

Will taping help prevent my child from reinjuring the ankle?

When can my child start competing again?

While you can't have all the answers, it helps to know those who can. That's where the other athletic health care team members can help. Let's look at the other members of the team, their roles, and your roles in interacting with them.

OTHER MEMBERS OF THE ATHLETIC HEALTH CARE TEAM

Your role on the athletic health care team is often defined by other members of the team. You can encourage athletes to take responsibility for their own health care. Parents not only need information from you (keeping them informed of preventive measures and injuries or illnesses their child has sustained), but they can also provide you with valuable support, such as ensuring that their child gets preseason physicals and follows your rules for injury and illness prevention. Finally, having good working relationships with athletic health care specialists can make for smooth baton passes from one leg of the relay to the next.

Athletes

First and foremost, the athletes must buy into their role in their own health care. They need to actively participate in preseason physicals, fitness screenings, conditioning, and also in their own injury assessment and care. It is also crucial that they understand the importance of reporting their injuries and illnesses to their parents, coaches, or other members of the athletic health care team. Finally, athletes must adhere to restrictions regarding their participation due to injury or illness.

Parents

Parents can assist other athletic health care team members by ensuring that their child participates in preseason physicals, fitness screenings, and conditioning. Parents can also watch for signs of injury or illness and ensure that their child reports such signs to coaches or other members of the athletic health care team. Finally, parents should support decisions by athletic health care team members to restrict their child's participation due to injury or illness.

Your role is to keep parents informed of possible injuries or illnesses that their child has sustained.

Emergency Medical Personnel and Paramedics

Emergency medical technicians (EMTs) and paramedics are specially trained to handle emergency medical problems. They are highly skilled in evaluating and monitoring urgent and serious medical problems, as well as in providing basic medical care. They are also experts in immobilizing serious injuries and providing swift and safe transportation to emergency medical facilities.

Try to become acquainted with the emergency medical personnel in your area. They may be willing to volunteer or contract their time and rescue vehicles to provide emergency care during tournaments and contests involving contact sports such as football or wrestling.

Once emergency medical personnel arrive on the scene of an injury, you should let them assume the care of the athlete. They handle health emergencies every day and are better trained than you. Your role is to assist them as needed by

1. providing information on how the injury occurred and what first aid care you have provided,
2. taking charge of crowd control, and
3. performing other tasks when asked.

If emergency personnel are not present when an athlete is injured, your role is to

1. protect the athlete from further harm,
2. send someone to call emergency medical personnel (if necessary),
3. evaluate the injury,
4. administer first aid, and
5. provide the EMTs with information on how the emergency occurred and what first aid care was provided.

Physicians

Physicians are the only members of the athletic health care team who are qualified to diagnose athletic injuries and illnesses. The physician can also prescribe illness and injury treatment and rehabilitation.

Types of Physicians

Which type of physician should an injured athlete see—a family practitioner, pediatrician, orthopedist, podiatrist? The athlete's parents or legal guardian (or the athlete's insurance plan) ultimately dictate the answer, but they may ask for your advice. To respond knowledgeably, it helps to know the various types of physicians.

Family practitioners specialize in general medicine for families. This includes infants to senior citizens.

Pediatricians specialize in providing medical care for infants through teenagers.

Orthopedists are trained to diagnose and provide medical and surgical care for injuries to bones, muscles, and other joint tissues such as cartilage, tendons, ligaments, and nerves.

Ophthalmologists are physicians specializing in the medical and surgical care of the eyes and in the prevention of eye disease and injury.

Physiatrists are physicians that specialize in diagnosing, treating, and prescribing rehabilitation for all forms of conditions that affect the musculoskeletal system.

Podiatrists, or foot doctors, provide medical and surgical care for leg and foot problems. They can also make special shoe inserts to correct alignment problems of the feet and legs.

Many of the physician specialty groups, such as orthopedics and pediatrics, offer special sports medicine training courses to their members. Physicians who have received this training are particularly sensitive to the special needs of athletes. They will do all they can to get athletes back to full participation as quickly and as safely as possible.

If you cannot find a physician with sports medicine training, then a physician who is personally active in sports and exercise may also be sensitive to an injured athlete's unique needs.

Working With Physicians

As a coach, you should try to establish a close working relationship with a physician. You may ask the physician for assistance in conducting team physicals and preseason screenings, or in teaching sports medicine basics to your coaching staff. Some physicians may volunteer or contract to provide medical coverage for home games.

Once a physician has examined an athlete, it's important that you support the physician's recommendations. This includes following any restrictions on sports participation. If the parent or legal guardian is not satisfied with the physician's diagnosis and treatment, seeking a second opinion may be warranted. However, it is unethical for the parents or guardians, or you, to send an athlete to numerous physicians in an attempt to get permission for the athlete to resume activity.

After a physician has evaluated an injured athlete, you should urge the athlete to seek follow-up care with an athletic trainer or physical therapist. These professionals are trained to analyze strength, joint motion, flexibility, coordination, and other physical attributes, and then instruct the athlete in an individualized rehabilitation program. They are also trained in administering modalities such as whirlpools, massage, ultrasound and muscle stimulation, and therapies such as joint mobilization. These modalities are important to help ease pain, decrease swelling, promote tissue healing, and restore function for a safe return to sports participation.

You should advise the athlete to obtain a referral from a physician. The athlete can then make an appointment with an athletic trainer (if one is not available at your school) or a physical therapist at a local sports medicine clinic, physical therapy clinic, or hospital physical therapy department.

Certified Athletic Trainers

Athletic trainers (ATCs) are nationally certified allied health professionals trained specifically in the prevention, evaluation, treatment, and rehabilitation of athletic injuries. During practices and competitions, athletic trainers can immediately evaluate and provide care for injuries, plus determine if an injured athlete can participate. They are trained to rehabilitate injuries so that athletes can safely return to sports. These individuals are also qualified to fit athletes with protective padding and equipment and provide supportive taping and protective bandaging.

Athletic trainers must work under the supervision or referral of a physician. In the high school setting, athletic trainers may work exclusively as an athletic trainer or work as a teacher during the day and as an athletic trainer before and after school. Sometimes athletic trainers who work in a sports medicine, orthopedic, or physical therapy facility are contracted or "loaned" to high schools to provide services. If your school does not employ an athletic trainer, you may want to suggest investigating these avenues for hiring one. Having an athletic trainer on site will ensure quicker and more thorough evaluations and care of injured athletes, and it can also free up the coaching staff to concentrate primarily on coaching.

Athletic trainers can also help to prevent injuries by screening athletes and developing and implementing preseason conditioning programs. Specifically, they evaluate the athletes' strength, flexibility, and coordination, and then develop individualized conditioning programs. Finally, athletic trainers can offer valuable tips on proper exercise technique for your athletes.

When an athlete has been injured, your role in working with an athletic trainer is to

- provide information on how the injury occurred,
- support the athletic trainer's decisions regarding the athlete's care and ability to participate, and
- encourage the athlete to be compliant in doing rehabilitation exercises.

Physical Therapists

Physical therapists (PTs) are health professionals who rehabilitate individuals suffering from disease or injury. They are trained to handle a wide variety of medical problems, including cerebral palsy, strokes, heart problems, paraplegia, burns, and athletic injuries.

Some PTs specialize in the evaluation, care, and rehabilitation of sports injuries. To do so, they must complete 2,000 hours of clinical sports medicine experience and successfully pass a sport physical therapy examination. Such individuals are then recognized as sport physical therapists.

When an athlete has been injured, your role in working with a physical therapist is the same as working with an athletic trainer:

- Provide information on how the injury occurred.
- Support the physical therapist's decisions regarding the athlete's care and ability to participate.
- Encourage the athlete to be compliant in doing rehabilitation exercises.

Dentists or Oral Surgeons

Both dentists and oral surgeons are trained to evaluate and treat conditions and injuries of the mouth, teeth, and jaw. Dentists have three or more years of undergraduate education plus four years of dental school. Oral surgeons are dentists who have completed a hospital surgical residency program for further training in the surgical treatment of conditions affecting the mouth, teeth and jaw, and portions of the face.

Your role is to encourage athletes in contact sports to wear appropriate protective mouthpieces or face protectors.

Optometrists

Although not a medical doctor, optometrists receive specialized training and certification in diagnosing vision problems and eye disease. They are also trained to prescribe eyeglasses, contact lenses, and drugs to treat eye disorders.

Your role is to encourage athletes in contact sports to wear appropriate protective eyewear or face protectors.

Strength and Conditioning Coaches

Strength and conditioning coaches can save you valuable time and energy by performing fitness assessments and developing and supervising specialized conditioning programs for athletes. The programs emphasize the fitness needs for specific positions (e.g., balance beam specialist or linebacker) and specific sports (e.g., golf or wrestling). The best-trained strength and conditioning coaches have completed certifications through national organizations such as the National Strength and Conditioning Association and the American College of Sports Medicine.

Your role is to insist that athletes attend fitness assessments and participate in all conditioning workouts.

Equipment Managers

Equipment managers can take on the role of overseeing the inspection, cleaning and maintenance, and storage of equipment, as well as equipment fitting. In working with the equipment manager, your role is to assist as needed with equipment fitting and maintenance, and to enforce proper equipment use by your athletes. You should also help watch for equipment wear and tear.

Table 1.1 summarizes the common roles of each member of the athletic health care team.

Table 1.1   Athletic Health Care Team Roles

Team member	Leg 1 – Prevention	Leg 2 – Recognition and first aid care	Leg 3 – Assessment and treatment	Leg 4 – Rehabilitation
Athlete	• Submit to preseason screening and physical • Participate in conditioning programs • Wear appropriate protective equipment • Abide by safety rules	• Inform parent, coach, or athletic trainer of illness or injury • Submit to injury or illness assessment by physician, athletic trainer, or sports physical therapist	Submit to first aid care or physician treatment	• Perform rehabilitation and conditioning exercises exactly as instructed • Only return to activities when instructed
Parent	• Ensure athlete participates in preseason screening and physical • Ensure athlete participates in conditioning programs • Ensure athlete wears appropriate protective equipment	• Watch for injuries and illnesses • Ensure athlete's injury or illness is thoroughly evaluated and receives proper treatment	Ensure athlete submits to appropriate first aid or physician treatment	• Encourage athlete to exactly follow rehabilitation and conditioning instructions • Don't allow athlete to participate until given clearance
Coach	• Ensure athlete participates in preseason screening and physical • Ensure athlete participates in conditioning programs • Ensure athlete wears appropriate protective equipment • Enforce safety rules	• Watch for injuries and illnesses • Act as first responder in providing first aid assessment and care • Recommend athlete's injury or illness be thoroughly evaluated and receives proper treatment	Act as first responder in providing first aid care	• Encourage athlete to exactly follow rehabilitation and conditioning instructions • Don't allow athlete to participate until given clearance
Physician	Conduct preseason physicals	• Volunteer or contract to provide on-site emergency medical assistance at sporting events • Evaluate athlete by conducting or ordering appropriate diagnostic tests	• Prescribe appropriate treatment • Refer injured athlete to athletic trainer or physical therapist for rehabilitation	• May recommend or prescribe specific rehabilitation exercises • May provide final clearance for return to full participation
Dentist or oral surgeon	Recommend and fit mouth guards	Evaluate dental injuries	Treat dental injuries	Provide final clearance for return to full activity after dental injury

Role				
Optometrist	Recommend and fit appropriate protective eyewear			
Emergency medical technician or paramedic		Volunteer or contract to provide on-site emergency medical assessment, care, and transportation at sporting events		
Athletic trainer	• Provide preseason fitness and injury risk assessment screening • Assist with scheduling and conducting preseason physicals • Recommend or develop conditioning programs • Inspect condition of equipment and playing areas • Recommend replacement or refurbishing of faulty equipment or playing areas • Ensure proper equipment fitting for each athlete • Recommend preventative bracing or taping as needed	• Watch for injuries and illnesses • Act as first responder in providing first aid assessment and care • Assist emergency medical technicians or paramedics in preparing an athlete for transportation to a medical facility • Recommend physician diagnosis as needed	Provide injury treatments (such as ultrasound) as prescribed by a physician	• Assess athlete's symptoms and ability to function • Develop individualized rehabilitation program • Maintain athlete's fitness during rehabilitation • Safely progress athlete back into full activity • Develop and fit protective braces or pads to prevent reinjury
Physical therapist	**Sports physical therapist—** • Provide preseason fitness and injury risk assessment screening • Recommend preventative bracing or taping as needed	**Sports physical therapist—** • Watch for injuries and illnesses • Act as first responder in providing first aid assessment and care • Recommend physician diagnosis as needed	Provide injury treatments (such as ultrasound) as prescribed by a physician	• Assess athlete's symptoms and ability to function • Develop individualized rehabilitation program • Maintain athlete's fitness during rehabilitation • Safely progress athlete back into full activity **Sports physical therapist—** Develop and fit protective braces or pads to prevent reinjury
Equipment manager	• Inspect condition of equipment • Replace or oversee refurbishing of faulty equipment • Ensure proper equipment fitting for each athlete			
Strength and conditioning coach	• Provide preseason fitness screening • Develop and supervise conditioning programs			Encourage athlete to exactly follow rehabilitation and conditioning instructions

Chapter 1 *REPLAY*

- ☐ Do you minimize the risk of injury to your athletes by doing the following?
    - ☐ Properly plan the activity. (p. 4)
    - ☐ Provide proper instruction. (pp. 4-5)
    - ☐ Warn of inherent risks. (p. 5)
    - ☐ Provide a safe physical environment. (p. 5)
    - ☐ Provide adequate and proper equipment. (p. 5)
    - ☐ Match your athletes appropriately. (p. 5)
    - ☐ Evaluate athletes for injury or incapacity. (p. 5)
    - ☐ Supervise the activity closely. (p. 5)
    - ☐ Provide appropriate emergency assistance. (pp. 5-6)
- ☐ Are you ready to provide information regarding how an injury occurred? Do you support the decisions of the athletic health care team and encourage athletes during rehabilitation? (p. 6)
- ☐ Have you become acquainted with the emergency personnel, physicians, athletic trainers, and physical therapists in your area? Do you have a list of various types of local physicians to refer athletes to? (p. 7)
- ☐ Have you developed a working relationship with a local physician? The physician may be used as a resource and may conduct team physicals or preseason screenings. (p. 8)

RECOMMENDED READING

McCaskey, A.S., and K.W. Biedzynski. 1996. A guide to the legal liability of coaches for a sports participant's injuries. *Seton Hall Journal of Sport Law* 6(1):7-125.

Spengler, J.D., Connaughton, D.P., and A.T. Pittman. 2006. *Risk Management in Sport and Recreation*. Champaign, IL: Human Kinetics.

CHAPTER 7

Sport First Aid Game Plan

IN THIS CHAPTER, YOU WILL LEARN:

- ▸ How to keep yourself educated about sport first aid.
- ▸ What health records you should keep for each athlete.
- ▸ How to develop and initiate a weather emergency plan.
- ▸ What to look for when checking facilities for hazards and equipment for proper fit and usage.
- ▸ What to include in a first aid kit.
- ▸ Why you should incorporate preseason physicals, fitness screenings, and conditioning programs into your game plan.
- ▸ How to develop a medical emergency plan.

To get your team ready for competition, you plan practices, develop playing strategies, and prepare your players. Through experience you know that this pregame planning process is essential to success. The same is true for sport first aid. To handle injuries effectively, you have to plan for them. You don't want to be caught unprepared for a critical health situation involving blood loss, unresponsiveness, or breathing difficulties. This chapter shows you how to prepare by gathering athletes' health records, developing emergency plans, stocking your first aid kit, and incorporating physical screening and conditioning into your overall program.

SPORT FIRST AID EDUCATION

ASEP strongly recommends that you supplement what you learn from this book (and from the Sport First Aid course) with certification in cardiopulmonary resuscitation (CPR) and automated external defibrillator (AED) use. You can obtain certification through the American Red Cross or the American Heart Association. These programs are recognized nationally as standards for providing first aid care. Upon achieving certification, you will be expected to provide the standard of care taught in the certification program.

Keeping Current

Because improvements are constantly being made in sports medicine, you need to keep yourself up-to-date on the latest in sport first aid. The sport first aid techniques used in the future will be very different and much better than the methods advocated now. Following are ways to keep up with these changes:

- Read current sports medicine books and articles to learn the newest techniques.
- Keep your first aid training and CPR certification current. Some CPR certifications only last for one to two years.
- Attend sports medicine and sport first aid seminars and clinics. The Sport First Aid course will be updated as advances in this area warrant, so plan to attend another course in the next few years (see appendix B for more information).

Recognizing Limitations

Even if you educate yourself extensively in sport first aid, do not attempt the duties of a physician. Recognize your limitations. Only provide the care that you are qualified to provide. An athlete may suffer for many years from the damage you can cause by overstepping the limits of your training. And if you do act irresponsibly and harm an athlete, you may end up the target of a lawsuit. If medical personnel are present, give them complete control to handle any illnesses or injuries, but assist them if requested.

KEEPING ATHLETES' HEALTH RECORDS

Like most coaches, you probably keep statistical records of your athletes' performances. Are you also familiar with each athlete's health information? If not, collect the following information from each player:

- Consent form
- Health history form
- Emergency information card

Consent Form

Remember, you cannot give first aid care to a minor unless you have consent. Before the season, you must have parents or legal guardians complete and return an explicitly worded consent form for their children. A form similar to the one shown in figure 2.1 informs the parents or guardians, and the athlete, of the inherent risks of sport and requests permission from the parent or guardian to treat the child for an emergency illness or injury.

Health History Form

It is very important to know whether any of your athletes have health problems that could affect their sports participation. Diabetes, asthma, epilepsy, heart murmurs, and skin conditions are among these problems. If a physician clears an athlete with a health problem for participation, you should have a record of the following:

- The health problem
- Special medications the athlete may need to take
- Activity restrictions for the athlete

A health history form (figure 2.2) will give you this information.

Emergency Information Card

In the event of an emergency, you must be able to contact the athlete's parents or guardian and physician. An emergency information card (figure 2.3, page 17) will provide their names and numbers. It should also alert you to informa-

Informed Consent Form

I hereby give my permission for _____ to participate in _____ during the athletic season beginning in _____. Further, I authorize the school to provide emergency treatment of any injury or illness my child may experience if qualified medical personnel consider treatment necessary and perform the treatment. This authorization is granted only if I cannot be reached and a reasonable effort has been made to do so.

Date _____ Parent or guardian _____

Address _____ Phone (   )_____

Cell phone (   )_____ Beeper number (   )_____

Family physician _____ Phone (   ) _____

Medical conditions (e.g., allergies or chronic illnesses) _____

_____

Other person to contact in case of emergency _____

Relationship with person _____ Phone (   ) _____

My child and I are aware that participating in _____ is a potentially hazardous activity. We assume all risks associated with participation in this sport, including, but not limited to, falls, contact with other participants, the effects of the weather, traffic, and other reasonable risk conditions associated with the sport. All such risks to my child are known and appreciated by my child and me.

We understand this informed consent form and agree to its conditions.

Child's signature _____ Date _____

Parent's or guardian's signature _____ Date _____

Figure 2.1 Informed consent form.

tion on any preexisting medical problems that may influence the treatment of an athlete. The athlete's parents must complete this card before the season. When the team practices or competes away from your school, you should take a copy of the card with you.

Remember that an athlete's health history and injury status are confidential pieces of information. Therefore, respect your athletes by keeping this information in a secure location and also by not speaking about the athlete's condition (to fans, players, media, and so forth) unless you have written permission from the athlete and the athlete's parent or guardian.

DEVELOPING A WEATHER EMERGENCY PLAN

Lightning, tornadoes, floods, hail, hurricanes, and other weather emergencies can create chaos during outdoor practices and competitions. To eliminate the chaos and prevent injuries to athletes, staff, and spectators, you should develop and implement a weather emergency plan. Here are some key elements to include (Walsh et al. 2000):

- *Weather decision maker*—Name of the individual who is responsible for deciding when to cease practices and competitions.
- *Specific criteria for when to suspend activities*—For example, to prevent lightning injuries, seek shelter if thunder occurs within 30 seconds of a lightning strike. Or, just the occurrence of thunder, without lightning, is enough to stop activities (Walsh et al. 2000).
- *Weather watcher*—Name of the individual who is responsible for monitoring weather reports for watches and warnings, and notifying the decision maker of serious weather conditions.
- *Method for monitoring weather conditions*—A weather radio, for example.

Athletic Medical Examination for _____
(sport)

Name _____ Age _____ Birth date _____

Address _____ Phone _____
       (street)   (city)   (zip)

Instructions

All questions must be answered. Failure to disclose pertinent medical information may invalidate your insurance coverage and may cancel your eligibility to participate in interscholastic athletics. Any further health problems must be discussed with the physician at the time of this examination.

Medical History

Have you ever had any of the following? If "yes," give details to the examining doctor.

	No	Yes	Details (if answered yes)
1. Head injury or concussion	___	___	_____
2. Bone or joint disorders, fractures, dislocations, trick joints, arthritis, or back pain	___	___	_____
3. Eye or ear problems (disease or surgery)	___	___	_____
4. Heat illness	___	___	_____
5. Dizzy spells, fainting, or convulsions	___	___	_____
6. Tuberculosis or bronchitis	___	___	_____
7. Heart trouble or rheumatic fever	___	___	_____
8. High or low blood pressure	___	___	_____
9. Anemia, leukemia, or bleeding disorder	___	___	_____
10. Diabetes, hepatitis, or jaundice	___	___	_____
11. Ulcers, other stomach trouble, or colitis	___	___	_____
12. Kidney or bladder problems	___	___	_____
13. Hernia (rupture)	___	___	_____
14. Mental illness or nervous breakdown	___	___	_____
15. Addiction to drugs or alcohol	___	___	_____
16. Surgery or advised to have surgery	___	___	_____
17. Taking medication regularly	___	___	_____
18. Allergies or skin problems	___	___	_____
19. Menstrual problems; LMP	___	___	_____
20. Diagnosed as having sickle cell trait	___	___	_____

Signature _____ Date _____

Figure 2.2 Health history form.

Emergency Information Card

Athlete's name _____ Age _____

Address _____

Home phone _____ Cell phone _____

Sport _____

List two persons to contact in case of emergency:

Parent's or guardian's name _____ Home phone _____

Address _____ Work phone _____

Second person's name _____ Home phone _____

Address _____ Work phone _____

Relationship to athlete _____

Insurance co. _____ Policy no. _____

Physician's name _____ Phone _____

Are you allergic to any drugs? _____ If so, what? _____

Do you have any allergies (e.g., bee stings or dust)? _____

Do you have _____ asthma, _____ diabetes, or _____ epilepsy? (Check any that apply)

Do you take any medications? _____ If so, what? _____

Do you wear contact lenses? _____

Other _____

Signature _____ Date _____

Figure 2.3 Emergency information card.

- *Designated safe place*—Area to seek shelter from serious weather conditions. For lightning protection, buildings are the best form of shelter. Do not allow anyone to use telephones connected to lines or to use showers, tubs, or pools. If shelter is not available, vehicles with metal roofs and closed windows are another option. For hail, tornadoes, hurricanes, and damaging winds, seek shelter in a basement, inner room, or hallway that is away from windows.

- *Guidelines for resuming activity*—Outline of specific criteria that have to be met before activity can resume. For example, in cases of lightning, do not leave the shelter until 30 minutes after the last lightning strike or clap of thunder.

Educate staff, athletes, and spectators regarding your emergency weather plan.

CHECKING FACILITIES AND EQUIPMENT

Although preparation and care of the playing area may be the responsibility of a groundskeeper or janitor, you are responsible for checking its safety. Litter, slippery floors, broken goals, worn playing surfaces, and countless other problems can lead to injury. Be sure to check for any hazards and have them fixed before the season (figure 2.4).

Check sports equipment before every season. Inspect sticks, rackets, bats, gymnastics apparatus, protective helmets and pads, and other equipment for damage. Be sure that goalposts, net standards, landing pits, and gymnastics apparatus are well padded and secured.

You'll also need equipment and supplies for handling injuries. A first aid kit and ice cooler

Facilities Inspection Checklist

Name of inspector _____ Date of inspection _____

Name and location of facility _____

_____

Note: This form is an incomplete checklist provided as an example. Use it to develop a checklist specific to your facilities.

Facility Condition

Circle Y (yes) if the facility is in good condition or N (no) if it needs something done to make it acceptable. In the space provided, note what needs to be done.

Gymnasium

Y N Floor (water spots, buckling, loose sections)	Y N Mats (clean, properly stored, no defects)
Y N Walls (vandalism free and padded, if appropriate)	Y N Uprights or projections (padded)
	Y N Wall plugs (covered)
Y N Lights (all functioning)	Y N Light switches (all functioning)
Y N Windows (secure)	Y N Heating or cooling system (temperature control)
Y N Roof (adverse impact of weather)	
Y N Stairs (well lighted)	Y N Ducts, radiators, and pipes
Y N Bleachers (support structure sound)	Y N Thermostats
Y N Exits (lights working)	Y N Fire alarms (regularly checked)
Y N Basketball rims (level, securely attached)	Y N Directions posted for evacuating the gym in case of fire
Y N Basketball backboards (no cracks, clean)	Y N Fire extinguishers (regularly checked)

Other (list) _____

_____

Locker rooms

Y N Floor	Y N Benches
Y N Walls	Y N Lockers
Y N Lights	Y N Exits
Y N Windows	Y N Water fountains
Y N Roof	Y N Toilets
Y N Showers	Y N Athletic trainer's room
Y N Drains	

Other (list) _____

_____

Figure 2.4   Facilities inspection checklist.

Adapted from Human Kinetics, 1985, *American Coaching Effectiveness Program Level 2 Sport Law Workbook* (Champaign, IL: Author), 40-41, and J.R. Olson, "Safety checklists: Making indoor areas hazard-free," *Athletic Business*, November 1985, 36-38.

Field or outside playing area

Y N	Stands	Y N	Sprinklers	Y N	Goal posts
Y N	Pitching mound	Y N	Garbage	Y N	Net
Y N	Dugouts	Y N	Security fences	Y N	Net standards
Y N	Track and fences	Y N	Water fountain		
Y N	Sidelines	Y N	Storage sheds		

Other (list) _____

_____

Pool

Y N   Equipment in good repair   Y N   Chemicals safely stored

Y N   Sanitary   Y N   Regulations and safety rules posted

Y N   Slipperiness on decks and diving board
       controlled

Lighting—adequate visibility

Y N   No glare

Y N   Penetrates to bottom of pool

Y N   Exit light in good repair

Y N   Halls and locker rooms meet code
       requirements

Y N   Light switches properly grounded

Y N   Has emergency generator to back up
       regular power source

Ring buoys

Y N   20-inch diameter

Y N   50-foot rope length

Safety line at break point in the pool grade (deep end)

Y N   Bright color floats

Y N   3/4-inch rope

Exits—accessible and secure

Y N   Adequate size, number

Y N   Self-closing doors

Y N   Self-locking doors

Y N   Striker plates secure

Y N   No obstacles or debris

Y N   Office and storage rooms locked

Guard chairs

Y N   Unobstructed view

Y N   Tall enough to see bottom of pool

First aid kit

Y N   Inventoried and replenished regularly

Stretcher, two blankets, and spine board

Y N   Inventoried and in good repair

Track

Y N   Throwing circles

Y N   Fences

Y N   Water fountain

Surface

Y N   Free of debris

Y N   Free of holes and bumps

Other (list) _____

_____

Recommendations/observations _____

_____

_____

_____

Stocking the First Aid Kit

A well-stocked first aid kit includes the following items:

- Antibacterial soap or wipes
- Arm sling
- Athletic tape—one and a half inch
- Bandage scissors
- Bandage strips—assorted sizes
- Blood spill kit
- Cell phone
- Contact lens case
- Cotton swabs
- Elastic wraps—three inch, four inch, and six inch
- Emergency blanket
- Examination gloves—latex free
- Eye patch
- First aid cream or antibacterial ointment
- Foam rubber—one-eighth inch, one-fourth inch, and one-half inch
- Insect sting kit
- List of emergency phone numbers
- Mirror
- Moleskin
- Nail clippers
- Oral thermometer (to determine if an athlete has a fever due to illness)
- Penlight
- Petroleum jelly
- Plastic bags for crushed ice
- Prewrap—underwrap for tape (for taping)
- Rectal thermometer (for use in cases of suspected heat illness)
- Safety glasses—for first aiders
- Safety pins
- Saline solution for eyes
- Sterile gauze pads—three-inch and four-inch squares (preferably non-stick)
- Sterile gauze rolls
- Sunscreen—sun protection factor (SPF) 30 or greater
- Tape adherent and tape remover
- Tongue depressors
- Tooth saver kit
- Triangular bandages
- Tweezers

must be available on the sidelines at every competition and practice.

When stocking your first aid kit, include only the items necessary for administering basic sport first aid. Omit all medicines, both over-the-counter (such as aspirin, pain medications, or decongestants) and prescription drugs. It is illegal for you to give any kind of medicine to athletes. Also, don't include iodine; some athletes are allergic to it.

→ Playing It Safe...
When Administering Medicine

It is illegal for you to give athletes any kind of medicine, including over-the-counter medicine such as aspirin, pain medications, and decongestants.

GETTING PLAYERS READY TO PERFORM

Athletes who are not in shape are more likely to be injured. To ensure that players are ready, institute these methods:

- Preseason physical exam
- Preseason screening
- Preseason conditioning
- Proper warm-up and cool-down
- Protective equipment, bracing, and taping
- Correct skill instruction
- Sound nutritional guidance
- Ban on horseplay

Disqualifying Medical Conditions

Some common problems found by the examining physician that could disqualify athletes from competition or limit their participation include the following:

- Uncontrolled diabetes
- Uncontrolled asthma
- Heart conditions
- Uncontrolled high blood pressure
- Epilepsy
- Previous head injuries
- Previous spinal injuries
- Chronic orthopedic problems (e.g., unstable knees, ankles, or shoulders)

In the past, individuals with the sickle cell trait were often disqualified from athletic participation because it was believed that carrying the trait put them at particular risk for sudden death. However, in a large-scale study of military recruits, Eckart et al. (2004) showed that the risk of sudden death was actually higher in those without the sickle cell trait than in those with the sickle cell trait. This doesn't mean that carrying the sickle cell trait is without risk in sports, but it does mean that it is not a condition that should disqualify athletes from sport participation.

Preseason Physical Exam

The first step in preparing an athlete for participation in sports is to require a preseason physical. A physician should conduct a very thorough examination that includes a general health exam as well as circulatory, respiratory, neurological, orthopedic, vision, and hearing examinations. Routine blood and urine analyses should also be performed. The physician should note and consider any preexisting or potential health problems when deciding whether an athlete is cleared to participate.

All athletes must turn in their physical exam forms prior to the season. Familiarize yourself with the records of athletes who have specific conditions that could affect their participation, such as asthma, diabetes, severe allergies, and epilepsy. Keep all forms in a secure file for future reference.

Preseason Screening

Although the physical exam will detect specific health problems, it does not provide insight about an athlete's fitness. A preseason screening can provide this information.

Preseason screening should be conducted in the off-season by a specially trained health professional, such as an athletic trainer, or by a fitness professional such as a certified strength and conditioning coach. Depending on the sport, each athlete should be evaluated for the following:

- *Strength* in the muscle groups most often used in the particular sport—for example, a football player's neck strength or a basketball player's ankle strength.
- *Flexibility* or tightness in the major muscle groups and tendons—hamstrings, quadriceps, shoulder, calf, and Achilles tendon.
- *Endurance* in muscles that undergo repetitive or sustained contraction.
- *Cardiovascular endurance* (especially for endurance athletes such as cross country runners, track athletes, triathletes, and cyclists).
- *Body composition* or percent body fat (especially important for wrestlers, gymnasts, and track athletes who severely restrict their diets to control their weight).
- *Upper and lower body coordination* to determine if an athlete's muscles fire quickly enough to protect a joint from injury. An example is a one-leg balance test where an athlete is timed to see how long the athlete can stand on one leg without wobbling or putting the other foot down.

These tests pinpoint potential fitness problems that can lead to injury. Coaches or athletic trainers should teach athletes conditioning exercises to help them improve these problems before the season.

Preseason Conditioning

Get athletes in shape by starting them on a conditioning program at least six weeks before the season. Conditioning exercises should focus on muscle strength, endurance, flexibility, power, and speed needed for the sport.

To improve strength, athletes need to perform at least two sets of six to eight repetitions of each exercise, 3 days a week. Postpubescent athletes should lift at least 70 percent of their maximum to gain strength. Although well-supervised resistance training has proven safe for prepubescent athletes, you can avoid weightlifting-related injuries by emphasizing activities that require these athletes to support their own body weight (e.g., push-ups). Training 3 days a week for at least 20 continuous minutes is necessary to improve cardiovascular endurance. And to improve flexibility, athletes should perform stretching exercises at least 5 days a week.

These are just basic guidelines for training athletes. For more information on preseason screening and conditioning, consult ASEP's *Successful Coaching* (Martens 2012).

Proper Warm-Up and Cool-Down

Be sure that your athletes warm up before workouts, practices, and competitions. This doesn't mean going out 5 minutes before practice and hitting or throwing a few balls. A proper warm-up is an exercise routine that prepares the body for vigorous physical activity. Athletes should warm up at least 15 minutes prior to activity using this sequence:

1. *General body warm-up.* Athletes jog or bike at a low intensity for 5 to 10 minutes. The intensity of the general warm-up should cause a slight increase in the heart and breathing rates. It should also cause the athlete to break into a light sweat. This helps to prepare the heart, lungs, muscles, and tendons for vigorous activity. Ultimately it helps to prevent injury as well as improve performance.

2. *Light calisthenics exercises.* After a general warm-up, athletes continue to warm up specific areas with appropriate calisthenic exercises such as

    • push-ups,
    • jumping jacks,
    • abdominal crunches,
    • lunges,
    • carioca (cross-over run).

3. *Sport-specific drills.* These are drills that allow athletes to practice the skills of their particular sport. For example, sport-specific softball drills include batting and throwing. In tennis and racquetball drills, players practice serves as well as backhand and forehand shots.

At the end of each practice, workout, or competition, athletes should gradually cool their bodies down. In other words, they should slowly reduce the intensity of their activity until their heart and breathing rates drop to near normal resting levels. Suddenly stopping exercise inhibits recovery from activity and can lead to problems such as fainting. Cool-down activities may include walking or light jogging for 5 to 10 minutes.

Athletes should conclude the cool-down with stretching. Since the muscles are very warm after activity, they will stretch more easily and maintain the stretched position longer. That's why the cool-down period is a prime time for athletes to achieve long-term improvements in their flexibility. The athletes should stretch each muscle group, appropriate to their sport, for a total of 2 to 3 minutes. For example, some muscle groups are

• shoulders and chest;
• arms and forearms;
• trunk (back and abdominal areas);
• hips and thighs; and
• lower legs.

In general, muscles need to be stretched for a total of 2 to 3 minutes a day to obtain lasting improvements in length. Stretches for each muscle group can be broken down into 15- to 30-second repetitions.

Protective Equipment, Bracing, and Taping

As a coach, you should become an expert on how to properly fit and use your sport's protective equipment. Also, you must instruct athletes how to correctly fit and wear the equipment. This is especially true in football, where helmets must be specially fitted and the athletes are required to wear all of their protective pads. Conduct surprise inspections to ensure that athletes adequately maintain and fit their equipment. To minimize the risk of broken equipment, particularly in football, consider conducting a regular inspection and having shoulder pads and helmets refurbished and retested on a regular basis.

Two often neglected but important pieces of equipment are safety glasses (figure 2.5), or goggles, and mouthpieces. If there is any chance of eye injury, particularly in contact or racket sports, athletes should wear safety eyewear. Mouth guards (figure 2.6) help prevent dental injuries.

What about protective bracing and taping? You may have heard about coaches who require certain football players to wear preventative knee braces or require basketball players to tape their ankles, even though the athletes have not suffered injuries. The coaches feel that braces or tape will help prevent injury.

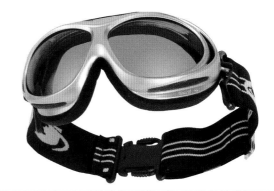

Figure 2.5 Sport safety glasses.
© Bolle Eyewear, Inc.

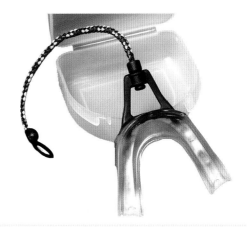

Figure 2.6 Sport mouth guards.

To Brace or Not to Brace?

Are protective bracing and taping all they're cracked up to be? They are certainly no substitute for being in shape. Remember that strength, flexibility, endurance, and power are the keys to preventing injury. Bracing and taping are of secondary importance. With the exception of some types of ankle braces, other protective bracing or taping has not been shown to conclusively prevent injuries. It is very difficult to prove whether a decrease in injuries can be attributed to wearing a protective brace. Ultimately the issue of preventive bracing and taping needs to be decided by the athlete and parents. Also, in some states, a physician's note justifying the need for wearing the brace may be required in order for the athlete to participate with a brace or splint.

Correct Skill Instruction

Many athletes are injured because they use incorrect technique. Since spear tackling was ruled illegal in football, the number of head and neck injuries among players has decreased. Baseball or softball players who dive headfirst into a base instead of sliding feet first are prone to tooth, head, and neck injuries. Many tennis players suffer from tennis elbow because they use incorrect backhand techniques.

You can help prevent these and other injuries by teaching your athletes safe and proper skill techniques. Also, keep an eye out for athletes who use potentially harmful techniques. Warn them of the possible injuries they could suffer, and then reinstruct them in the appropriate skills.

Sound Nutritional Guidance

Encourage your athletes to eat balanced meals according to the MyPlate guidelines (figure 2.7). You can help athletes and their parents determine nutrient needs by recommending that they go to the MyPlate website (www.choosemyplate.gov) and click on the SuperTracker link. Athletes can create individual profiles, and the SuperTracker will help them determine their nutrient needs based on their size, gender, age, and activity level.

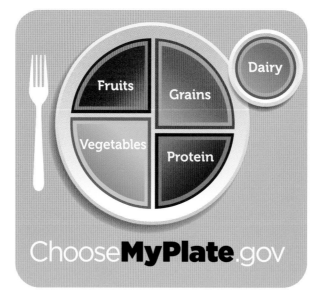

Figure 2.7 MyPlate.
U.S. Department of Agriculture.

Also encourage athletes to drink plenty of fluids to maintain adequate hydration. Specifically, the National Athletic Trainers' Association (Casa et al. 2000) recommends

- 17 to 20 ounces of fluid at least 2 hours before workouts, practice, or competition;
- another 7 to 10 ounces of water or sports drink 10 to 15 minutes before workouts, practice, or competition;
- 7 to 10 ounces of cool (50 to 59 degrees Fahrenheit) water or sports drink every 10 to 20 minutes during workouts, practice, or competition; and
- after workouts, practices, and competitions, 16 to 24 fluid ounces of water or sports drink for every pound of water lost through sweat (Manore, Barr, and Butterfield 2000).

For activities lasting over 60 minutes, athletes may benefit from a sports drink, which is generally a combination of a carbohydrate source, the electrolytes potassium and sodium, and water. A sports drink with the proper carbohydrate content of 6 to 7 percent (14 to 17 grams of carbohydrate per 240 milliliters) may enhance fluid absorption and provide carbohydrates for energy to working muscles. See chapter 11 for more information on hydration.

Contrary to popular belief, healthy athletes do not need to take vitamin, mineral, protein, or carbohydrate supplements. By following a balanced diet outlined by the MyPlate website, they will get all of the nutrients they need for competition.

Eating on the Road

An adequate, high-carbohydrate, moderate-protein, low-fat (20 to 25 percent of total calories) diet can be obtained on the road with a little planning and organization (Manore, Barr, and Butterfield 2000). If budgets allow, bring along dried fruits, juices, low-fat granola bars, and other snacks that offer healthy alternatives to vending machines. In addition, many restaurants will honor special requests for teams, such as pasta bars, low-fat sandwich options, and fresh fruits and vegetables. Encourage athletes to consume juices and skim milk products as opposed to soft drinks; baked, broiled, or boiled meats instead of fried meats; and plenty of carbohydrate-rich foods such as potatoes, rice, pasta, breads, bagels, fruits, and vegetables. Portions must be appropriate, and be sure to plan meals to allow adequate time for digestion before a competition (digestion takes anywhere from two to five hours, depending on what is eaten).

An adequate diet for an athlete is similar to gasoline for an automobile. It's fuel for performance. To better inform your athletes about the "octane" in their diets, and to learn more about sports drinks and other nutritional issues, read *Nancy Clark's Sports Nutrition Guidebook, Fifth Edition* (Clark 2013).

Eating for Performance

To help prevent upset stomachs during competition, athletes should

- eat at least three to four hours before practices, workouts, and competitions;
- avoid foods that are high in fat such as french fries, potato chips, and peanut butter;
- avoid foods that are high in fiber such as lettuce, beans, cabbage, spinach, and nuts;
- avoid foods that are high in sugar such as candy bars, cakes, doughnuts, and honey;
- eat plenty of high-carbohydrate foods that are easily digested, such as pasta, breads, low-fiber cereals, fruit juices, potatoes, and bananas; and
- eat foods that are familiar to the athlete—the pregame meal is no time to try new foods.

Ban on Horseplay

Although joking and kidding are basically harmless, physical horseplay such as "wrestling around," pushing, and hitting can lead to unnecessary injury. Establish the rule of "no horseplay" at the start of the season and enforce it at all times.

DEVELOPING A MEDICAL EMERGENCY PLAN

The final step in preparing for sports injuries is to develop a medical emergency plan. To conduct a thorough evaluation of an injured athlete, activate the emergency medical system (EMS), and provide effective first aid, use the following response plan adapted from the American Safety & Health Institute:

- Assess—How do I evaluate the scene and the injured athlete?

- Alert—How do I activate the EMS?
- Attend—How will first aid care be provided?

Assess

First, your plan needs to specify how you will evaluate an injured athlete. This plan should address issues such as

- what to do first when you arrive at an injured athlete's side,
- how to evaluate the safety at the scene for the injured athlete, and
- steps for evaluating responsive and unresponsive athletes.

Chapters 4 and 5 provide more detailed guidelines for evaluating injuries and illnesses.

Alert

Next, your plan should indicate how to activate the EMS. If medical personnel are not present, how do you send for medical assistance while evaluating and providing first aid care to an athlete? To help everything go more smoothly in the event of a health emergency, you should develop a plan, before the season begins, for activating the emergency medical system. Here's an example of an effective step-by-step approach:

1. *Delegate the responsibility of seeking medical help.* The person can be an assistant coach, a parent, or an athlete. But it must be someone who is calm and responsible. Make sure that this person is on-hand during every practice and game.

2. *Make a list of emergency telephone numbers.* Save the list in your mobile phone and put a printed copy in your first aid kit and take it to every practice and game. Include the following phone numbers:
   - Rescue unit
   - Hospital
   - Team physician (if applicable)
   - Police
   - Fire department

   Before traveling to an away game, talk to the host coaches about emergency services.

3. *Take each athlete's emergency information card to every practice and game.* This is especially important if an athlete is unresponsive and unable to tell you who you should contact or to give you that person's phone number.

4. *Give an emergency response card (figure 2.8) to the contact person calling for emergency assistance.* This will prompt the caller to provide critical information to the emergency care staff. It will also help calm the caller by providing everything the caller needs to communicate to emergency personnel.

5. *Complete an injury report form and keep it on file for any injury that occurs.* This form should provide the information requested in the sample shown in figure 2.9.

Attend

Finally, your plan needs to indicate how first aid care will be provided. If medical personnel are on-hand at the time of the injury, assist them as needed while they assume the care of the injured athlete. If medical personnel are not present, provide first aid care to the extent of your qualifications. Chapters 4, 5, and 6 cover first aid basics and the proper way to move an injured athlete. Part III discusses care of specific injuries.

Handling Minor Injuries

Many injuries don't require emergency medical attention. An athlete who slightly twists an ankle or suffers a minor bruise is not in serious condition. However, sometimes noncritical injuries or illnesses can severely impair performance. Therefore, you should evaluate and monitor them closely to ensure that no further complications exist.

For these so-called "minor" injuries, you should

1. assess injury,

2. attend to the injury (first aid),

3. remove the athlete from participation if the athlete is in a great deal of pain or suffers from a loss of function (e.g., can't walk, run, jump, or throw),

4. contact the athlete's parents to discuss the injury,

5. suggest that the athlete see a physician to rule out a serious injury, and

6. complete an injury report form while the incident is still fresh in your mind.

Handling Serious Injuries

If a serious injury or illness does occur, initiate your emergency plan in this sequence:

1. Assess the safety of the scene and the athlete's level of responsiveness.

2. Send a contact person to **alert** emergency medical personnel and the athlete's parents.

3. Send someone to wait for the rescue team, help them open doors and gates, and direct them to the injured athlete.

4. Assess the injury.

5. Attend to the injury (first aid).

6. Assist emergency medical personnel in preparing the athlete for transportation to a medical facility.

7. Appoint someone to go with the athlete if the parents are not available. This person should be responsible, calm, and familiar with the athlete. Assistant coaches or parents are best for this job.

8. Complete an injury report form while the incident is still fresh in your mind.

Information for Emergency Call

(Be prepared to give this information to the EMS dispatcher.)

1. Location

   Street address _____

   City or town _____ Zip code _____

   Directions (e.g., cross streets or landmarks) _____

2 Telephone number from which the call is being made _____

3. Caller's name _____

4. What happened _____

5. How many persons injured _____

6. Condition of victim(s) _____

   _____

7. Help (first aid) being given _____

Note: Do not hang up first. Let the EMS dispatcher hang up first.

Figure 2.8 Emergency response card.

Injury Report

Name of athlete _____

Date _____ Time _____

First aider (name) _____

Mechanism of injury _____

_____

_____

Type of injury _____

Anatomical areas involved _____

First aid administered _____

_____

_____

Other treatment administered _____

_____

Referral action _____

_____

First aider (signature)

Figure 2.9 Injury report form.

Chapter 2 *REPLAY*

☐ Do you regularly study sports medicine literature and attend sports medicine seminars? (pp. 13-14)

☐ Are you currently certified in CPR? (p. 14)

☐ Have all of your athletes filled out an informed consent form for emergency medical treatment, a health history form, and an emergency information card? (p. 14)

☐ Have you prepared and implemented a weather emergency plan? (pp. 15-17)

☐ Do you regularly inspect the condition of playing areas and equipment? (pp. 17-20)

☐ Do you find and repair any defects in playing equipment before the start of each season? (pp. 17-20)

☐ Do you have a well-stocked first aid kit? (pp. 17, 20)

☐ Do you require athletes to undergo extensive physical examinations and preseason screening to pinpoint any potential health or fitness problems? (p. 21)

☐ Do you have a preseason conditioning plan, and do you incorporate warm-up and cool-down exercises into every practice and competition to help prevent injuries? (pp. 21-22)

☐ Do you enforce policies that require athletes to wear protective equipment and refrain from physical horseplay? (pp. 22-25)

☐ Do you teach athletes correct sport skill techniques and repeatedly warn them against techniques that are potentially dangerous? (p. 23)

☐ Do you provide sound nutritional guidance, sufficient hydration, and nutritional eating opportunities? (pp. 23-25)

☐ Have you developed an emergency plan, including who is responsible for what duties, how a duty should be carried out, when certain actions should be taken, and what paperwork needs to be completed? (pp. 25-27)

REFERENCES

American Safety & Health Institute. 2006. *CPR and AED for the Community and Workplace.* Holiday, FL: American Safety & Health Institute.

Casa, D.E., S.K. Hillman, S.J. Montain, R.V. Reiff, B.S.E. Rich, W.O. Roberts, and J.A. Stone. 2000. National Athletic Trainers' Association position statement: Fluid replacement for athletes. *Journal of Athletic Training* 35(2):212-224.

Clark, N. 2013. *Nancy Clark's Sports Nutrition Guidebook, Fifth Edition.* Champaign, IL: Human Kinetics.

Eckart, R.E., et al. 2004. Sudden death in young adults: A 25-year review of autopsies in military recruits. *Annals of Internal Medicine* 141:829-34.

Manore, M.M., S.I. Barr, and G.E. Butterfield. 2000. Nutrition and athletic performance: Position of the American Dietetic Association, Dietitians of Canada, and the American College of Sports Medicine. *Journal of the American Dietetic Association* 100:1543-1556.

Martens, R. 2012. *Successful Coaching, Fourth Edition.* Champaign, IL: Human Kinetics.

Walsh, K.M., B. Bennett, M.A. Cooper, R.L. Holle, R. Kithil, and R.E. Lopez. 2000. National Athletic Trainers' Association position statement: Lightning safety for athletics and recreation. *Journal of Athletic Training* 35(4):471-477.

PART II

Basic Sport First Aid Skills

"Achieving success and personal glory in athletics has less to do with wins and losses than it does with learning how to prepare yourself so that at the end of the day, whether on the track or in the office, you know that there was nothing more you could have done to reach your ultimate goal."

Jackie Joyner-Kersee

Preparation is the key to eliminating the anxiety and uncertainty over performing sport first aid. Just like your athletes, you'll be more confident and successful if you master the basic skills and learn the basic rules and strategies.

Chapter 3 will help you develop a basic knowledge of anatomy, which is essential to your becoming a competent sport first aider. Also, the glossary (pages 303 to 306) explains sport first aid terms that you'll commonly encounter.

Once you've developed a sound knowledge base, in chapter 4, you'll learn basic strategies for evaluating and caring for life-threatening conditions.

Tactics for evaluating and caring for bleeding, shock, unstable injuries, and local tissue damage are outlined in chapter 5. You'll be able to apply these basic skills and guidelines to all sport first aid injuries and illnesses that are of secondary importance to the life-threatening conditions covered in chapter 4.

Finally, in chapter 6, you'll learn ways to assist in safely moving an injured or ill athlete. The emphasis here is on caution and proper technique.

The information in these chapters will help you take the guesswork out of evaluating and caring for injured or ill athletes.

Anatomy and Sport Injury Terminology

IN THIS CHAPTER, YOU WILL LEARN:

- ▶ What the roles of the musculoskeletal, neurological, digestive, respiratory and circulatory, and urinary systems are.
- ▶ How most injuries and illnesses occur.
- ▶ What distinguishes acute and chronic injuries.
- ▶ How to recognize the main types of acute and chronic injuries.

Winning takes precise execution of plays, stunts, or maneuvers. A 6-4-3 double play will never fly if a second baseman isn't in position to field the shortstop's toss and nail the throw to first base. The body functions in a similar way—one system or organ can directly affect another. If one part is broken, other parts may not work correctly.

To provide appropriate first responder care to a broken part, you must know the body's systems, anatomy, and common malfunctions (injuries and illnesses). Then, you'll be able to better recognize injuries and effectively communicate an athlete's symptoms and problems to emergency personnel, sports medicine professionals, and parents or guardians.

Perhaps you are wondering whether knowing anatomy terminology is really all that important. If so, consider this: You have likely worked with athletes who have torn tendons or sprained ligaments. But do you know the difference between a tendon and a ligament? Do

you know what a sprain really is, compared to a strain or fracture? And do you know how long it takes ligaments to heal? If you are unsure of answers to questions such as these, this chapter is for you.

To get a better grasp of sport first aid terminology, let's review basic human anatomy. The body is divided into several systems, each with unique organs and tissues. All are vital to supporting life and promoting top sports performance.

MUSCULOSKELETAL SYSTEM

The musculoskeletal system is made up of bones, joints, muscles, tendons, and other tissues.

Bones

The skeleton (bones) is the body's foundation. It serves to

- shape and support the body, and
- protect important organs such as the brain, lungs, and heart.

Figure 3.1 illustrates the anatomical names for some of the bones.

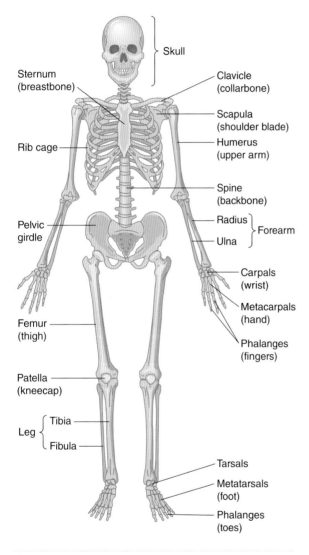

Figure 3.1   Skeletal system.

Joints

When two bones meet, they form a joint. Joints are also made up of ligaments, tendons, cartilage, and bursas (figure 3.2). Without joints, the body would be unable to move. Primary joints include the hip, knee, ankle, shoulder, elbow, and wrist.

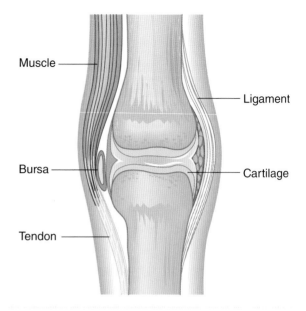

Figure 3.2   Joint structure.

Ligaments

Ligaments connect bones at a joint. This function is critical to maintaining joint stability. Without ligaments, bones and joints would constantly move out of position and prevent any purposeful movement.

Cartilage

Cartilage is a gristly type of tissue found on the ends of bones. There are several different types of cartilage, and they function primarily to absorb shock when bones hit each other and reduce friction when bones rub together.

Muscles

Muscles are elastic tissues that move bones. The muscle groups that are important in sports, and commonly injured, are the rotator cuff, quadriceps, hamstrings, and gastrocnemius (figure 3.3):

Rotator cuff—Located on the shoulder blade, these muscles are involved in throwing, swimming, and hitting (volleyball and racquet sports). The rotator cuff also plays a major role in helping to

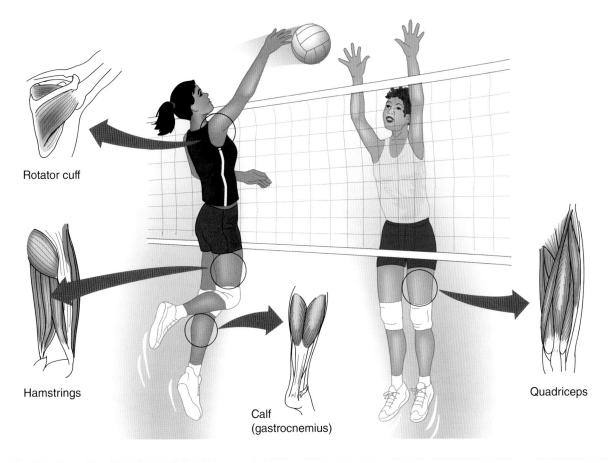

Figure 3.3 Four of the major muscle groups.

hold the upper arm bone (humerus) in the shoulder socket.

Quadriceps—Located on the front of the thigh, these muscles straighten the knee and move the thigh forward. They help provide the power to jump and run.

Hamstrings—Located on the back of the thigh, these muscles bend the knee and extend the thigh backward. They help generate the force needed to propel the body forward from the landing phase of running.

Gastrocnemius (calf)—Located on the back of the lower leg, these muscles point the foot down and also help bend the knee. They are especially active when pushing off to jump or run.

Tendons

Tendons attach muscle to bone. They are somewhat elastic to allow for stretching or pulling by the muscles. Common tendons injured in sport (figure 3.4) include the Achilles (heel), patellar (knee), biceps (upper arm), and rotator cuff (shoulder). Tendon fibers are covered by several types of sheaths. One type, the synovial sheath, secretes and absorbs a fluid that acts as a lubricant between tendon fibers and bundles.

Bursa

Bursas are small, fluid-filled sacs located between bones, muscles, tendons, and other tissues. These sacs help reduce rubbing between tissues, for example, between tendons and bones.

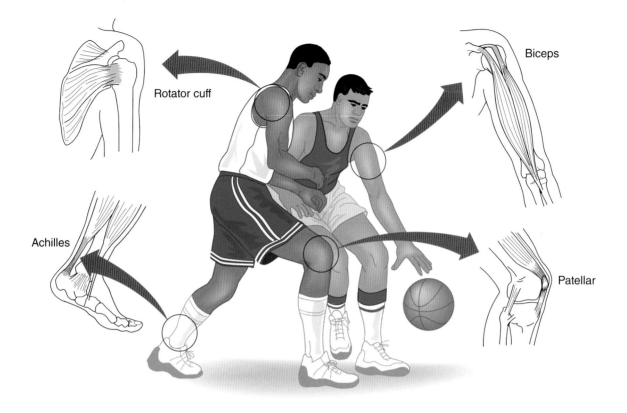

Figure 3.4 Four tendons commonly injured in sport.

NEUROLOGICAL SYSTEM

The neurological system is the body's control center (figure 3.5). It is made up of the brain, spinal cord, and a network of nerves. The brain coordinates the functioning of all systems and tissues. Digestion, breathing and heart rates, muscle contraction, and most other bodily functions depend on signals from the brain. Nerves relay these signals from the brain and also carry feedback from the tissues to the brain.

The spinal cord is the main trunk from which the nerves branch. It is protected by the spine. The vertebrae (bones) of the spine are held together by ligaments and are separated by cartilage discs (figure 3.6).

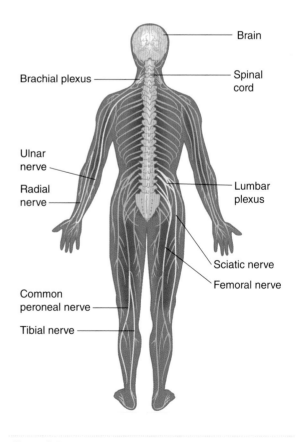

Figure 3.5 Neurological system.

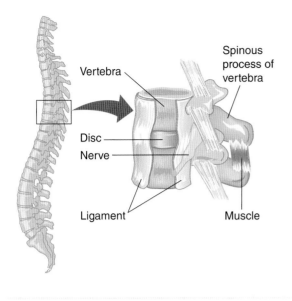

Figure 3.6 Spine structures.

DIGESTIVE SYSTEM

The digestive system is the body's energy supply center. Its organs assist in breaking down food into energy substances that fuel the muscles and other tissues (figure 3.7). Once swallowed, food travels down a long tube, called the esophagus. From the esophagus, food enters the stomach where it is partially digested. It continues on through the small and large intestines where nutrients are further broken down and absorbed for use in the body. Also during this process, waste products accumulate and eventually exit from the large intestines through the rectum. The liver assists in the process by excreting a fluid (bile) that helps break down fats. The gallbladder acts as an extra reservoir for bile. The pancreas excretes fluids that aid in digestion as well as insulin, a hormone, which helps regulate sugar levels within the body. The appendix is a part of the small intestine but has no known function in humans.

RESPIRATORY AND CIRCULATORY SYSTEMS

With the digestive system as the energy supplier, the circulatory and respiratory systems serve as energy releasers. These two systems work together

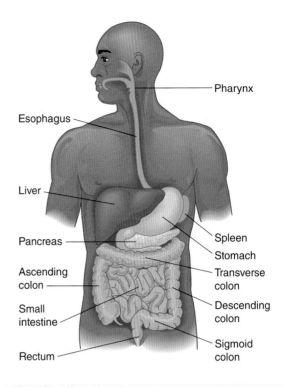

Figure 3.7 Digestive system.

to supply the oxygen the body needs to sustain life. Oxygen helps release the energy from food to fuel the tissues.

The respiratory system is the body's oxygen-transporting network. The respiratory organs are located in the head and chest (figure 3.8).

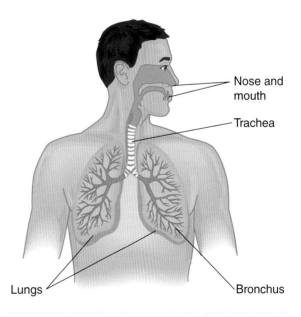

Figure 3.8 Respiratory system.

The circulatory system consists of the blood-transporting network shown in figure 3.9. The heart pumps the blood throughout the body via blood vessels.

The Respiratory and Circulatory Systems at Work

A person breathes in oxygen-filled air through the nose, mouth, or both. This air travels down the windpipe or trachea until it reaches the lungs. Inside the lungs, the oxygen passes through tiny sacs called alveoli and into thin blood vessels called capillaries. The capillaries join together into large blood vessels called pulmonary veins, which take the oxygen-filled blood to the heart.

The heart pumps the oxygen-filled blood through the arteries to the rest of the body. In the tissues, oxygen (O_2) is used to release energy and is broken down to a waste product called carbon dioxide (CO_2). The capillaries pick up the carbon dioxide, and this blood, called venous or low-oxygen blood, returns to the heart via the veins. The heart pumps the low-oxygen blood to the lungs, which breathe out the carbon dioxide and breathe in new supplies of oxygen.

A synopsis of this circulatory cycle is illustrated in figure 3.10.

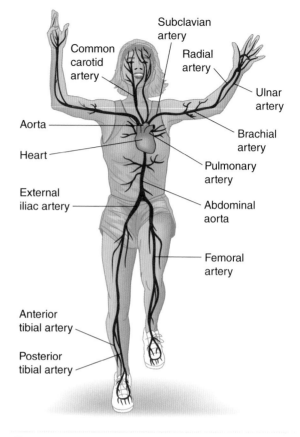

Figure 3.9 Circulatory system.

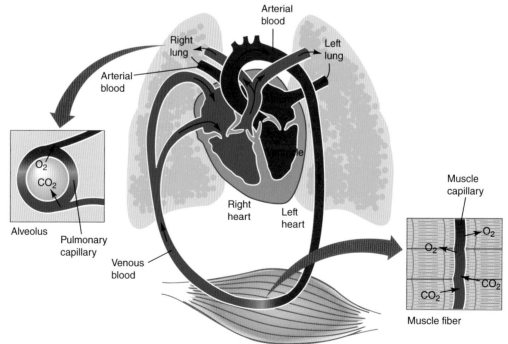

Figure 3.10 Circulorespiratory system.

URINARY SYSTEM

After energy is supplied (by digestion) and then released for the body to use (by circulation and respiration), by-products result. The urinary system gets rid of these waste products from energy breakdown. The organs shown in figure 3.11 participate in this process.

Waste products are brought to the kidneys through the blood (circulatory system). The kidneys filter out the waste products from the blood and combine them with water to make urine. Urine is released from the kidneys and travels through the ureter to the bladder. The bladder stores the urine until it is released from the body.

Athletes perform their best when all of these systems are working correctly. But what happens when an injury or illness occurs?

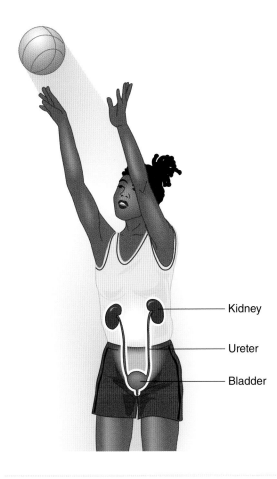

— Kidney

— Ureter

— Bladder

Figure 3.11 Urinary system.

HOW INJURIES AND ILLNESSES OCCUR

Injuries and illnesses are often classified according to what causes them and how long it takes for them to occur.

Causes

Injuries result from several causes: compression, tension or stretching, and shearing.

Compression—An impact injury to a specific body part that causes bleeding, superficial or deep tissue bruising, broken bones, or joint injuries. Colliding with another athlete or with sports equipment, and falling on a hard surface, are examples of a compression mechanism.

Tension—An injury that occurs when a tissue is stretched beyond its normal limits. This can occur when landing from a jump, overstriding when running, or landing on an outstretched hand.

Shearing—A friction injury caused by two surfaces rubbing together. Contact between the skin and the ground can cause a shearing injury to the skin (for example, when sliding into a base). Although shearing usually causes skin injuries, it can also affect other tissues, such as cartilage.

Length of Time to Develop

Injuries or illnesses can occur suddenly or develop slowly over time.

Acute injuries and illnesses occur suddenly as a result of a specific injury mechanism such as falling or coming into contact with another player or equipment. Examples include broken bones, cuts, bruises, and kidney injuries.

Chronic injuries and illnesses develop over a period of several weeks and are typically caused by repeated injury. Examples include shin splints, tennis elbow, diabetes, and epilepsy.

ACUTE INJURIES

Let's look at some specific acute injuries and how these may occur. Acute injuries occur suddenly and are caused by one specific injury mechanism. Common acute injuries include the following:

- Contusions
- Abrasions
- Punctures
- Cuts—incisions, lacerations, and avulsions
- Sprains
- Strains
- Cartilage tears
- Dislocations and subluxations
- Bone fractures

Contusions

Contusions, or bruises, result from a direct blow. Tissue and capillaries are damaged and lose fluid and blood. This causes pain, swelling, and discoloration. Superficial (skin) contusions (figure 3.12) are minor, but deep contusions to bone or muscle can cause loss of function. If a direct blow contuses the heart, lungs, brain, or kidneys, it can cause the damaged tissue to bleed heavily, thus reducing blood flow to the organ. These types of contusions can be life threatening. Contusions accounted for 15% of all types of injuries for boys and girls in a high school injury study (Comstock, Collins, and Yard 2008).

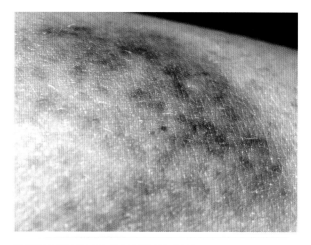

Figure 3.12 Contusion.
© Bruce Coleman Inc./Photoshot.

Abrasions

Abrasions occur when tissue is injured by friction or scraping. Most abrasions, like turf burns and strawberries, injure the skin (figure 3.13). However, the cornea (outer layer of the eye) can also be abraded or scratched by dust and other objects.

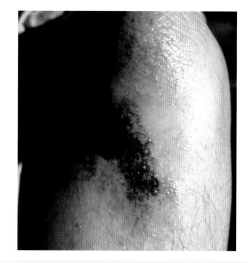

Figure 3.13 Abrasion.
© Bruce Coleman Inc./Photoshot.

Punctures

Punctures are narrow stab wounds to the skin and internal organs. In sports, they're often caused by track spikes or wood splinters (figure 3.14). Although superficial skin punctures may

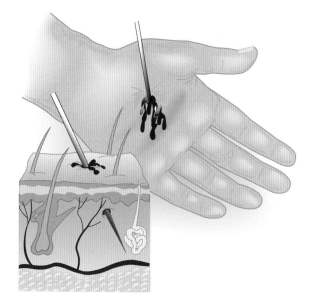

Figure 3.14 A puncture is a narrow stab wound.

not bleed much, they are a breeding ground for infection because bacteria can be pushed deep into the wound. Javelins and other sharp implements used in sports can puncture internal organs like the lungs. These injuries are life threatening and require prompt treatment.

Cuts

Tissue may be cut or torn several ways:

Lacerations—Jagged, soft-tissue cuts (figure 3.15) caused by a blow from a blunt object. They are deeper than abrasions and cause steady bleeding. For example, a basketball player can suffer a laceration above the eye after catching an elbow to the face.

Incisions—Smooth cuts caused by very sharp objects like glass or metal (figure 3.16). These injuries usually bleed heavily and quickly. Most situations where incisions occur can be prevented by simply conducting regular and thorough inspections of facilities and equipment.

Avulsions—Complete tissue tears, such as tearing off the end of the ear lobe (figure 3.17). Wearing rings can sometimes cause finger avulsions if the ring gets caught in something and is forcefully pulled. It's obvious that most of these injuries could be avoided if athletes were forbidden from wearing jewelry.

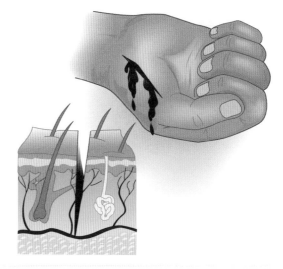

Figure 3.16 An incision is a smooth cut and usually bleeds heavily and quickly.

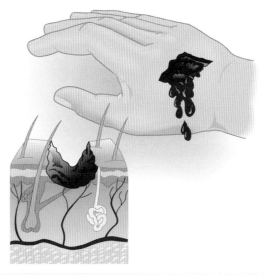

Figure 3.17 An avulsion is a complete tissue tear.

Sprains

Sprains are stretching or tearing injuries to ligaments and are classified from minor to serious as Grade I, II, or III (figure 3.18). They are typically caused by compression or a twisting or torsion mechanism. In a 2005-06 and 2006-07 high school sports injury study, ligament sprains were by far the most common type of injury reported, accounting for 32.6 percent of injuries (Comstock, Collins, and Yard 2008). See table 3.1 for a breakdown of sprains by sport.

In minor or Grade I sprains, some of the ligament fibers will be stretched and a few may be

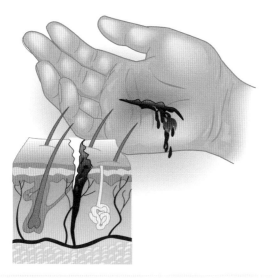

Figure 3.15 A laceration is jagged and deep and causes steady bleeding.

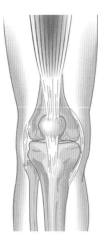

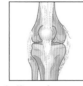

Grade I sprain
Ligament(s) stretched slightly
with a few fibers possibly torn

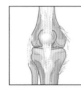

Grade II sprain
Ligament(s) stretched and
partially torn

Grade III sprain
Ligament(s) torn completely

Figure 3.18 Sprains.

Table 3.1 Frequency of Sprains Out of All Reported Types of Injury

Sport	Percentage
Volleyball – Girls	55.3
Basketball – Boys	44.6
Basketball – Girls	44.3
Soccer – Girls	35.1
Football	29.2
Softball – Girls	27.4
Soccer – Boys	26.4
Wrestling	25.4
Baseball	22.5

Data from Comstock, Collins, and Yard 2008.

torn. This results in mild pain, minimal to no swelling, and no loss of motion. Grade II or moderate sprains involve some ligament fiber stretching and more fiber tearing; however,

portions of the ligament are still intact. These injuries will cause some pain, swelling, and loss of joint function. In severe or Grade III sprains, a ligament tears completely. The athlete will likely experience extreme pain with any joint movement and therefore may be unable to move the joint. There will also be widespread swelling in the joint (particularly in ankle, elbow, finger, knee, and toe sprains).

Since ligaments support joints by holding bones together, sprains can cause serious joint instability. And, once stretched or torn, ligaments may not heal as tight as before the injury. This leads to looseness in the ligament and the joint and can result in numerous reinjuries (sprains). Even if ligaments heal to their original length, they can take anywhere from 6 to 12 weeks to fully heal.

Strains

If a muscle or tendon is forcefully and excessively shortened or stretched, it can become strained. A strain, like a sprain, is a stretching or tearing injury (figure 3.19); strains, however, occur in muscles and tendons. In a study of high school sports injuries (Comstock, Collins, and Yard 2008), strains were the second-most common type of injury reported, at a frequency of 17.6 percent. See table 3.2 for a breakdown of strains by sport.

Also like sprains, strains are classified as Grade I (minor), Grade II (moderate), and Grade III (severe). In minor or Grade I strains, some of the muscle or tendon fibers will be stretched, but very few may be torn. This results in mild pain, minimal to no swelling, and no loss of motion. More muscle or tendon fibers are torn in Grade II or moderate strains, but again, some portions of the muscle or tendon are still intact. These injuries cause some swelling, pain, loss of muscle or joint function, and possible *indentation* over the site of the injury. In severe or Grade III strains, a muscle or tendon tears completely. The athlete will likely experience extreme pain and will be unable to move the joint that is attached to the affected muscle or tendon. Torn muscles and tendons will roll up, causing a lump.

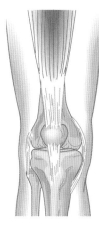

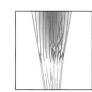

Grade I strain
Muscle or tendon stretched slightly

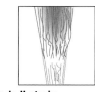

Grade II strain
Muscle or tendon stretched and partially torn

Grade III strain
Muscle or tendon torn completely

Figure 3.19 Strains.

Table 3.2 Frequency of Strains Out of All Reported Types of Injury

Sport	Percentage
Baseball	23.5
Soccer – Boys	21
Soccer – Girls	20.7
Wrestling	19.7
Softball – Girls	18.5
Volleyball – Girls	18.1
Football	15.3
Basketball – Girls	13.5
Basketball – Boys	12.7

Data from Comstock, Collins, and Yard 2008.

Cartilage Tears

As you'll remember, cartilage covering and between bones reduces shock and friction. If a joint's bones are twisted or compressed, they can bruise, or pinch and tear, the cartilage. This occurs most often in the knee (figure 3.20).

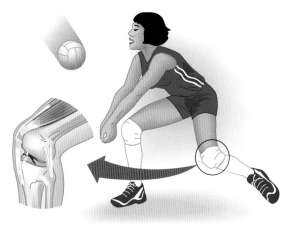

Figure 3.20 Knee cartilage tear.

Dislocations and Subluxations

Sometimes when a joint is hit or twisted, the bones move out of position. In a dislocation, the bones stay out of place until a physician repositions them. If the bones "pop out" of place but immediately "pop" back in, a subluxation has occurred. In sports, dislocations and subluxations occur most frequently to the shoulder (figure 3.21), elbow, finger, and kneecap.

Clavicle (collarbone)

Scapula

Humerus

Figure 3.21 Shoulder dislocation.

41

Dislocations and subluxations also injure the soft tissues around a joint. For example, ligaments are often sprained during dislocations and subluxations because they are stretched or torn when the bones move out of place. Other times, bones break and cartilage tears during these injuries.

Fractures

Bones that are compressed, twisted, or hit too hard can break or fracture. In recent studies of high school sports injuries (Comstock, Collins, and Yard 2008; Yard and Comstock 2006), fractures were the second-most common type of injury reported, at 9.4 percent. See table 3.3 for a breakdown of fractures by sport. Figure 3.22 shows the two main categories of fractures: closed and open.

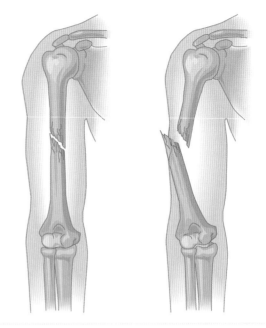

Figure 3.22   Closed and open fractures.

Table 3.3   Frequency of Fractures Out of All Reported Types of Injury

Sport	Percentage
Lacrosse – Females	21.4
Softball – Girls	16.5
Field Hockey – Girls	14.5
Baseball	13.9
Wrestling	11.8
Basketball – Boys	11.3
Football	10.2
Lacrosse – Boys	8.3
Soccer – Boys	7.9
Soccer – Girls	6.4
Basketball – Girls	6.2
Ice Hockey – Girls	6.2

Data from Comstock, Collins, and Yard 2008, and Yard and Comstock 2006.

Closed Fractures

Closed fractures result when a bone breaks but does not protrude through the skin. They are the most common type of fracture in sport. Sometimes they cause a noticeable deformity, although not always. The two types of closed fractures prevalent in sport are avulsion and epiphyseal fractures:

Avulsion fractures occur when sprained ligaments pull off a piece of bone. This often takes place in the ankle (figure 3.23) and finger.

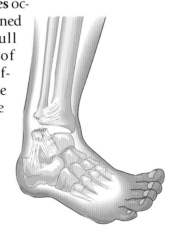

Figure 3.23   Avulsion fracture of the ankle.

Epiphyseal (growth plate) fractures result when the soft growth plates at the ends of bones are injured. These fractures most often occur to athletes before age 18 and can affect the bone's growth. Growth plate fractures typically occur in the elbow of baseball pitchers, as shown in figure 3.24.

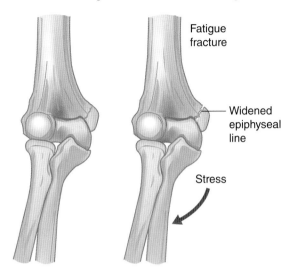

Figure 3.24 Epiphyseal (growth plate) fracture.

Open Fractures

Open fractures occur when a broken bone pierces the skin. These wounds must be carefully covered with sterile gauze to help prevent infection in the exposed bone and muscle tissues. Fortunately, open fractures are rare in most sports.

CHRONIC INJURIES

Chronic injuries occur over time and are often caused by repeated blows, overstretching, repeated friction, or overuse. Such repeated trauma can cause injuries to the muscles, tendons, bursas, and bones. These injuries typically occur in athletes who have a muscle strength and flexibility imbalance, or in athletes who exercise excessively.

Chronic Muscle Strain

If a muscle is repeatedly overworked or overstretched, a chronic strain can result. This type of injury develops over a period of weeks or months. These strains are different from acute strains because they are not caused by one specific episode of injury (such as sprinting to first base).

Bursitis

A bursa can become swollen and sore if it suffers from repeated blows or irritation. Bursitis can also be caused by tendons rubbing back and forth across the bursa. Elbow (figure 3.25) and kneecap bursitis are the most common types in sports.

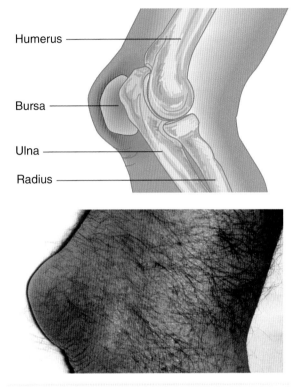

Figure 3.25 Bursitis occurs when the bursa becomes swollen and sore.
© Custom Medical Stock Photo.

Tendinosis, Tenosynovitis, and Paratendinitis

Just as bursas become irritated, tendons can also be irritated by repeated overstretching or overuse, especially if they are weak or tight. There are several types of tendon injuries. Although often known simply as tendinitis, these injuries are more accurately classified by different names based on the part of the tendon that is affected. For example, tendinosis is a condition in which microtears occur in the tendon. Tenosynovitis is an inflammation of the synovial sheath that surrounds the tendon. Paratendinitis is an inflammation or thickening of the tendon sheath (not a synovial sheath).

Like sprains and strains, tendinitis can also be classified as mild, moderate, and severe. In mild cases, symptoms include slight pain that occurs with specific skills or activities during extreme exertion. The pain subsides once the painful activity stops. There is minimal to no swelling and no loss of motion. Moderate tendinitis may cause some swelling. Pain occurs with more activities and skills, limits extreme muscle exertion, and continues up to several hours after the activity stops. In severe tendinitis, the pain intensifies, occurring with any level of exertion, extending into daily activities, and lasting longer (sometimes more than 24 hours after activity stops). Pain also limits muscle and joint function. Swelling or thickening of the tendon (particularly the Achilles or patellar tendon) will be more prominent. Chapters 12 and 13 describe the signs and symptoms, as well as the proper first aid care, for tendinitis at various locations on the body.

The tendons of the biceps, patella (kneecap), Achilles (heel), and rotator cuff (shoulder) are especially prone to repeated microtrauma in sports. Inflexible and weak patellar and Achilles tendons can be overstressed by repeated running and jumping activities (figure 3.26). The biceps

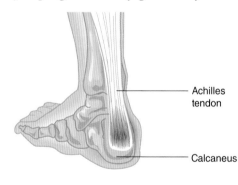

Achilles tendon

Calcaneus

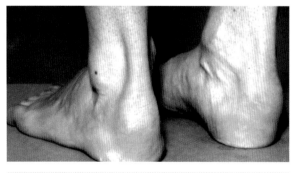

Figure 3.26 Tendinitis results when tendons are irritated.
© Custom Medical Stock Photo.

and rotator cuff tendons are usually overstressed when an athlete throws with a weak and inflexible shoulder. These types of injuries can also be caused by increasing an athlete's workout or practice regimen too quickly. Generally, increasing the intensity and duration of specific exercises and workouts by 10 to 15 percent per week is considered a safe progression.

Chronic Bone Injuries

Repeated and long-term wear and tear can cause bones to crack or grow abnormally. Two of the more prevalent types of chronic bone injuries are osteoarthritis and stress fractures.

Osteoarthritis

Osteoarthritis typically results from long-term wear over many years, but it can also develop in a shorter period (a few years) as a result of one traumatic injury such as a joint dislocation. Since they take several years to develop, these injuries are more common in postpubescent athletes. However, injuries that are ignored or left untreated in young athletes can lead to osteoarthritis in just a few years. For example, repeated ankle or knee sprains can cause cumulative joint trauma and lead to osteoarthritis.

Stress Fractures

Repeated stress or shock can eventually cause a bone to crack (stress fracture). Athletes involved in high-impact sports (running, basketball, soccer, and gymnastics) and high-velocity activities (baseball pitching) are especially prone to these injuries.

PUTTING IT ALL TOGETHER

This chapter has introduced some of the injuries that you may encounter as a coach. Common injuries and their mechanisms of injury are listed in table 3.4. For an overview of what injuries affect what body parts, check out table 3.5. Also, for more information on specific injuries, see the chapters in part III.

Table 3.4 Injuries and Their Mechanisms

Acute injuries	Compression	Tension	Shearing
Contusions	X		
Abrasions			X
Punctures	X		
Lacerations	X		X
Incisions	X		
Avulsions	X	X	X
Sprains		X	X
Acute strains		X	
Cartilage tears	X		X
Dislocations and subluxations	X	X	
Bone fractures	X		
Epiphyseal fractures	X	X	
Chronic injuries			
Chronic muscle strain		X	
Bursitis	X	X	X
Tendinosis, tenosynovitis, and paratendinitis		X	
Osteoarthritis	X		X
Stress fractures	X		

Table 3.5 Examples of Injuries That Affect Specific Body Tissues

Tissue	Injury	Type of injury
Bone	Closed fracture	Acute
	Open fracture	Acute
	Avulsion fracture	Acute or chronic
	Osteoarthritis	Chronic
	Stress fracture	Chronic
Cartilage	Tear	Acute or chronic
	Contusion	Acute
Ligament	Sprain	Acute
Muscle	Strain	Acute or chronic

(continued)

Table 3.5 Examples of Injuries That Affect Specific Body Tissues *(continued)*

Tissue	Injury	Type of injury
Tendon	Strain Tenosynovitis Tendinosis Paratendinitis	Acute Chronic Chronic Chronic
Bursa	Bursitis Contusion	Chronic Acute
Skin	Laceration Incision Abrasion Puncture Avulsion (example: earlobe)	Acute Acute Acute Acute Acute
Eye	Puncture Abrasion (corneal)	Acute Acute
Other organs (e.g., heart, kidney)	Puncture Contusion	Acute Acute

Chapter 3 *REPLAY*

☐ Are you familiar with each of the body systems and its organs? Think about the musculoskeletal, neurological, digestive, circulatory and respiratory, and urinary systems. (pp. 31-37)

☐ What tissues do muscles connect to, and how do those tissues help us to move? (pp. 32-33)

☐ What tissues make up a joint? (p. 32)

☐ Where are ligaments found and what role do they play in joint stability? (p. 32)

☐ What are the three mechanisms that result in most injuries? (p. 37)

☐ What terms are used to indicate the length of time it takes an injury to develop? (p. 37)

☐ Can you describe the meanings of compression, tension, and shearing? (p. 37)

☐ What are some common acute injuries and how do they occur? (pp. 38-42)

☐ What are three types of cuts and how can you distinguish between them? (p. 39)

☐ Can you define what causes sprains and what tissue they occur in? (pp. 39-40)

☐ Can you define what causes strains and what tissues they occur in? (pp. 40-41)

☐ Can you classify and describe three types of acute bone fractures? (pp. 42-43)

☐ What causes chronic injuries to occur and what distinguishes them from acute injuries? (p. 43)

☐ What are some common chronic injuries and how do they occur? (pp. 43-44)

REFERENCES

Comstock, R.D., C.L. Collins, and E. E. Yard. National high school sports-related injury surveillance study, 2005-06 and 2006-07 school years (Personal communication, February 1, 2008).

Yard, E.E. and R.D. Comstock. 2006. Injuries sustained by pediatric ice hockey, lacrosse, and field hockey athletes presenting to United States emergency departments. *Journal of Athletic Training*, 41(4): 441-449.

Emergency Action Steps

IN THIS CHAPTER, YOU WILL LEARN:

- How to perform the emergency action steps.
- What to do if an athlete stops breathing, including checking breathing, performing cardiopulmonary resuscitation, and using an automated external defibrillator.
- How to recognize and respond to airway blockage, including how to perform the Heimlich maneuver.

INJURIES AND TECHNIQUES IN THIS CHAPTER

Imagine lining up behind your center, ready to take the snap. It's late in the fourth quarter, you're on the 30-yard line, it's fourth down, and you're down by two points. Suddenly, three hungry linebackers are staring you down from across the line. You realize your play is doomed against a blitz. You've got seven seconds left on the play clock. What do you do?

If you're able to think and react quickly, you call an audible that could save the game.

The need to recognize serious problems and react to them quickly and correctly is not unique to football. The same holds true for assessing an athlete's breathing and providing basic life support. Both require an ability to analyze what's going on. And both require split-second thinking and reacting.

In this chapter, you'll learn how to conduct emergency action steps for an injured or ill athlete. This will include assessing the scene; assessing the athlete for level of responsiveness; checking for breathing; and responding appropriately with life-saving first aid. Correctly assessing an athlete can help you more accurately provide first aid care and communicate with emergency medical personnel.

EMERGENCY ACTION STEPS

Your initial assessment of the athlete will consist of the Emergency Action Steps: Assess (the scene and the athlete), Alert, and Attend to breathing. These steps will help you spot and care for life-threatening problems in an injured or ill athlete. Perform these steps quickly—in a minute or less.

Assess the Scene

When an athlete goes down because of injury or illness, the first thing to consider is safety. Your immediate goal is to protect the athlete—and yourself—from harm. First, you or an assistant should instruct all other players and bystanders to leave the athlete alone. They can cause further injury by trying to move the athlete.

Second, consider the environment. Is the athlete in danger from downed power lines, lightning, traffic, cold, or heat exposure? Are you in danger from any of these conditions? If so, you will need to carefully consider how to minimize the risk of injury to yourself and evaluate if the athlete may need to be immediately moved to prevent the environment from worsening the athlete's condition. See "Playing It Safe When Moving an Injured or Ill Athlete" and chapter 6 for instructions on when and how to safely move an injured athlete.

Third, try to calm the athlete and keep him or her from rolling around or jumping up and down, which can cause further injury.

Finally, think about whether the athlete is lying in a position or wearing equipment that will prevent you from evaluating his or her condition or from providing first aid for a life-threatening condition. You may need to move the athlete or remove the specific equipment that is hindering the assessment or first aid care.

→ Playing It Safe...
When Moving an Injured or Ill Athlete

In almost every case, you should let emergency medical personnel move a seriously injured athlete. Move a critically injured or ill athlete to another site only if

- the area is unsafe (e.g., lightning, downed electrical lines, traffic, or other runners in a road race),
- the athlete's position prevents you from providing CPR or life-saving first aid, or
- the athlete is suffering from exertional heat syndrome (see chapter 11)

See chapter 6 for proper techniques for moving an athlete.

Reposition a critically injured or ill athlete only when necessary to perform CPR, control profuse bleeding, or prevent the athlete from choking on vomit or secretions.

Assess the Athlete

As you approach the athlete, review in your mind how the injury or illness occurred. Was there a direct hit to a certain area of the body? Was a joint or body part twisted? Was the athlete stung by an insect? This information gives you insight into what type of injury you're dealing with.

Also review in your mind what you may know about the athlete's medical history. Does the athlete have a history of asthma, heart problems, kidney disorders, neurological problems, diabetes, or seizures? Has the athlete ever suffered this injury or condition before? This information provides additional clues to what may be wrong with the athlete that may guide the care you provide.

When you reach the athlete, quickly check whether the athlete is responsive or unresponsive. Gently tap or squeeze the athlete's shoulder and ask, "Are you all right, (athlete's name)?"

➜ Playing It Safe...
Working Around a Face Mask

Rescue breaths are not required with compression-only CPR. Therefore, it is not necessary to take the time to remove the face mask if an athlete is wearing a helmet.

NOTE: Do not remove an unresponsive athlete's helmet. If you suspect a serious injury to the head or spine, place your hands on both sides of the athlete's helmet to keep the head, neck, and spine in line.

Alert

If the athlete doesn't respond, or he or she responds but is badly hurt, looks or acts very ill, or quickly gets worse, alert EMS (Call 9-1-1) or activate your facility's emergency action plan.

Attend to Breathing

After determining the athlete is responsive or unresponsive and alerting EMS or your emergency action plan, attend to the athlete's breathing.

Your objective is to see if the athlete needs CPR and to check for any other life-threatening conditions that require immediate attention, such as severe bleeding. If you don't find any conditions that are immediately life-threatening, do a more thorough physical assessment to determine the course of treatment. This assessment is described in the next chapter.

For a Responsive Athlete

1. First identify yourself and ask the athlete's permission to help.
2. Ensure that the athlete is fully responsive and breathing normally without making gasping, noisy, snorting, or gurgling sounds. The athlete should be able to talk and keep the airway open and clear.
3. Move the athlete only if the athlete is in an area that may cause further harm; the athlete is at risk for breathing in fluid, vomit, or blood; or you must leave the athlete alone to get help. If any of these are true, then you may need to move the athlete using the techniques outlined here. For an uninjured athlete, use the recovery position. For an injured athlete, automatically assume he or she may have a head or spine injury and use the HAINES position or the four- or five-person rescue (see chapter 6). Remember: Move an athlete only if it is necessary to protect the athlete from further harm or to provide life-saving first aid.
4. Look for and control any severe bleeding with direct pressure (see next chapter for more on this).
5. Look for normal tissue color and body temperature. If skin is bluish or ashen or if it feels cool, this may indicate the athlete has had reduced circulation for at least a few minutes.
6. While waiting for medical assistance, continue to monitor the athlete's alertness and make sure he or she continues breathing normally.
7. Continue to control bleeding, monitor tissue color and temperature, and help maintain the athlete's normal body temperature.

See page 259 in appendix A for a summary of how to attend to a responsive athlete.

For an Unresponsive Athlete

1. Alert EMS and retrieve an automated external defibrillator (AED). If other people are present, have them do this while you attend to the athlete.
2. Check the athlete for breathing. If an unresponsive athlete is lying facedown, look to see if the ribs are rising and falling, indicating that the athlete is breathing. You can also check for breathing by placing your hand in front of the athlete's nose and mouth and feeling for breaths. Look, listen, and feel for breathing for at least 5 seconds but no more than 10. Occasional gasps are not normal and are not capable of supplying the athlete with enough oxygen to sustain life. If the athlete is not breathing or is making gasping, noisy, snorting, or gurgling sounds, you may have to move the athlete onto his or her back to administer CPR.

Recovery Position for an Uninjured Athlete

1. Kneel beside the athlete; make sure both legs are straight.
2. Place the arm nearest to you out at a right angle to the body, elbow bent palm up.
3. Bring the far arm across the chest; hold the back of the hand against the athlete's cheek nearest you (figure 4.1a).
4. With your other hand, grasp the far leg just above the knee and pull it up (figure 4.1b).
5. Keeping the athlete's hand pressed against the cheek, pull on the far leg to roll the athlete toward you.
6. Adjust the upper leg so both the hip and the knee are bent at right angles (figure 4.1c).

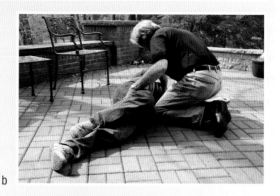
b

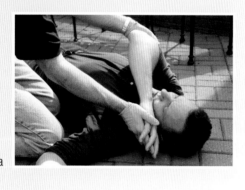
a

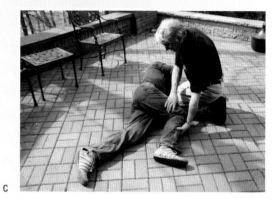
c

Figure 4.1 Recovery position. (a) Bringing the far arm across the athlete's chest. (b) Pulling up the far leg. (c) Bending the hip and knee at right angles.
Photos courtesy of American Safety & Health Institute.

If you are alone and the athlete is on his or her front, place the athlete's closest arm up over the head. Support the neck with your hand. Place your other hand on the athlete's hip and roll the athlete's body toward you until the athlete is on his or her back. As best as you can, roll the body and head all at once to minimize injury to the spine.

If other people are present and the athlete is on his or her front, use the four- or five-person rescue described in chapter 6.

3. Begin CPR. CPR uses chest compressions to help circulate blood with oxygen to the organs when the heart is not beating. Basic CPR is described as follows. However, it is not meant to take the place of certification offered through the American Red Cross, American Heart Association, or other nationally recognized organizations.

COMPRESSIONS

1. Expose the athlete's chest.
2. Place the heel of one hand in the center of the chest between the nipples. Put the other hand on top of the first. Your fingers can be either straight or fastened together, but they should be kept off the athlete's chest.
3. Position your body so your shoulders are directly over your hands. Straighten your arms and lock your elbows.
4. Use your upper-body weight to help compress the athlete's chest. Push forcefully straight down on the chest, approximately 2 inches (5 cm) for a normal-sized adult and one-third to one-half of chest depth for a child (1 to 8 years old).
5. Release pressure and completely remove your weight at the top of each compression

HAINES Position for an Injured Athlete Who Is Breathing

1. Kneel beside the athlete.
2. Place the athlete's closest arm above the head and the farthest arm across the chest (figure 4.2a).
3. Bend the athlete's nearest leg at the knee.

4. Place your hand under the hollow of the athlete's neck to help stabilize.
5. Roll the athlete toward you so that the head rests on the extended arm.
6. Bend both legs at the knees to stabilize the athlete (figure 4.2b).

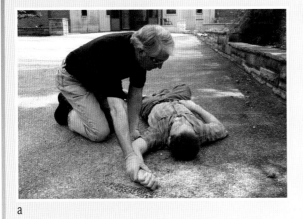
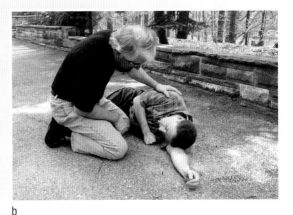

a

b

Figure 4.2 HAINES position. *(a)* Placing the athlete's closest arm above the head. *(b)* Bending both legs at the knees.
Photos courtesy of American Safety & Health Institute.

so the chest returns to its normal position and the heart can fill with blood.

6. Give chest compressions at a speed of about 100 per minute. Allow the athlete's chest to recoil completely. To get the most oxygenated blood to the athlete's brain and heart, minimize interruptions in chest compressions.

7. Continue chest compressions until someone with training equal to or better than yours takes over, an AED or the EMS providers arrive, the athlete shows signs of life, you are exhausted, or the scene becomes too dangerous to continue.

DEFIBRILLATION. In some cases an athlete's heart may be beating irregularly, so blood with oxygen is not effectively circulating to the body. So when performing CPR, use an automated external defibrillator (figure 4.3) to assess whether the heart is beating irregularly. If it is, then the AED will shock the heart in an attempt to establish a normal beating rhythm. If you are alone

and need to perform CPR, retrieve the AED and apply it before beginning compressions. If someone else is present, begin chest compressions and send that person to get the AED.

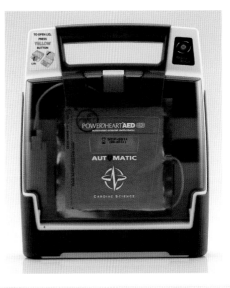

Figure 4.3 Automated external defibrillator (AED).
Courtesy of Cardiac Science Corporation (800-991-5465).

Once the AED arrives, if you are alone, do the following:

1. Turn on the AED.

2. Select and attach the adult pads if the athlete is an adult. If the athlete is a child and child pads are available, use them; if child pads are not available, use adult pads. (Note: AEDs are not used for infants.)

3. Listen to and follow the voice prompts on the AED.

4. Most AEDs will automatically begin to analyze the athlete's heart rhythm when the electrodes are fully attached. Ensure no one touches the athlete while the AED is analyzing the heart rhythm.

5. If a shock is indicated, make sure no one is touching the athlete. Stay clear of the athlete and press the shock button on the AED to give one shock.

6. Continue as directed by the AED until EMS arrives.

If another person is available, have him or her open and turn on the AED while you continue CPR. Stop CPR when the pads are ready to be attached to the athlete's chest.

Page 260 in appendix A summarizes how to attend to an unresponsive athlete and pages 263 and 264 summarize CPR and AED procedures. Next we will look at the procedures for a blocked airway due to choking.

Asthma or Other Conditions

Note: An athlete may have difficulty breathing due to injuries or to medical conditions such as asthma. Review the asthma first aid flow chart on page 271 in appendix A. It outlines the steps to take in the event of an asthma attack.

AIRWAY BLOCKAGE

In sports, an athlete's airway may become blocked due to

- breathing in a foreign object such as gum or food,
- the tongue falling back against the throat in an unresponsive athlete, or
- swelling from a direct blow or severe allergies.

In these cases the airway may have either mild or severe blockage. The first aid care that you provide will differ depending on the kind of blockage that occurs.

This chapter deals with first aid care for airway blockage caused by a foreign object such as food, gum, or the tongue (in an unresponsive athlete). Chapter 7 addresses first aid care for airway blockage caused by swelling from severe allergic reactions.

Mild Airway Blockage in a Responsive Athlete

The airway is partially blocked, allowing some, but not enough, air to pass through to the lungs.

Cause

- Foreign object such as gum or food lodges in the airway

Check for Signs

- Can breathe in and out and can speak

- Strong coughing or gagging as food/liquid "goes down the wrong pipe"
- May hear high-pitched squeaking or whistling noise (wheezing) between strong coughs

✚ FIRST AID

1. Ask, "Are you okay?" If the athlete says "yes" but has trouble breathing or grasps throat (the universal choking sign), the athlete may have a partially blocked airway.
2. Encourage the athlete to cough.
3. Monitor the athlete until (a) the object is dislodged and the athlete breathes normally, or (b) the airway becomes severely blocked (athlete is unable to cough or speak). If this happens, perform the Heimlich maneuver described in the next section. If the Heimlich maneuver does not dislodge the object or the athlete becomes unresponsive, have someone call for EMS and begin CPR.

Playing Status

- If the object dislodges and the athlete's breathing and color in lips, skin, and nail beds return to normal, the athlete can return to activity.

Severe Airway Blockage in a Responsive Athlete

Airway is totally blocked, preventing air from entering the lungs.

Cause

- Foreign object such as gum lodges in the airway

Checks for Signs

- Athlete grasping throat (universal choking sign)
- Cannot cough or make any sound
- Blue lips, nails, skin

✛ FIRST AID

1. Ask, "Are you choking?"
2. If the athlete shakes head "yes" or gives the universal choking signal, then ask, "Can I help?" If the athlete nods "yes" or is unable to speak, cough, or cry, immediately begin the Heimlich maneuver.

3. If the athlete shakes the head "no" to "Are you choking?" send for emergency medical assistance and check for other causes of the breathing difficulties. These are discussed in chapter 7.

Playing Status

- After undergoing the Heimlich maneuver, even if the object dislodges and the athlete's breathing returns to normal, the athlete cannot return to play until he has been evaluated by EMS and checked by a physician. Internal injuries can result from abdominal thrusts, even when they are performed correctly.

Heimlich Maneuver

Purpose: To dislodge an object causing severe blockage.

How It Works

- Uses compressions to force air out of the lungs to dislodge the blockage.

Technique

1. Stand behind the athlete if an adult, and kneel if a child.
2. Make a fist. Place the thumb side against the athlete's abdomen, just above the navel (see figure 4.4).
3. Give quick inward and upward thrusts.
4. Continue the compressions until
   a. the object is expelled; or
   b. the athlete loses responsiveness from lack of air, then do CPR.

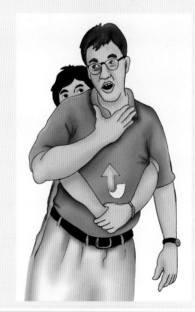

Figure 4.4 Heimlich maneuver hand position.
Courtesy of American Safety & Health Institute.

Page 261 in appendix A reviews the first aid procedures for treating airway blockage in a responsive athlete, and page 262 in appendix A summarizes first aid procedures for airway blockage in an unresponsive athlete.

Before you move on to the physical assessment in chapter 5, take time to review the emergency action steps as summarized in figure 4.5.

→ Playing It Safe...
When Performing the Heimlich Maneuver

If you place your fist too high, the thrusts can break the tip of the breast bone and cause internal injuries.

Severe Airway Blockage in an Unresponsive Athlete

Causes
- Foreign object such as gum lodges in the airway
- Back of tongue obstructs the airway

Check for Signs
- Unresponsive
- Not breathing

⊕ FIRST AID

If the athlete loses responsiveness from choking, do the following:

1. If possible, protect the athlete from falling when he or she loses consciousness.
2. Have someone immediately alert EMS.
3. If the athlete is not on his or her back, move the athlete onto the back using the HAINES technique if you are certain there are no head or neck injuries. Otherwise, use the four- or five-person technique outlined in chapter 6.
4. If you are certain that the athlete does not have a head or neck injury, open the mouth and remove the object if you see it. Also look to see if the tongue has slipped back and is blocking the airway. If it is, gently tilt the athlete's head back until the tongue has been cleared from the airway.
5. If the athlete still isn't breathing, continue CPR until the AED or EMS arrives or the object dislodges and the athlete shows signs of life. If this occurs, recheck the athlete's breathing. If the athlete is breathing (not gasping), continue to monitor breathing and monitor and care for shock as needed until EMS arrives.

Playing Status
- Cannot return to activity until examined and released by a physician.

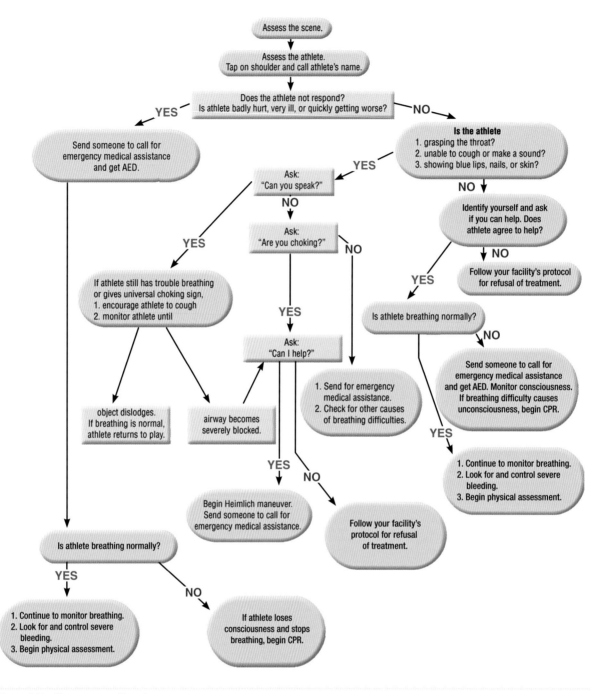

Figure 4.5 Emergency action steps.

Chapter 4 REPLAY

- ☐ What are the very first steps that should be taken when an athlete sustains an injury or sudden illness? (pp. 50-54)
- ☐ If an athlete is unresponsive, who should be called? (p. 51)
- ☐ What are the emergency action steps and how are they conducted? (pp. 50-54)
- ☐ If an athlete is responsive and has mild blockage of the airway, what should you do? (p. 55)
- ☐ If an athlete is responsive and has a severe blockage of the airway, what should you do? (p. 56)
- ☐ If an athlete is unresponsive and has a blockage of the airway, what should you do? (p. 57)
- ☐ Can you describe when and how to perform
  - ☐ the Heimlich maneuver? (p. 56)
  - ☐ cardiopulmonary resuscitation? (pp. 52-54)
  - ☐ CPR with an automated external defibrillator? (pp. 53-54)

REFERENCES

Berg, R.A., R. Hemphill, B.S. Abella, T.P. Aufderheide, D.M. Cave, M.F. Hazinski, E.B. Lerner, T.D. Rea, M.R. Sayre, and R.A. Swor. 2010. Part 5: Adult basic life support: 2010 American Heart Association Guidelines for Cardiopulmonary Resuscitation and Emergency Cardiovascular Care. *Circulation* 122: S685-S705

Markenson, D., J.D. Ferguson, L. Chameides, P. Cassan, K. Chung, J. Epstein, L. Gonzales, R.A. Herrington, J.L. Pellegrino, N. Ratcliff, and A. Singer. 2010. Part 17: First aid: 2010 American Heart Association and American Red Cross guidelines for first aid. *Circulation* 122: S934-46.

CHAPTER 5

Physical Assessment and First Aid Techniques

IN THIS CHAPTER, YOU WILL LEARN:

- ▸ How to conduct a physical assessment of an injured or ill athlete, using the HIT (history, inspection, and touch) method.
- ▸ How to control profuse bleeding.
- ▸ What methods to use to minimize widespread tissue damage.
- ▸ How to splint unstable injuries.
- ▸ How to control slow, steady bleeding.
- ▸ What to do to minimize local tissue damage.

INJURIES AND TECHNIQUES IN THIS CHAPTER

Flawlessly executing a difficult mount is only the beginning of a balance beam routine, just as the emergency action steps is only the start of sport first aid assessment and care. Both are pivotal skills but only a small portion of an entire routine. Beam specialists and sport first aiders alike must also be able to perform more common and basic but equally important skills. For a gymnast, these may be turns and jumps on the beam. For the sport first aider, these skills include conducting a physical assessment and corresponding first aid techniques.

PHYSICAL ASSESSMENT

After completing the emergency action steps and establishing that the athlete is breathing normally, you should begin the physical assessment to pinpoint the nature, site, and severity of an injury or illness. Do not begin the physical assessment until normal breathing has been established. As with the emergency action steps, follow a standard pattern, such as the following, to make the evaluation more thorough. The HIT acronym will help you remember these steps:

H—History

I—Inspection

T—Touch

History

In the physical assessment, the "history" step is a time to gather additional information about how the injury or illness happened. Your goal is to determine the location, mechanism, symptoms, and previous occurrences.

In taking an injury history, follow these steps:

1. Recall what you saw and heard.
2. Talk to the injured athlete—listen for symptoms that describe how the athlete is feeling, such as numb, pain, grating sensation, or cold.
3. Talk to other athletes, coaches, officials, or bystanders (if they witnessed the injury and if the athlete can't recall what happened).
4. Check the athlete's medical history card.

If the athlete is suffering from an injury, find out the following:

- What caused the injury (e.g., direct contact with another player, object, or the ground; or a twisting or turning motion)?
- Did the athlete hear a pop, crack, or other noise when the injury occurred?
- Where does it hurt?
- Did the athlete feel any unusual symptoms when the injury happened (e.g., pain, numbness, tingling, weakness, grating, or a snapping feeling)?
- Has the athlete suffered this injury before?

If the athlete is suffering from a sudden illness, find out the following:

- What symptoms the athlete is experiencing, such as nausea, dizziness, shortness of breath, and so on
- If the athlete is suffering from a chronic illness (e.g., diabetes, epilepsy, asthma, or allergies)
- Whether the athlete takes any medications for the illness
- What, if anything, seemed to bring on the illness (e.g., a bee sting, exposure to dust, or spoiled food)

The information that you gather during the history step will help guide your next step, which is the inspection.

Inspection

Use the information from the injury history to pinpoint where you should look for obvious signs (actual physical manifestations) of an injury or illness. For example, if an athlete reports hearing and feeling a pop in the ankle, you'll want to look for signs of an ankle injury such as a deformity or swelling. The following are other obvious signs that you should check for:

- *Bleeding*—Is it profuse or slow? Dark red or bright red?

- *Skin appearance*—Is the skin pale or flushed? Dry or sweaty? Is it blue or gray?

- *Pupils*—Compare the two pupils. Are they dilated (enlarged), constricted (small), or uneven in size? Also, use the penlight from your sport first aid kit to check whether each pupil reacts to light by constricting (figure 5.1). If the pupils are uneven or do not react to light, the athlete may be suffering from a head injury.

- *Deformities*—Do you see any indentations or bumps? If the deformity is on one side of the body, always compare it to the opposite side.

- *Signs of sudden illness*—Vomiting or coughing.

- *Swelling*—Is there any puffiness around the injured area or other areas?

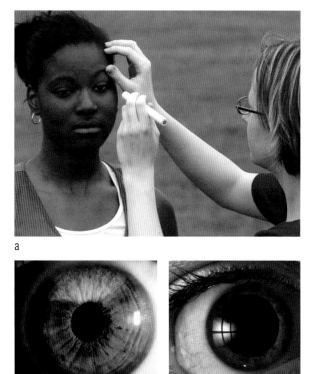

Figure 5.1 Comparing pupils: *(a)* Check whether each pupil reacts to light by constricting; *(b)* pupil with normal dilation; and *(c)* pupil that is dilated.

Photos (b) and (c) are © Custom Medical Stock Photo.

- *Discoloration*—Is there any bruising or other marks?

- *Ability to walk*—Does the athlete limp or is the athlete totally unable to bear weight?

- *Position of an upper extremity (arm, elbow, forearm, wrist, or hand)*—Is the athlete supporting the forearm with the other hand or is the arm held in an unusual position, such as out to the side?

For some illnesses and injuries, it's helpful to check the athlete's pulse (heart) rate. This can be done at either the wrist (radial pulse, figure 5.2) or neck (carotid pulse, figure 5.3). Always use your fingers to check the pulse because your thumb has its own pulse. The carotid pulse is easier to feel than the radial; however, be careful not to push too hard, or you may reduce blood flow to the athlete's brain. When taking the pulse, try to determine the rate, regularity, and strength of the heartbeat.

If the athlete has been active, pulse rate will be faster than the resting pulse rate. Table 5.1 provides normal resting heart rate per minute for various ages. If pulse rate doesn't return to resting levels within a few minutes, or if the rate feels irregular, you should suspect a potentially life-threatening injury or illness and send for emergency medical assistance.

Table 5.1 Heart Rates

Age group	Resting heart rate (beats per minute)
Children (5 to 12 years)	60-120
Adolescents (12 to 18 years)	75-85
Adults	60-100

The information gathered during the inspection should help to further pinpoint the exact nature of an illness or injury. This information, combined with what is learned in the history and in the "touch" portion of the assessment, which is performed next, will determine the first aid that you will provide.

Taking the Athlete's Pulse

RADIAL PULSE

1. Place your index and middle fingertips just below the athlete's thumb.

2. Slide your fingertips down until you feel a bony bump.

3. Move your fingers just to the inside of the bump, toward the middle of the wrist.

4. Apply slight pressure to feel the athlete's pulse (figure 5.2).

5. Check the pulse for no more than 10 seconds.

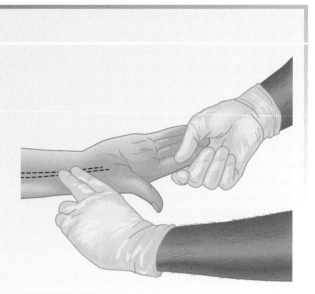

Figure 5.2 Taking the radial pulse.

CAROTID PULSE

1. Using the hand nearest the athlete's body, place your index and middle fingertips over the athlete's Adam's apple.

2. Slide your fingertips back and up in the groove along the side of the neck. Use the index and middle finger to gently apply pressure over the carotid artery (figure 5.3).

3. Check the pulse for no more than 10 seconds.

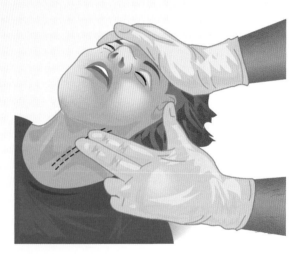

Figure 5.3 Taking the carotid pulse

Touch

Sometimes, looks can be deceiving. What appears to be an intact, fully functioning body part may in fact have severe internal damage. So, to get a better idea of the nature of the injury, gently touch the injured area with your fingertips. Start away from the injury, for example, start at the fingers and wrist if the hand is injured, and work your way toward the injury. Check for the following:

- *Point tenderness*—Is there an area that is extremely painful?

- *Skin temperature*—Is it hot? Cool? Sweaty? Dry?

- *Sensation*—Can the athlete feel you touching the area?

- *Deformity*—Can you feel any bumps or indentations that you did not see in the inspection?

Again, if one side of the body is injured (such as the ribs, arm, or leg), always compare it to the opposite side. After completing the physical assessment of history, inspection, and touch, you will be better able to focus your first aid techniques on the specific injury or illness that is affecting an athlete.

Take some time to review the procedures of the physical assessment, shown in figure 5.4.

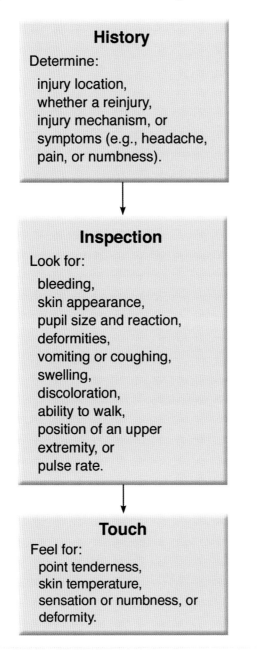

History

Determine:

injury location,
whether a reinjury,
injury mechanism, or
symptoms (e.g., headache,
pain, or numbness).

Inspection

Look for:

bleeding,
skin appearance,
pupil size and reaction,
deformities,
vomiting or coughing,
swelling,
discoloration,
ability to walk,
position of an upper
extremity, or
pulse rate.

Touch

Feel for:
point tenderness,
skin temperature,
sensation or numbness, or
deformity.

Figure 5.4 Physical assessment protocol.

Remember to continue to monitor breathing even after beginning to administer first aid to the site of the injury. You must continually observe any seriously injured athlete, even though the athlete's breathing may initially be normal.

BASIC SPORT FIRST AID TECHNIQUES

Upon completing the physical assessment, you may find that you have to control external bleeding, minimize systemic tissue damage (shock), splint injuries, and minimize local tissue damage. So let's discuss these basic first aid techniques, in order of priority.

Controlling Profuse Bleeding

Although not a common injury, profuse bleeding from an artery or vein can be life threatening. Bleeding can also occur internally, from injuries such as bruised muscles, ruptured spleens, and bruised kidneys. Details on bleeding internal organs and how to care for them are explained in chapter 9.

Before administering first aid for bleeding, be sure to protect yourself against exposure to infected blood.

Preventing Blood-Borne Pathogen Transmission

Don't let a fear of human immunodeficiency virus (HIV), hepatitis B, or other blood-borne pathogens keep you from administering first aid to injured athletes. Learn more about these diseases and how they can be transmitted. Contact your state athletic association for specific sports rules and policies regarding blood-borne pathogens. For example, some sports require athletes to change a bloody uniform before returning to competition.

Precautions to Protect Against Blood-Borne Pathogens

If care of an injured athlete involves handling

- bloody wounds or dressings,
- mouth guards,
- body fluids,
- bloody linen or clothing, or
- bloody playing surfaces and equipment,

then follow these guidelines:

1. Wear disposable examination gloves (latex free, to avoid allergic reactions).
2. Wear safety glasses or a face shield if your face will be exposed to blood or body fluids.
3. Immediately wash any portion of your skin that comes in contact with blood or body fluid.
4. Bag contaminated linens or clothing, and then wash them in hot water and detergent.
5. Clean contaminated floors, equipment, and other surfaces with a 1:10 solution of bleach and water. Wiping up the solution reduces its effectiveness, so you should let the surface air dry after the solution is applied.
6. Remove your contaminated gloves properly (see Proper Removal of Contaminated Gloves). Place contaminated gloves and bandages in a biohazard waste bag.
7. Immediately wash your hands with soap and water after removing the examination gloves. You can clean with an alcohol-based hand rub, but if your hands are visibly soiled, wash with soap and water.

Taking these steps all the time, regardless of who the athlete is, is called "taking Universal Precautions." This means that you treat all human blood and most body fluids as if they were infectious for blood-borne pathogens, even if you think perhaps they aren't.

Review your school district's plan for

- disposing of contaminated waste;
- handling athletes who are infected with blood-borne pathogens;
- reporting employee (coaches, teachers, and others) exposure to blood-borne pathogens; and
- protecting employees against the transmission of blood-borne pathogens (i.e., policies, procedures, equipment, and possibly hepatitis B vaccinations).

PROPER REMOVAL OF CONTAMINATED GLOVES

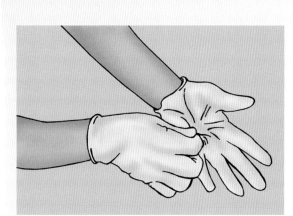

1. Without touching the bare skin, grasp either palm with the fingers of the opposite hand.

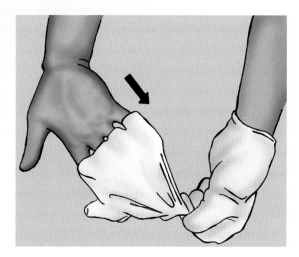

2. Gently pull the glove away from the palm and toward the fingers, removing the glove inside out. Hold on to the glove with the fingers of the opposite hand.

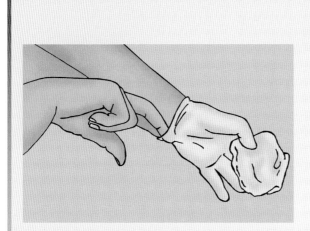

3. Without touching the outside of the contaminated glove, carefully slide the ungloved index finger inside the wristband of the gloved hand.

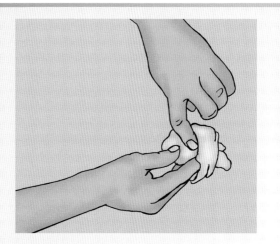

4. Gently pulling outward and down toward the fingers, remove the glove inside out.

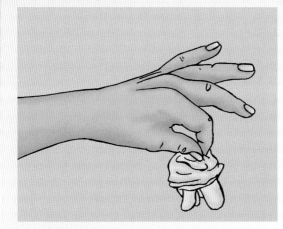

5. Throw away both gloves in an appropriate container.

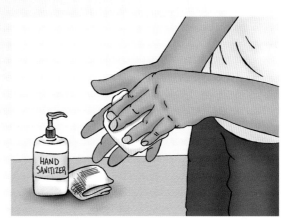

6. Use an alcohol-based hand rub to clean your hands and other exposed skin.

Courtesy of American Safety & Health Institute.

➥ Playing It Safe...
With Bleeding Injuries

- Do not attempt to pull out embedded objects.
- Do not remove blood-soaked bandages from a wound. This may cause bleeding to resume. For example, if you put gauze over an athlete's hand to stop bleeding, don't remove the gauze to see whether the wound has stopped bleeding. You'll know if it's still bleeding because blood will continue to seep through the bandages.
- Do not give aspirin to the athlete. Aspirin can cause increased bleeding.

Arterial and Venous Bleeding

Profuse bleeding caused by a cut to a limb.

Once you have protected yourself from infected blood, you need to quickly determine the extent of the bleeding. A cut to a limb artery or vein can cause profuse bleeding. The first aid steps for arterial and venous bleeding are identical. However, the causes and signs of each are slightly different.

Causes of Arterial Bleeding

- Very deep incision, laceration, or puncture of an artery

Check for Signs of Arterial Bleeding

- Bright red blood
- Rapid or spurting bleeding

Causes of Venous Bleeding

- Deep incision, avulsion, or puncture of a vein

Check for Signs of Venous Bleeding

- Dark red blood
- Rapid bleeding

FIRST AID

1. Put on gloves and goggles or mask, if you haven't already done so, to protect yourself against blood-borne pathogens.
2. Send for emergency medical assistance.
3. Cover the wound with sterile gauze pads.
4. Apply firm, direct pressure over the wound with your hand.
5. Apply elastic roller gauze or elastic bandage over the gauze pads. Make sure it's not so tight that a finger cannot be slipped under the bandage.
6. If the initial dressings become soaked with blood, place additional gauze pads and roller gauze over the existing dressings.
7. Monitor breathing and provide CPR as needed.
8. Monitor and treat for shock as needed (addressed later in this chapter).

Playing Status

- The athlete cannot return to activity until examined and released by physician.

Page 267 in appendix A summarizes the first aid techniques for profuse bleeding.

➡ Playing It Safe...
When Treating for Shock

Do not give fluids to an athlete who is suffering from shock. Doing so can cause vomiting or choking.

Minimizing Systemic Tissue Damage

Injury, illness, or dehydration can cause the body to shift into life-saving mode. The body attempts to preserve life-sustaining blood, water, and oxygen to the brain, heart, lungs, and other vital organs by diverting them from the skin, limbs, and other noncritical tissues. This is called shock. If not treated, shock can cause extensive and irreversible tissue damage and even death.

Table 5.2 summarizes what was discussed in the previous chapter about positioning an ill or injured athlete and adds positioning for shock from severe bleeding.

Systemic Tissue Damage (Shock)

A condition in which the body diverts blood, water, and oxygen from the skin, limbs, and other noncritical tissues to the brain, heart, lungs, and other vital organs.

Causes
- Trauma, heat, allergic reactions, severe infection, dehydration, poisoning, low pain tolerance, bleeding

Ask if Experiencing Symptoms
- Weakness
- Fatigue
- Dizziness
- Nausea
- Thirst
- Anxiety

Check for Signs
- Cool and clammy skin
- Pale or grayish skin
- Weak and rapid pulse
- Slow and shallow breathing
- Dilated pupils
- Blank stare
- Confusion
- Possible unresponsiveness
- Sweating
- Shaking or shivering
- Bluish lips and fingernails

✚ FIRST AID

1. Send for emergency medical assistance if you haven't already done so.
2. Position the athlete appropriately, depending on his or her condition (see table 5.2).
3. Monitor breathing and provide CPR if needed.
4. Maintain normal body temperature by covering the athlete as needed.
5. Provide first aid care for bleeding and other injuries.
6. Reassure the athlete.

Playing Status
- The athlete cannot return to activity until examined and released by physician.

Table 5.2 Positions for Ill or Injured Athletes

Condition	Position	Rationale
Responsive athlete with suspected spinal injury	Manually stabilize the head so that the head, neck, and spine do not move and are kept in line (see figure 5.5).	Pain and loss of function usually accompany a spinal injury, but the absence of pain does not mean that the athlete has not been significantly injured. If you suspect an athlete could possibly have a spinal injury, assume he or she does.
Unresponsive, uninjured athlete who is breathing, but having difficulty with secretions or vomiting	Recovery position	Protects airway by allowing fluid to drain easily from the mouth.
Unresponsive, injured athlete who is breathing, but having difficulty with secretions or vomiting OR who you must leave unattended to get help	Modified recovery position (HAINES)	Protects airway by allowing fluid to drain easily from the mouth. Using the HAINES position, there is less neck movement and less risk of spinal-cord damage
Unresponsive athlete who is not breathing (or you are unsure)	Flat on the back for CPR	Occasional gasps are not normal and are not capable of supplying the athlete with enough oxygen to sustain life.
Responsive or unresponsive athlete with signs and symptoms of shock from severe bleeding	Flat on the back	It is best to leave the athlete lying flat. If athlete is having difficulty with secretions or vomiting, place in the recovery position. If spinal injury is suspected, use the HAINES position.

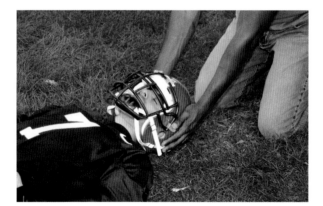

Figure 5.5 Potential head and spine injury—position face up and flat on ground, while stabilizing the head.

Splinting Unstable Injuries

To prevent further tissue damage, bone fractures, joint dislocations and subluxations, and Grade II and III ligament sprains should be stabilized. Remember, the hallmark of first aid care is to prevent further injury and to do no harm. With this in mind, follow these guidelines for applying splints:

1. Do not move the athlete until all unstable injuries are splinted, unless the athlete is in danger of further injury or requires repositioning for CPR or control of profuse bleeding or shock.

2. Contact emergency medical personnel and let them splint the following:

- Large joint dislocations (shoulder, hip, knee, kneecap, elbow, wrist, and ankle)

- Injuries where bones create an obvious deformity

- Compound fractures

- Fractures of the spine, pelvis, hip, thigh, shoulder girdle, upper arm, elbow, kneecap, or shin

- Displaced rib fractures or displaced clavicle from a severe sternoclavicular joint sprain (see page 151 in chapter 12)

- Any musculoskeletal injuries that result in loss of circulation or nerve damage signified by numbness, blue or grayish skin, cold skin, inability to move fingers or toes of affected limb, or significant weakness of the affected limb

- Any musculoskeletal injuries in which the athlete is also suffering from shock

Prevent the athlete from moving until emergency medical personnel arrive. If emergency medical assistance will arrive in 20 minutes or less, stabilize the injured limb with your hands. Place one hand above and the other below the injured area and limit movement while you wait for emergency personnel to arrive.

3. If the arrival of emergency medical help will take longer than 20 minutes, splint the injury in the position in which you found it. However, for spine fractures, simply stabilize the head, prevent the athlete from moving, and wait for emergency medical personnel to arrive.

4. Cover the ends of exposed bones with sterile gauze.

5. Splint with rigid or bulky materials that are well padded. You don't need expensive manufactured splints. Tongue depressors, boards, cardboard, bats, magazines, blankets, and pillows can be used as splints.

6. For fractures or for severe joint sprains, immobilize the bones above and below the joint. For example, if the lower leg is broken just below the knee, immobilize the thighbone and the lower leg bones. For fractures that occur in the middle of a bone, stabilize the joints above and below the fracture. For instance, if the upper arm bone is broken in the middle, apply a splint and then use a sling to immobilize the elbow and shoulder.

7. Secure the splint with ties or an elastic wrap. Place ties above and below the injury, but not directly over it. Apply light, even pressure with the wrap, so as not to press directly upon the injury.

8. Periodically check the skin color, temperature, and sensation of the hand and fingers or foot and toes of the splinted limb. Splints that are too tight can compress nerves or arteries. If an athlete complains of numbness, if the skin appears blue or gray or feels cold, or if the nail beds appear blue, then the splint is too tight.

For a summary of splinting techniques, see page 268 in appendix A.

Pages 72 and 73 show proper splinting techniques for the upper arm (figure 5.6), elbow (figure 5.7, a and b), forearm and wrist (figure 5.8), finger (figure 5.9), thigh (figure 5.10), kneecap (figure 5.11), lower leg (figure 5.12), and ankle and foot (figure 5.13).

Playing It Safe... With Splinting

- Do not attempt to reposition fractured or dislocated bones. This could sever nerves and arteries as well as cause further damage to the bones, ligaments, cartilage, muscles, and tendons.

- Do not attempt to push exposed bones back under the skin.

SPLINTING TECHNIQUES

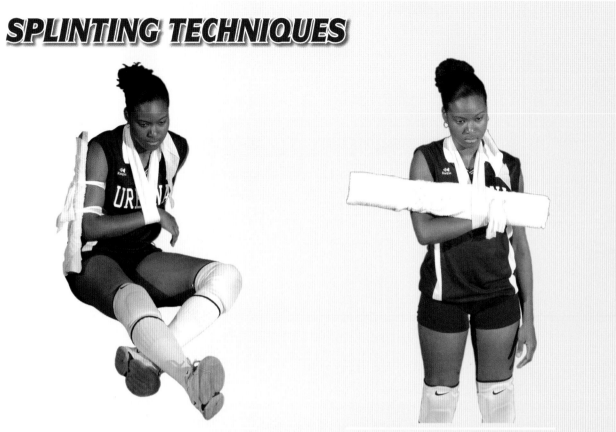

Figure 5.6 Proper splint for the upper arm.

Figure 5.7a Proper splint for the elbow.

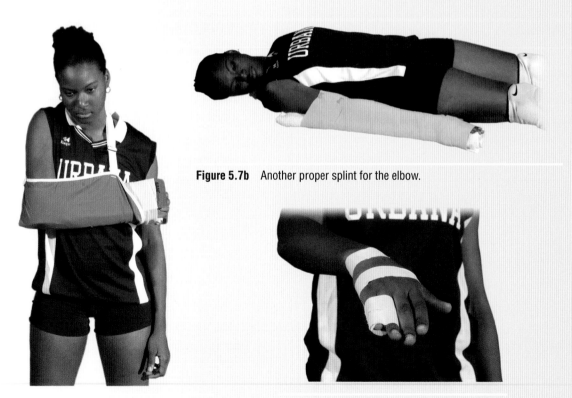

Figure 5.7b Another proper splint for the elbow.

Figure 5.8 Proper splint for the forearm or wrist.

Figure 5.9 Proper splint for the finger.

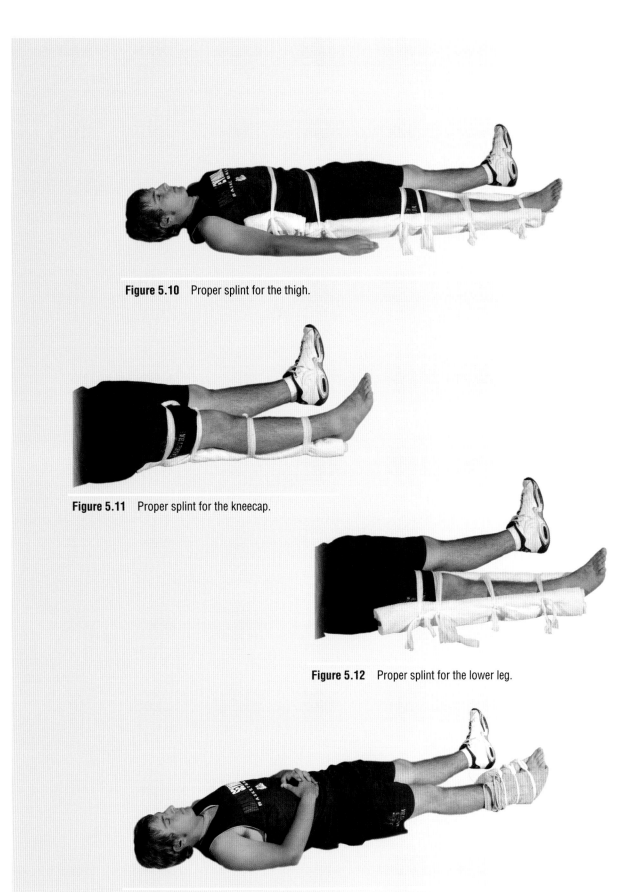

Figure 5.10   Proper splint for the thigh.

Figure 5.11   Proper splint for the kneecap.

Figure 5.12   Proper splint for the lower leg.

Figure 5.13   Proper splint for the ankle and foot.

Controlling Slow, Steady Bleeding

After all the unstable injuries are splinted, you should administer first aid for any slow, steady (capillary) bleeding of superficial wounds.

See chapter 14 for additional information and first aid procedures for abrasions and superficial lacerations.

Capillary Bleeding

Slow, steady bleeding caused by superficial wounds.

Causes
- Superficial skin abrasion or laceration

Check for Signs
- Slow, oozing blood

⊕ FIRST AID

1. Put on gloves and goggles or mask as needed, if you haven't already done so, to protect yourself against blood-borne pathogens.
2. Apply sterile gauze, then firm, direct pressure over the wound with your hand.
3. Once bleeding stops, do the following:
   a. Gently clean the wound.

b. Cover the wound with sterile gauze or bandage.
c. If you are unable to clean all debris from the wound, or if the wound edges gape open and do not touch (may need stitches), send the athlete to a physician.

Playing Status
- The athlete can return to activity if bleeding stops and the athlete was not sent to a physician. The wound must be covered to protect it as well as to protect other athletes from the possible transmission of blood-borne pathogens.

Minimizing Local Tissue Damage

If part of the body is injured, the body's local tissue reaction can cause damage to the surrounding tissues. For example, in an ankle sprain, not only does the injured ligament bleed and swell, but the tissues around it do as well. That's why you see discoloration and swelling all around the ankle joint.

Injury or infection to a particular area can cause the following localized tissue reactions:

- Bleeding from the injured blood vessels
- Fluid leakage from damaged tissue cells
- Swelling
- Temperature increase
- Pain
- Loss of function (inability to use a body part)

Bleeding and fluid leakage from the damaged tissue cells can disrupt blood flow not only to the injured tissues but also to surrounding tissues. This can delay healing. The best way to minimize local tissue damage is to apply the PRICE principle:

P—Protection
R—Rest
I—Ice
C—Compression
E—Elevation

All of the components of PRICE work to reduce the chance of further injury to the area. In addition, they minimize swelling, which helps prevent further tissue damage.

Protection

Protect the athlete from further injury by preventing the athlete from moving and by keeping other athletes and hazards clear of the athlete.

Rest

Rest the athlete from any activity that causes pain. If simple movements such as bending, straightening, reaching overhead, or walking are painful, "rest" means immobilizing the injured limb by splinting or preventing weight bearing with crutches. Do not allow the athlete to return to participation until the athlete is examined and released by a physician and is able to play without pain or loss of function (e.g., no limping, no decrease or adjustments in arm movements). If pain only occurs during strenuous workouts or sports participation, rest the athlete from the painful exercises, drills, and sport skills and refer the athlete to a physician.

Ice

During the first 72 hours following an injury, ice can help minimize pain and control swelling caused by bleeding and fluid loss from the injured tissues. There are several different ways ice can be applied, such as with an ice bag (figure 5.14a), ice massage (figure 5.14b), gel cold pack, ice whirlpool, chemical cold pack, and ice water bucket. No matter which method is used, athletes will typically experience cold, pins and needles, dull aching, and numbness sensations when ice is applied. These sensations are normal and to be expected. Table 5.3 discusses the application, indications, problems, and precautions of each method.

Ice helps control swelling after the initial injury by helping reduce blood flow (bleeding). Compression and elevation are also valuable in helping to reduce initial blood loss, and once the bleeding has stopped, they are needed to get rid of the swelling that has already occurred.

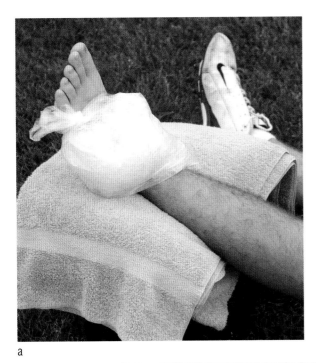

a

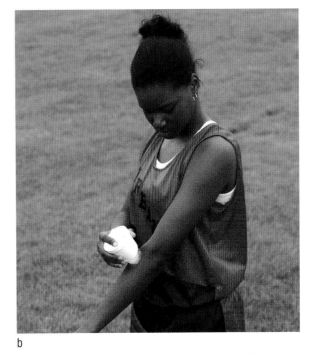

b

Figure 5.14 *(a)* Ice bag and *(b)* ice massage.

Table 5.3 Types of Ice Applications

Type	Applications	Indications	Problems	Frequency	Precautions
Ice bag (figure 5.14a)	Place crushed ice (conforms the best to the body) in a plastic bag directly over injury.	Large areas such as the back, shoulder, thigh, upper arm, chest, knee, and ankle		15-20 minutes or until area feels numb. Can be reapplied every 2 hours as needed for pain and swelling.	Do not apply over open wounds or if athlete is allergic to cold. Apply a thin cloth between the skin and the ice bag.
Ice massage (figure 5.14b)	Rub ice cube or ice frozen in a paper cup directly over injury.	Small bony areas, such as elbows, wrists, hands, and feet		5-10 minutes or until area feels numb. Can be reapplied every 2 hours as needed for pain and swelling.	Do not apply over open wounds or if athlete is allergic to cold.
Gel cold pack	Place cooled pack over injury.	Small areas, depending on size of pack		15-20 minutes or until area feels numb. Can be reapplied every 2 hours as needed for pain and swelling.	Packs have a tendency to freeze the skin, so apply a thin cloth between the skin and the pack.
Ice whirlpool	Submerse foot, leg, hand, or arm into icy water.	Limbs	1. Athletes typically do not tolerate well 2. Since injured area is placed down into whirlpool, does not allow for concurrent elevation 3. Inconvenient	10-15 minutes or until area feels numb. Can be repeated every 2 hours as needed for pain and swelling.	Do not place athletes with open wounds in a whirlpool. This can increase risk of infection.
Chemical cold pack	Place cooled pack over injury.	Small areas, depending on size of pack	May not remain cold long enough	15-20 minutes or until area feels numb. Can be reapplied every 2 hours as needed for pain and swelling.	Chemicals may cause skin burns if pack is punctured.
Ice water bucket	Submerse ankle, foot, wrist, or hand into icy water.	Limbs	1. Athletes typically do not tolerate well 2. Since injured area is placed down into bucket, does not allow for concurrent elevation 3. Inconvenient	10-15 minutes or until area feels numb. Can be repeated every 2 hours as needed for pain and swelling.	Do not place limbs with open wounds in a bucket. This can increase risk of infection.

Playing It Safe...
When Applying Ice

In some instances, ice can be harmful. Following are some contraindications, or reasons, for which ice should not be applied.

- Do not apply ice if the athlete lacks feeling in the area.
- Do not apply ice if the athlete is allergic to cold. Allergic reactions to ice include blisters, red skin, and rashes.
- Do not ice for longer than 20 minutes. This can minimize the ability of the ice to restrict blood flow to the area.

- Do not apply a tight compression wrap in combination with ice. This may result in nerve damage.
- Do not apply ice directly over an open wound.
- Do not apply ice directly over a superficial nerve, like the ulnar nerve (figure 5.15) at the elbow or the peroneal nerve (figure 5.16) on the outside of the knee.

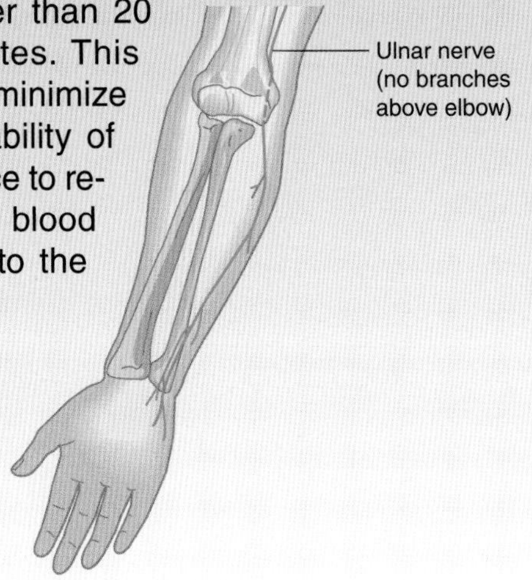

Ulnar nerve (no branches above elbow)

Figure 5.15 Do not apply ice directly over the ulnar nerve.

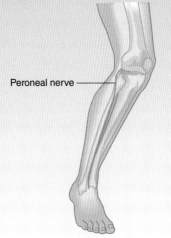

Peroneal nerve

Figure 5.16 Do not apply ice directly over the peroneal nerve.

Compression

To control initial bleeding of joint or limb tissues, or to reduce residual swelling, apply an elastic wrap to an injured limb, especially the foot, ankle, knee, thigh, hand, or elbow. Follow these steps to apply an effective compression wrap:

1. Start several inches below the injury (farthest from the heart). For example, for the ankle, start the wrap just above the toes (figure 5.17a).
2. Wrap upward (toward the heart), in an overlapping spiral, starting with even and somewhat snug pressure, then gradually wrapping looser once above the injury (figure 5.17b).
3. Periodically check the skin color, temperature, and sensation of the injured area to make sure that the wrap isn't compressing any nerves or arteries. (For example, for a forearm wrap, check the fingers and nail beds for blue or purplish tint and for coldness.) Wraps that are too tight can reduce blood flow to the area and cause tissue damage.

Figures 5.18 to 5.21 illustrate compression wraps for other parts of the body.

COMPRESSION WRAPS

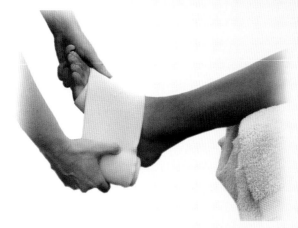

Figure 5.17a Start wrap farthest away from the heart.

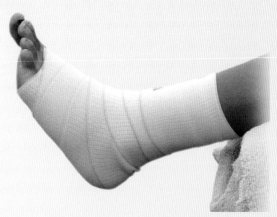

Figure 5.17b Wrap in a spiral fashion with even pressure.

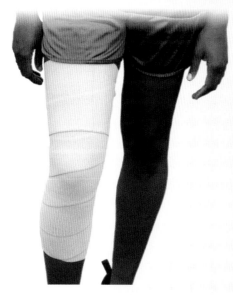

Figure 5.18 Knee compression wrap.

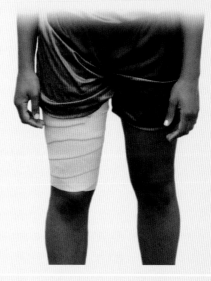

Figure 5.19 Thigh compression wrap.

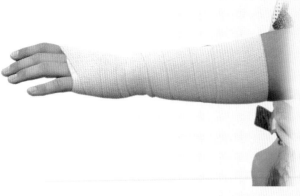

Figure 5.20 Forearm compression wrap.

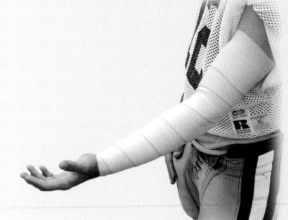

Figure 5.21 Elbow compression wrap.

Playing It Safe...
With Applying Heat

If swelling from an acute injury is still present, do not apply heat. Heat causes increased blood flow to the area and can increase swelling. Heat therapy is generally reserved for warming up chronic muscle strains or tendinitis injuries prior to exercise or activity. So do not apply or recommend heat unless a medical professional prescribes it.

Elevation

Used in combination with ice and compression, elevation can also minimize internal tissue bleeding and subsequent swelling (figure 5.22). Elevate the injured part above the heart as much as possible for the first 72 hours, or longer if swelling persists.

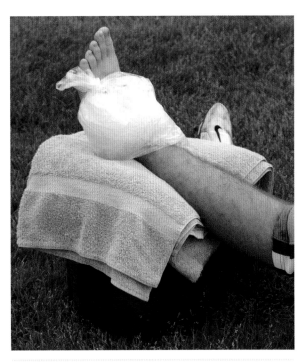

Figure 5.22 Elevate the injured part above heart level.

Chapter 5 REPLAY

- ☐ What two criteria should be met before performing a physical assessment? (p. 62)
- ☐ When doing a physical assessment, what does the HIT process mean? (pp. 62-65)
- ☐ What is the difference between arterial and venous bleeding? (p. 68)
- ☐ How do you stop profuse bleeding? (pp. 65-68)
- ☐ What are the signs and symptoms of shock? (p. 69)
- ☐ When is it acceptable to splint an unstable injury? (pp. 70-71)
- ☐ How should a splint be applied for fractures or for severe sprains? (p. 71)
- ☐ What are the signs that a splint is applied too tight? (p. 71)
- ☐ When can an athlete who has a wound that is bleeding slow and steady return to activity? (p. 74)
- ☐ What does PRICE stand for? (pp. 74-79)
- ☐ What are the cons of using cold whirlpools and ice bucket immersion? (p. 76)
- ☐ How do you correctly apply a compression wrap on the thigh? (p. 78)
- ☐ What is the technique for effective elevation? (p. 79)

REFERENCES

Berg, R.A., R. Hemphill, B.S. Abella, T.P. Aufderheide, D.M. Cave, M.F. Hazinski, E.B. Lerner, T.D. Rea, M.R. Sayre, and R.A. Swor. 2010. Part 5: Adult basic life support: 2010 American Heart Association Guidelines for Cardiopulmonary Resuscitation and Emergency Cardiovascular Care. *Circulation* 122: S685-S705

Markenson, D., J.D. Ferguson, L. Chameides, P. Cassan, K. Chung, J. Epstein, L. Gonzales, R.A. Herrington, J.L. Pellegrino, N. Ratcliff, and A. Singer. 2010. Part 17: First aid: 2010 American Heart Association and American Red Cross guidelines for first aid. *Circulation* 122: S934-46.

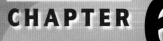

CHAPTER **6**

Moving Injured or Sick Athletes

IN THIS CHAPTER, YOU WILL LEARN:

▸ When to call for emergency medical assistance to move an athlete.

▸ When it may be acceptable to move an athlete yourself.

▸ What moving techniques you should use.

▸ How to do the one-person drag, four- or five-person rescue, the one-person walking assist, the two-person walking assist, the four-handed carrying assist, and the two-handed carrying assist.

In golf, knowing when to use a particular club for a particular situation is critical to winning. For example, a driver is used for hitting a long ball off the tee. A wedge is used to make a short, arcing shot to the green, and a putter is used for precision shots on the green.

This same theory can be used when determining when and how to move an injured athlete. You must carefully select which move to do at which time or you could further harm an athlete.

Perhaps the most difficult decisions in giving first aid care are when to move an athlete and when to call for emergency medical assistance. As with all first aid procedures, the basic rule for moving injured athletes is to err on the side of caution. Chapter 1 discussed the legal system's expectation of you as a coach, which is to minimize the risk of injury to athletes under your supervision. This includes the risk of further injury by moving.

MOVING CRITICALLY INJURED ATHLETES

For life-threatening or serious injury or illness, keep the athlete still and call for emergency medical assistance to move the athlete. Critical conditions include

- breathing difficulties;
- head, neck, or back injuries;
- shock;
- profuse bleeding;
- internal injuries;
- unresponsiveness;
- large joint dislocations (shoulder, hip, knee, kneecap, elbow, and ankle);
- compound fractures;
- fractures of the spine, pelvis, hip, thigh, shoulder girdle, upper arm, kneecap, or shin;

- displaced fracture of the ribs or Grade III sternoclavicular joint sprain;
- first-time seizures; and
- serious eye injuries.

However, it may be necessary for you to move an athlete in these situations if (a) the athlete is in danger of further harm, or (b) it is necessary to move or reposition the athlete to provide first aid for a life-threatening condition.

Danger of Further Harm

Following are incidents in which an athlete may need to be moved because of the potential for further harm:

- Environmental emergencies—Lightning, tornado, hurricane, fire, downed electrical lines, or flooding.

- Dangerous scene—Traffic, other runners, cyclists, uncontrolled animals, or insect swarms (particularly in road races).

Unable to Provide First Aid for Life-Threatening Conditions

Following are occasions in which repositioning an athlete is necessary to provide appropriate first aid:

- Unresponsive athlete lying on stomach or side who needs CPR.
- Athlete suffering from heatstroke who must be quickly cooled with water and ice.

Different techniques for moving a critically injured or ill athlete include the one-person drag, and the four- or five-person rescue.

One-Person Drag

Purpose: **To move an unresponsive athlete from a dangerous environment by yourself.**

Technique

1. Squat down just beyond the athlete's head.
2. Place your hands under the athlete's armpits and cradle the head with your forearms (figure 6.1).
3. Partially straighten your knees to protect your back.
4. Slowly drag the athlete to a safe location.

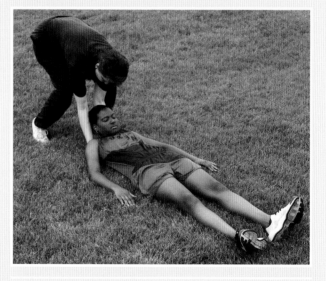

Figure 6.1 One-person drag.

➡ Playing It Safe...
When Moving Critically Injured, Unresponsive Athletes

Suspect that an unresponsive athlete may have a head or spine injury if the injury was caused by a sudden and forceful movement (direct blow), compression, or twisting of the spine. Manually stabilize the head, neck, and back before repositioning the athlete to provide CPR or moving the athlete.

Four- or Five-Person Rescue

Purpose: To turn over a responsive or unresponsive athlete who is face down breathing normally and who MUST be moved or placed on a spine (back) board. This technique may also be used to roll unresponsive victims into the recovery or the HAINES position to allow vomit to drain from the mouth.

Technique

1. A formally trained first aid provider goes to the athlete's head and directs the other rescuers.
2. This individual grasps the head, holding on to both sides of the head and jaw (figure 6.2*a*).
3. The lead rescuer commands the other rescuers to position themselves at the shoulder, hips, and legs, as shown in figure 6.2*b*.
4. A fifth rescuer places the spine board (if available) next to the athlete.
5. The lead rescuer uses the command "ready" then "up" to instruct everyone to roll the athlete (facing away from the board, toward the rescuers) as a unit, being sure to keep the head, neck, shoulders, trunk, hip, and legs in alignment (figure 6.2*b*).
6. The fifth rescuer slides the board next to the athlete's back.
7. The lead rescuer, using the "ready" and "down" commands, instructs everyone to slowly roll the athlete onto the board as a unit (figure 6.2*c*).

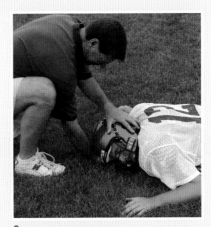

a

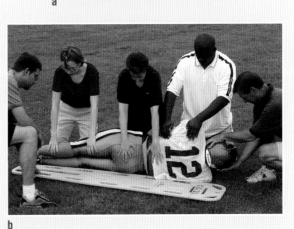

b

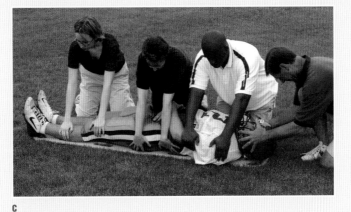

c

Figure 6.2 The five-person rescue. *(a)* A trained first aider holds sides of head and jaw, *(b)* the group rolls the athlete toward the rescuers, and *(c)* the group rolls the athlete onto the board.

MOVING NONCRITICALLY INJURED ATHLETES

A common situation you may face is one in which an athlete has a minor or moderate injury such as a muscle pull or arm contusion. When this type of situation arises, you will use one of several types of assists.

Less severely injured athletes can be more readily moved, but you must still exercise ex-treme caution. If necessary, you may move an athlete suffering from these conditions:

- Sprains and strains
- Solar plexus injury ("wind knocked out")
- Contusions
- Facial injuries
- Closed and nondisplaced (no gross deformity) fractures of the finger, hand, wrist, forearm, ankle, and foot
- Finger dislocations

➡ Playing It Safe...
When Moving Noncritically Injured Athletes

Before moving a noncritically injured athlete, you should

- control profuse bleeding and
- immobilize or splint all unstable injuries.

One-Person Walking Assist

Purpose: **To walk a dazed or slightly injured athlete off the playing area by yourself.**

Technique

1. Instruct the athlete to place an arm around you and hold on to your shoulder.
2. Grasp the athlete around the waist with your free hand.
3. Instruct the athlete to lean on you as needed when walking (figure 6.3).

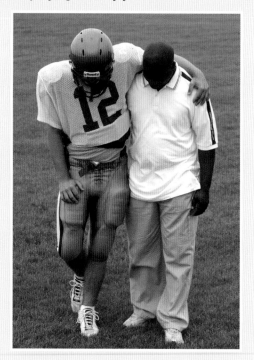

Figure 6.3 One-person walking assist.

Two-Person Walking Assist

Purpose: To walk a dazed or slightly injured athlete off the playing area with the help of another person.

Technique

1. Instruct the assistant to follow your directions, so as not to endanger the well-being of the athlete.
2. Stand on opposite sides of the athlete.
3. Place the athlete's arms around you (and your assistant) and instruct the athlete to hold on to your shoulders.
4. Hold the athlete around the waist.
5. Slowly walk to the sidelines, supporting the athlete with your arms and shoulders (figure 6.4).

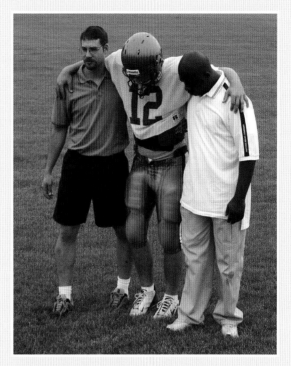

Figure 6.4   Two-person walking assist.

Four-Handed Carrying Assist

Purpose: To move (with the help of another person) a responsive and coherent athlete who is not able to walk but is able to assist you in moving himself or herself, by holding on to the rescuers' shoulders. This carry is especially useful if it is too far or too difficult for the athlete to move with the two-person walking assist.

Technique

1. Instruct the assistant to follow your directions, so as not to endanger the well-being of the athlete.
2. Stand behind the athlete and face each other.
3. Grasp your right forearm with your left hand.
4. Then grasp each other's left forearm with your right hand (figure 6.5a).

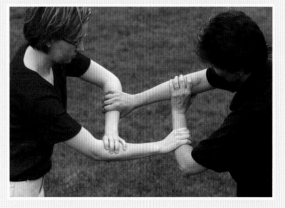

Figure 6.5a   Four-handed carrying assist hand positions.

(continued)

Four-Handed Carrying Assist *(continued)*

5. Instruct the athlete to sit on your arms and to place arms around your shoulders (figure 6.5*b*).

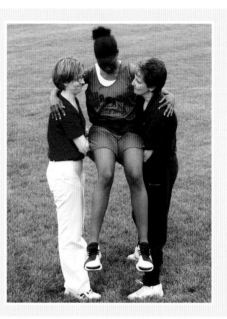

Figure 6.5b Four-handed carrying assist athlete position.

Two-Handed Carrying Assist

Purpose: **To move (with the help of another person) a slightly dazed athlete who is not able to walk and needs additional support from the rescuers.**

Technique

1. Instruct the assistant to follow your directions, so as not to endanger the well-being of the athlete.
2. Stand behind the injured athlete, facing your partner.
3. Grasp each other's forearms nearest the athlete.
4. Instruct the athlete to sit on your and your assistant's arms and to put his or her arms around your shoulders.
5. Support the athlete's back with your free arms (figure 6.6).
6. Slowly lift the athlete by straightening your legs.

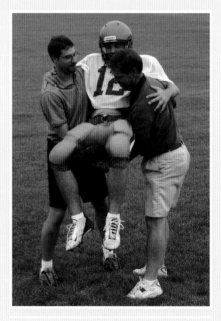

Figure 6.6 Two-handed carrying assist.

Page 269 in appendix A summarizes the guidelines for moving sick or injured athletes, and table 6.1 matches the type of transfer to use with certain injury conditions.

If you have a history of back or leg problems, or if you are considerably smaller than the athlete, do not attempt the four-handed carrying assist or the two-handed carrying assist.

Table 6.1 Type of Transfer to Use for Injury Conditions

Situation	Number of rescuers	Type of transfer
Unresponsive athlete in danger of further injury if left in present location	1	One-person drag
Need to move unresponsive athlete in order to assess or to provide life-saving first aid	4 or more	Four- or five-person rescue
Walking a dazed or slightly injured athlete off the playing area	1 2	One-person walking assist Two-person walking assist
Moving a responsive and coherent athlete who is not able to walk but is able to assist in moving himself or herself	2	Four-handed carrying assist
Moving a slightly dazed athlete who is not able to walk and needs additional support from the rescuers	2	Two-handed carrying assist

Chapter 6 *REPLAY*

☐ What injuries are considered so serious that an athlete should not be moved until emergency medical assistance arrives? (pp. 81-82)

☐ Under what two conditions may you move a critically injured athlete? (p. 82)

☐ If an athlete is injured and you suspect head, neck, or back injuries, and yet the athlete must be moved, what guidelines must be followed? (p. 82)

☐ What two methods can be used to move a critically injured athlete? (pp. 82-83)

☐ What two things must be done before moving an athlete with a closed, nondisplaced fracture, or a strain or sprain? (p. 84)

☐ What four methods can be used to move a noncritically injured athlete? (pp. 84-87)

☐ Can you describe the steps of the
    ☐ one-person drag? (p. 82)
    ☐ four- or five-person rescue? (p. 83)
    ☐ one-person walking assist? (p. 84)
    ☐ two-person walking assist? (p. 85)
    ☐ four-handed carrying assist? (pp. 85-86)
    ☐ two-handed carrying assist? (p. 86)

PART III

Sport First Aid for Specific Injuries

"I won't accept anything less than the best a player's capable of doing . . . and he has the right to expect the best that I can do for him and the team."

Lou Holtz

Being the best at sport first aid involves appropriately applying the basics of sport first aid to specific injuries and illnesses. So before proceeding to the next chapters, you may want to review what you learned about your athletic health care teammates, your first aid responsibilities, basic anatomy, and evaluation and first aid procedures. After all, you wouldn't expect your athletes to run a play during a game without reviewing it in practice.

Once you're confident about your comprehension of the material, you are ready to learn how to apply it to specific injury and illness situations. Part III covers more than 110 different conditions. The chapters are ordered according to priority, from life-threatening conditions to serious then minor problems. Chapters 7 through 11 will familiarize you with potential life-threatening problems such as respiratory conditions, head and spine injuries, internal organ injuries, sudden illnesses, and temperature-related illnesses. Although you may never face these life-threatening situations during your coaching career, it's vital that you are prepared—an athlete's life may depend on it. Upper body and lower body musculoskeletal injuries, face and scalp injuries, and skin conditions are covered in chapters 12 through 15.

In each chapter, specifics of each condition are outlined including the

- name of the condition,
- definition,
- possible causes,
- symptoms (sensations that the athlete felt or is experiencing), and
- signs (actual physical manifestations that you can directly observe).

Plus, each condition includes strategies for the following:

First Aid: How to care for the condition

Playing Status: Determining when it is safe to allow an athlete to resume participation

Prevention: How to best avoid future occurrences of an injury or illness

By no means will these chapters teach you all you need to know about evaluating and caring for all sport injuries and illnesses. However, they will give you basic guidance on how to act in the event of certain injuries and illnesses and can serve as a resource that you can refer to when needed.

As a coach, you are often the initial caregiver, so you owe it to your athletes to be prepared to help them when they need it.

Respiratory Emergencies and Illnesses

IN THIS CHAPTER, YOU WILL LEARN:

- ▸ How to identify the signs and symptoms of anaphylactic shock, asthma, collapsed lung, throat contusion, pneumonia or bronchitis, solar plexus spasm ("wind knocked out"), and hyperventilation.
- ▸ What first aid care to provide for each of these conditions.
- ▸ How to prevent allergies, asthma, bronchitis, and pneumonia from progressing into life-threatening emergencies.

INJURIES AND ILLNESSES IN THIS CHAPTER

You're down by one, there are six seconds left on the clock, you have no time-outs left, and your team is inbounding the ball from under your opponent's basket. There is precious little time to waste. If your team doesn't have a set play to handle the full-court press and get the ball to your best scorer, time is going to run out. The same holds true for respiratory illnesses. They can quickly turn into emergency situations. So if you don't have a set plan for handling them, time could run out for an athlete with a respiratory emergency.

Choking and respiratory arrest are obvious respiratory emergencies and were covered in chapter 4. But allergic reactions, contact injuries, sickness, and anxiety can also cause breathing problems in athletes. This chapter will help you prepare to deal with these additional respiratory emergencies and illnesses.

Anaphylactic Shock

A severe allergic reaction to a substance causing the body to respond with swelling of the throat, lips, or tongue.

Causes

- Exposure to an allergy-causing substance such as insect venom, pollen, molds, latex, certain foods (such as peanuts and seafood), and drugs.

Ask if Experiencing Symptoms

- Chest tightness
- Difficulty breathing
- Dizziness
- Anxiety

Check for Signs

- Wheezing or gasping noises
- Swollen tongue, lips, and throat
- Bluish or gray skin, fingernails, or lips
- Hives
- Swollen eyes
- Abdominal cramping
- Nausea
- Vomiting
- Mental confusion

⊕ FIRST AID

If the athlete has antidotal medicine, do the following:

1. Send someone to retrieve the athlete's medicine. It may be in an injectable form of epinephrine (Epi-Pen).
2. If necessary, you may assist the athlete in injecting the medicine.*

3. Alert emergency medical assistance.
4. Monitor breathing and provide CPR if needed.

If the athlete does not have antidotal medicine, do the following:

1. Send for emergency medical assistance.
2. Monitor breathing and provide CPR if needed.

Playing Status

- If CPR or emergency medical personnel were necessary, the athlete cannot return to activity until examined and released by a physician.
- Athletes who recover without needing life-saving first aid or emergency medical assistance should get clearance from their physician before returning to activity.

Prevention

- Check playing area for insect nests.
- Be aware of athletes with severe allergies.
- Remind athletes to bring an auto-injector to every practice and competition.

*Administer an Epi-pen when a victim is unable to do so only if you have been trained to use it properly, the medication has been prescribed by a physician, and such administration is allowed by state law.

See pages 270 and 271 in appendix A for an overview of first aid protocol for anaphylactic shock and asthma (described on page 94).

Collapsed Lung

Lung partially collapses due to air or fluid pressure (figure 7.1).

Causes

- Direct blow to the ribs that compresses or tears the lung
- Spontaneous collapse of a lung, not caused by an injury
- Puncture by a sharp object such as a broken rib, an arrow, or a javelin

Ask if Experiencing Symptoms

- Shortness of breath
- Chest pain

Check for Signs

- Bruise or open wound in the chest
- Sucking noise coming from an open chest wound
- Gasping for air
- Increased breathing rate

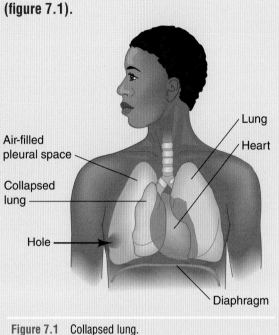

Figure 7.1   Collapsed lung.

⊕ FIRST AID

1. Send for emergency medical assistance.
2. Reassure the athlete.
3. Place the athlete in a semireclining position as long as this doesn't cause further injury.
4. Cover any open, sucking wound with a non-porous material such as aluminum foil or multiple layers of sterile gauze.
5. Monitor breathing and provide CPR if needed.

Playing Status

- The athlete cannot return to activity until examined and released by a physician.

Prevention

- Enforce safety regulations during archery or javelin practice or competition.
- Require athletes to wear rib protectors for appropriate contact sports.

93

Asthma

Condition in which the air passages in the lungs constrict (figure 7.2) and interfere with normal breathing.

Causes

- Allergic reaction to dust, molds, pet dander, or other substances
- Exposure to cold environments such as ice-skating rinks
- Exposure to smoke or other inhaled substances
- Adverse response to strenuous exercise

Ask if Experiencing Symptoms

- Tightness in the chest
- Shortness of breath

Check for Signs

- Trouble exhaling
- Wheezing noises when breathing
- Increased respiratory rate (normally 12-20 breaths per minute at rest)
- Fingernails, lips, or skin may turn blue or gray
- Pulse rate may increase to 120 beats per minute or more
- Athlete is noticeably frightened

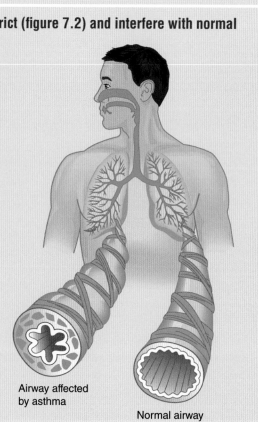

Airway affected by asthma

Normal airway

Figure 7.2 Constricted breathing passages caused by asthma.

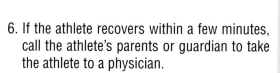

If the athlete has an asthma inhaler or medicine, do the following:

1. Send someone to retrieve the athlete's inhaler or medicine and have the athlete use the medicine when it arrives.
2. If necessary, you may assist the athlete in using the inhaler or taking the medicine.*
3. Monitor breathing and provide CPR if needed (if either is needed, send for emergency medical assistance).
4. Monitor the athlete's skin and lip color. If either changes to blue or gray, send for emergency medical assistance.
5. Call for emergency medical assistance if the athlete shows no signs of improvement a few minutes after administering the medication.

6. If the athlete recovers within a few minutes, call the athlete's parents or guardian to take the athlete to a physician.

If asthma medicine is not available or the athlete does not respond to medication, do the following:

1. Send for emergency medical assistance.
2. Monitor breathing and provide CPR if needed.
3. Place the athlete in a seated or semireclining position.
4. Monitor and treat for shock as needed.
5. Reassure the athlete.

*Administer an Epi-pen when a victim is unable to do so only if you have been trained to use it properly, the medication has been prescribed by a physician, and such administration is allowed by state law.

Playing Status

- If CPR or emergency personnel were necessary, the athlete cannot return to activity until examined and released by a physician.
- Athletes who recover without needing lifesaving first aid or emergency medical assistance should get clearance from their physician before returning to activity.

Prevention

- Be aware of all athletes who have asthma. Keep an asthma action card on file (see figure 7.3).
- Encourage athletes with asthma to take an active role in managing their condition.
- Remind athletes with asthma to bring their medication to all practices and games.
- Monitor athletes with asthma who compete in cold or dusty environments.
- Give athletes with asthma frequent rests during activity.
- If an athlete with asthma suffers daily signs and symptoms, send the athlete to a physician.

Hyperventilation

Rapid breathing that creates a deficit of carbon dioxide in the bloodstream which upsets the oxygen and carbon dioxide balance.

Causes

- An overexcited athlete breathes too rapidly
- A blow to the solar plexus

Ask if Experiencing Symptoms

- Shortness of breath
- Numbness or tingling around the mouth or on the arms, hands, and feet
- Dizziness or light-headedness

- Weakness
- Chest pain
- Panic or anxious feeling

Check for Signs

- Rapid breathing
- Increasing pulse rate
- If the athlete doesn't recover, the athlete may faint

⊕ FIRST AID

1. Talk calmly and reassure the athlete.
2. Place the athlete in a seated or semireclining position.
3. Encourage the athlete to breathe normally.
4. Instruct the athlete to inhale slowly, hold one second, then exhale slowly through pursed lips.

5. If the athlete does not recover within a few minutes, send for emergency medical assistance, monitor breathing, and provide CPR as needed. Also, check for other injuries that could be contributing to the problem.

Playing Status

- The athlete can return to activity once breathing returns to normal.
- Monitor the athlete for signs of recurrence.
- If CPR or emergency personnel were necessary, the athlete cannot return to activity until examined and released by a physician.

Prevention

- Try to calm an excitable athlete.
- Teach anxious or excitable athletes correct breathing techniques.

Asthma and Allergy Foundation of America

STUDENT ASTHMA ACTION CARD

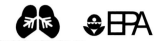
National Asthma Education and Prevention Program

Name:_____ Grade:_____ Age:_____

Homeroom Teacher:_____ Room:_____

Parent/Guardian   Name:_____ Ph: (h):_____

                 Address:_____ Ph: (w):_____

Parent/Guardian   Name:_____ Ph: (h):_____

                 Address:_____ Ph: (w):_____

Emergency Phone Contact #1_____

                         Name   Relationship   Phone

Emergency Phone Contact #2_____

                         Name   Relationship   Phone

Physician Treating Student for Asthma:_____ Ph:_____

Other Physician:_____ Ph:_____

EMERGENCY PLAN

Emergency action is necessary when the student has symptoms such as, _____ , _____ ,

_____ , _____ or has a peak flow reading of _____ .

• Steps to take during an asthma episode:

1. Check peak flow.
2. Give medications as listed below. Student should respond to treatment in 15-20 minutes.
3. Contact parent/guardian if _____

_____

4. Re-check peak flow.
5. Seek emergency medical care if the student has any of the following:
    ✔ Coughs constantly
    ✔ No improvement 15-20 minutes after initial treatment with medication and a relative cannot be reached.
    ✔ Peak flow of _____
    ✔ Hard time breathing with:
        • Chest and neck pulled in with breathing
        • Stooped body posture
        • Struggling or gasping
    ✔ Trouble walking or talking
    ✔ Stops playing and can't start activity again
    ✔ Lips or fingernails are grey or blue

} **IF THIS HAPPENS, GET EMERGENCY HELP NOW!**

• Emergency Asthma Medications

Name	Amount	When to Use
1.		
2.		
3.		
4.		

Figure 7.3   Asthma action card.

© 2008 The Asthma and Allergy Foundation of America. For more information, visit www.aafa.org.

Solar Plexus Spasm

The solar plexus is a nervous system structure located just below the rib cage (figure 7.4).

In this condition, the diaphragm, which causes the lungs to expand with air, spasms because of signals sent to it from the solar plexus. It is commonly described as "having the wind knocked out."

Cause
- Direct blow to the area below the rib cage

Ask if Experiencing Symptoms
- Inability to breathe in (inhale)
- Pain just below the breastbone

Check for Signs
- Possible temporary unresponsiveness
- Labored breathing or hyperventilation

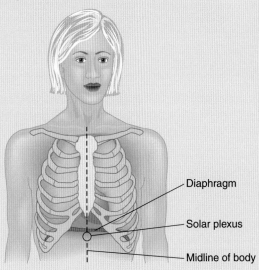

Figure 7.4 Location of the solar plexus, which when hit hard can temporarily paralyze the diaphragm.

⊕ FIRST AID

1. Reassure the athlete.
2. Loosen constricting clothing.
3. Encourage the athlete to relax.
4. Instruct the athlete to take a short breath followed by a slow, deep breath.
5. Monitor breathing and provide CPR if needed (if CPR is needed, send for medical assistance).
6. If the athlete still has pain or does not recover in a few minutes, call for emergency medical assistance.
7. Monitor for signs and symptoms of other internal injuries. Signs and symptoms to watch for include shock, vomiting, or coughing up blood.

Playing Status
- The athlete can return to activity if breathing returns to normal and there is no deformity or pain in the affected area.
- If CPR or emergency personnel were necessary, the athlete cannot return to activity until examined and released by a physician.

Prevention
- Require athletes to wear appropriate protective padding in contact sports such as football and ice hockey.

Pneumonia or Bronchitis

An inflammation, or viral or microorganism infection, of the lungs that can cause fluid or mucus to collect in the lungs.

Causes

- Infection by a microorganism
- Irritation by an inhaled substance such as dust or chemicals
- Chronic respiratory problems (e.g., asthma or bronchitis)

Ask if Experiencing Symptoms

- Shortness of breath
- Chest tightness
- Chest pain
- Fatigue
- Chills
- Muscle aches

Check for Signs

- Possible fever
- Labored breathing
- Coughing, possibly with mucus
- Possible wheezing during expiration

➕ FIRST AID

1. Send the athlete to a physician if the athlete is suffering from a fever, coughing, and congestion.

Playing Status

- If the athlete is suffering from a fever, coughing, and congestion, the athlete cannot return to activity until examined and released by a physician.
- The athlete can return to activity if there is no fever, and coughing and congestion are under control.

Prevention

- Prevent indirect contact with an infected athlete via shared water bottles, towels, and the like.
- Emphasize the importance of washing hands to help prevent the transmission of infectious illnesses.

Throat Contusion

Contusion to the throat that may interfere with air passing to the lungs.

Causes

- Direct blow to the throat area (e.g., getting hit with a baseball, softball, or hockey puck, or getting hit by an elbow in basketball or football)

Ask if Experiencing Symptoms

- Pain in the throat
- Pain with swallowing
- Shortness of breath

Check for Signs

- Gasping for air
- Breathing rate may increase
- Swelling or discoloration where the object hit the throat
- Deformity in the throat area
- Crunchy or grating sound when touched
- Voice changes—may vary from hoarseness to total inability to speak
- Difficulty swallowing
- Wheezing
- Coughing
- Coughing up or spitting blood

1. Reassure the athlete.
2. Place the athlete in a seated or semireclining position.
3. Apply ice to the injured area to help reduce swelling (see chapter 5 for more details on the use of ice).
4. Monitor breathing and provide CPR if needed (if CPR is needed, send for medical assistance).
5. Within a few minutes, if breathing does not return to normal, or if the athlete's throat is swollen or deformed and the athlete is having difficulty talking or swallowing, send for medical assistance.
6. Treat for shock if necessary (see chapter 5) and send for medical assistance if it occurs.

Playing Status

- The athlete may return to activity if breathing, pulse, swallowing, and voice return to normal and there is no pain or deformity in the throat area.
- If CPR or emergency personnel were necessary, the athlete cannot return to activity until examined and released by a physician.

Prevention

- Require all field hockey, lacrosse, and ice hockey goalies and all baseball and softball catchers to wear throat protectors.

Chapter 7 REPLAY

☐ Define anaphylactic shock. (p. 92)

☐ What should you do if an athlete has a collapsed lung caused by a hole in the chest? (p. 93)

☐ How does asthma affect an athlete's lungs? (p. 94)

☐ What can an athlete do to help prevent asthma attacks? (p. 95)

☐ What causes hyperventilation? (p. 95)

☐ What should you do if an athlete is hyperventilating? (p. 95)

☐ How does having the "wind knocked out" affect the body? (p. 97)

☐ When should an athlete with bronchitis or pneumonia not participate in activity? (p. 98)

☐ What signs indicate when a throat contusion is potentially life threatening? (pp. 98-99)

Head, Spine, and Nerve Injuries

IN THIS CHAPTER, YOU WILL LEARN:

- ▸ How to recognize the signs and symptoms of head, spine, and nerve injuries.
- ▸ What type of first aid to provide for head, spine, and nerve injuries.
- ▸ Strategies to use in your sport first aid game plan to prevent head, spine, and nerve injuries.

INJURIES IN THIS CHAPTER

HEAD INJURIES

In the past, most head injuries were called concussions and rated by severity according to signs and symptoms. In sport, we used "dinged" or "getting his bell rung" to describe an athlete's minor concussion. These dings or bell-ringers didn't cause unconsciousness, and the typical signs and symptoms of disorientation, dizziness, headache, memory loss, and disrupted balance were short-term inconveniences. Mild concussions just temporarily stunned the brain. So once an athlete shook off the cobwebs and appeared oriented, he or she was good to go. Dings and bell-ringers were just part of the game in contact sports. A label of traumatic brain injury was reserved for the most severe injuries that caused permanent brain damage.

Now, more research is showing that dings and bell-ringers aren't so short term and minor, and they're not limited to contact sports like football and hockey. The brain injury these incidences can cause is very real and possibly long term or cumulative.

Mild blows to the head don't just stun the brain; they can disrupt blood flow, cause electrical and chemical imbalances, and possibly injure brain cells. These changes are microscopic and, more often than not, not visible on MRI brain images or skull x-rays. However, they can be detected by neurological tests that assess an athlete's cognition, memory, multitasking ability, emotional functioning, and motor (movement) skills like balance and reaction time. In addition, headaches, dizziness, nausea, and other signs and symptoms from minor hits are actually manifestations of microtrauma to the brain. So dings and bell-ringers are actually mild traumatic brain injuries, or MTBIs.

Researchers have found that MTBIs are not limited to athletes in contact sports. Injury records across various sports have revealed that sports typically considered noncontact are showing surprising rates of MTBIs. In one of the most comprehensive studies of sport injuries, Marar (2012) analyzed the rate of concussion (minor and severe traumatic brain injury) across 20 high school sports from 2008 through 2010. Not surprisingly, the highest occurrence was found in football, which accounted for 47.1 percent of reported concussions. More surprising was that noncontact sports like girls' soccer (8.2 percent), girls' basketball (5.5 percent), and boys' soccer (5.3 percent) each accounted for a higher percentage of concussions in the study than did contact sports like ice hockey and lacrosse. Wrestling concussions were 5.8 percent of the total number of reported concussions.

This MTBI injury data was obtained from research conducted by Comstock and colleagues (2011) at the Center for Injury Research and Policy at the Nationwide Children's Hospital. In a separate report by the Center during 2009-2010, the percentage of head injuries among all injuries across all sports was also recorded. Ankle injuries were first at 14.7%, and concussions were second at 14.6%. Surprisingly, when analyzed as a percentage of all injuries per sport, head injuries were high on the list of injuries for most of the 20 sports studied. For example, ice hockey players suffered more head injuries than any other injuries. Head injuries were also the top injury suffered in football, wrestling, softball, girls' field hockey, boys' and girls' lacrosse, and cheerleading. It was the second most common injury sustained by athletes in boys' and girls' basketball, girls' soccer, and girls' volleyball. Table 8.1 summarizes the findings of this study.

In a later study, Comstock and colleagues (2012) collected injury data from nine sports in U.S. high schools during 2011-2012. From their data, the researchers estimated injury rates for these sports across all U.S. high schools. Head injuries were the most common injury across all sports combined. Interestingly, head injuries reported for most sports have increased. This may be due to the increased media coverage and thus increased recognition of sport-related head injuries. The data from the Center for Injury Research and Policy appears to indicate that head injury prevention efforts need to be targeted across all of the sports studied. Table 8.2 summarizes the head injury estimates projected in the 2011-2012 injury surveillance study.

Most of these injuries are not so short term that an athlete will recover in a few minutes or even a day. In Marar's study, 40 percent of concussion symptoms (headache, dizziness, difficulty

Table 8.1   Frequency of Head Injury by Sport

Sport	Percentage of injuries in that sport
Boys' ice hockey	24.2
Cheerleading	20.3
Girls' lacrosse	19.4
Football	19.2
Boys' lacrosse	18.6
Girls' soccer	15.7
Softball	14.3
Boys' basketball	13.9
Girls' field hockey	13.4
Girls' basketball	12.1
Boys' soccer	10.8
Wrestling	10.3
Girls' volleyball	8.5
Baseball	5.0
Boys' track and field	4.1
Girls' gymnastics	3.4
Girls' swimming and diving	2.7

Data from Comstock, Collins, and McIlvain 2011.

Table 8.2   Estimated Frequency of Head Injury by Sport

Sport	Estimated percentage of injuries in that sport
Wrestling	24.6
Girls' soccer	23.8
Football	23.6
Boys' soccer	23.0
Softball	21.2
Girls' basketball	20.8
Girls' volleyball	16.3
Baseball	14.6
Boys' basketball	13.9

Data from Comstock et al. 2013.

with concentration, confusion, light sensitivity, and nausea) resolved in three days or fewer. But symptom resolution does not necessarily mean that the athlete is fully recovered. It can take a week, a month, six months, or longer in some cases. The length of time isn't dependent on how the athlete feels or looks. An athlete who looks and feels fine can still have impaired cognition, memory, multitasking ability, emotional functioning, and motor (movement) skills, which are indicative that the brain has not fully recovered. If an athlete is allowed to return to participation before the brain is fully recovered, the brain can suffer further injury if he or she is mildly bumped

or jarred too quickly. This is known as second-impact syndrome, which can cause excessive and life-threatening brain swelling.

Repeated blows, even minor ones, can lead to cumulative brain damage and long-term impairment of brain functioning. Reports of long-term health issues suffered by athletes after repeated blows to the head have brought MTBIs to the forefront of the media and to the attention of lawmakers. But for all the hype and all of the well-intentioned laws, the challenges are still the same. How do you recognize the signs of a brain injury and, more important, what can be done to prevent it? The following sections focus on causes, signs and symptoms, and first aid strategies you can use to minimize long-term or permanent brain injury.

Brain injuries are commonly caused by one of two mechanisms:

1. A direct blow to the head can injure the skull or brain tissue on the side of contact (figure 8.1) or the brain tissue on the side opposite the impact (figure 8.2). For example, if an athlete's head hits a goalpost, the athlete could potentially suffer a skull fracture at the site of impact or a brain injury on the same side or opposite side.

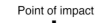
Point of impact

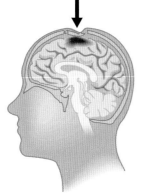

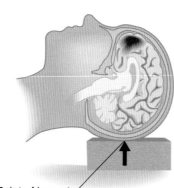

Point of impact

Figure 8.1 Skull injury from a direct blow.

Figure 8.2 Brain injury on opposite side of direct blow.

2. A sudden, forceful jarring or whipping of the head, without contact, can also injure the brain. This movement can cause the brain to bounce back and forth in the skull. It's been theorized that these jarring types of injuries may also cause fractures at the base of the skull.

Page 272 in appendix A summarizes how to assess and provide first aid care for head injuries.

Athlete With a Head Injury

If an athlete has suffered a blow to the head or a whipping of the head and neck, immediately evaluate for symptoms and signs of injury.

Causes

- Direct blow to the head
- Sudden, forceful jarring or whipping of the head

Ask if Experiencing Symptoms

- Headache
- Dizziness
- Ringing in the ears
- Grogginess
- Nausea
- Blurred or double vision

Check for Signs

- Confusion
- Unsteadiness
- Inability to multitask (unable to do several athletic skills at once or do a skill correctly when distracted)
- Short-term memory loss
- Emotional changes such as a short temper or depression
- Unresponsiveness to touch or voice (call out the athlete's name and tap on the shoulder)
- Irregular breathing
- Bleeding or a wound at the point of the blow
- Blood or fluid leaking from the mouth, nose, or ears
- Arm or leg weakness or numbness
- Neck pain with a decrease in motion
- Bump or deformity at the point of the blow
- Convulsions
- Abnormalities in pupils (unequal in size or failure to constrict to light)
- Vomiting

If an athlete exhibits any of the previously listed signs or symptoms, pull the athlete out of activity. Symptoms such as headache or ringing in the ears may be the early signs of a more serious injury. In these cases, do the following:

1. Continue to monitor the athlete and alert emergency medical services if signs and symptoms worsen.

2. Immediately contact the parent or guardian and have them take the athlete to a physician.

3. Give the parent or guardian a checklist of signs and symptoms (figure 8.3) to monitor.

For injuries with more severe signs such as confusion, unsteadiness, vomiting, convulsions, increasing headaches, increasing irritability, unusual behavior, arm or leg weakness or numbness, neck pain with a decrease in motion, pupil abnormalities, or unconsciousness, do the following:

1. Immediately call emergency medical services.

2. Stabilize the head and neck until EMS takes over. Leave an athlete's helmet on when stabilizing the head and neck. You don't want to jar the head or neck unnecessarily. This is especially true if the athlete is also wearing shoulder pads.

3. Monitor the athlete for breathing difficulty and perform CPR if necessary.

4. Control any profuse bleeding but avoid applying excess pressure over a head wound.

5. Monitor for shock and treat as needed.

6. Immobilize any fractures or unstable injuries as long as it does not jostle the athlete, which may worsen his or her condition.

Playing Status

When can an athlete return to a sport after a brain injury? In most cases, this decision has already been decided for you. Check your state law or the regulations of the National Federation of State High School Associations (NFHS) to ensure that your athletes are receiving mandated care and supervision. The NFHS prohibits athletes from returning to activity until examined and released by a physician. Many states are enacting laws with similar or stricter guidelines. Check your state for specific laws regarding brain injuries in athletes.

Prevention

- Educate yourself, your athletes, and their parents or guardians about concussions (see figure 8.3). Visit the CDC website at www.cdc.gov.

- During preseason physicals, screen for any history of head, spine, or nerve injuries. Have these athletes cleared by a physician, preferably a neurologist, before allowing them to participate.

- Use preseason brain testing. Numerous software programs or testing contractors can assess each athlete's normal brain function, including memory, cognitive functioning, motor (muscle and balance) control, and other functions before the beginning of a sport season. This information is then used as a baseline from which an athlete's brain function can be compared when an injury is suspected or has occurred. Doctors and athletic trainers can monitor this information while the athlete recovers and determine when an athlete is ready to progressively return to activity. These tests can also be used to monitor the athlete for any signs of decreasing brain function as he or she progresses back into full participation. A decrease in function signals that the athlete is not ready to proceed further and may need to actually decrease activity. This type of testing can be an important tool for you, your athletes, and their physicians in helping to more objectively determine the severity of a brain injury, the level of recovery, and the athlete's readiness to return to activity.

(continued)

- Incorporate neck strengthening exercises into your preseason and in-season conditioning programs. These can be done simply by providing resistance to the head with a hand against all of its normal movements (see figures 8.4 and 8.5).

For sports requiring helmets, ensure the following:

- Helmets are regularly checked for damage and replaced if necessary.
- Older helmets are regularly replaced.
- Helmets are properly fitted to each athlete.
- Athletes are instructed in effectively securing helmets in place. A well-fitted helmet isn't effective if chin straps are not snapped and snug.

- Athletes are repeatedly reminded not to use the top of the helmet as a point of contact when tackling or checking another player or lowering the head just before contacting another athlete. Enforce this rule as necessary by sidelining offending athletes and reinforcing proper technique.
- Prohibit diving into water less than 6 feet deep.
- Train and use spotters at all times during gymnastics and cheerleading.
- Monitor athletes for signs or symptoms of head injury.
- Educate athletes about the signs and symptoms of head injuries. Encourage athletes to report signs of suspected brain injury in teammates. Consider providing some sort of recognition to these athletes in order to encourage reporting.

Playing It Safe...
When an Athlete Is Wearing a Helmet and Shoulder Pads

1. Check for breathing by placing your hand next to the athlete's nose and mouth to feel for breaths or watching to see if the athlete's chest or abdomen rises and falls.
2. Stabilize the head and neck but leave the helmet and pads on—taking them off will move the neck.

Playing It Safe...
No Ammonia Caps or Smelling Salts

Using ammonia caps or smelling salts to rouse an athlete may cause him or her to suddenly jerk the head and worsen the condition.

HEADS×UP
CONCUSSION IN HIGH SCHOOL SPORTS

A FACT SHEET FOR **PARENTS**

What is a concussion?

A concussion is a type of traumatic brain injury. Concussions are caused by a bump or blow to the head. Even a "ding," "getting your bell rung," or what seems to be a mild bump or blow to the head can be serious.

You can't see a concussion. Signs and symptoms of concussion can show up right after the injury or may not appear or be noticed until days or weeks after the injury. If your child reports any symptoms of concussion, or if you notice the symptoms yourself, seek medical attention right away.

What are the signs and symptoms of a concussion?

If your child has experienced a bump or blow to the head during a game or practice, look for any of the following signs of a concussion:

SYMPTOMS REPORTED BY ATHLETE	SIGNS OBSERVED BY PARENTS/GUARDIANS
• Headache or "pressure" in head • Nausea or vomiting • Balance problems or dizziness • Double or blurry vision • Sensitivity to light • Sensitivity to noise • Feeling sluggish, hazy, foggy, or groggy • Concentration or memory problems • Confusion • Just "not feeling right" or "feeling down"	• Appears dazed or stunned • Is confused about assignment or position • Forgets an instruction • Is unsure of game, score, or opponent • Moves clumsily • Answers questions slowly • Loses consciousness (even briefly) • Shows mood, behavior, or personality changes

How can you help your child prevent a concussion or other serious brain injury?

- Ensure that they follow their coach's rules for safety and the rules of the sport.
- Encourage them to practice good sportsmanship at all times.
- Make sure they wear the right protective equipment for their activity. Protective equipment should fit properly and be well maintained.
- Wearing a helmet is a must to reduce the risk of a serious brain injury or skull fracture.
  - However, helmets are not designed to prevent concussions. There is no "concussion-proof" helmet. So, even with a helmet, it is important for kids and teens to avoid hits to the head.

What should you do if you think your child has a concussion?

SEEK MEDICAL ATTENTION RIGHT AWAY. A health care professional will be able to decide how serious the concussion is and when it is safe for your child to return to regular activities, including sports.

KEEP YOUR CHILD OUT OF PLAY. Concussions take time to heal. Don't let your child return to play the day of the injury and until a health care professional says it's OK. Children who return to play too soon—while the brain is still healing—risk a greater chance of having a repeat concussion. Repeat or later concussions can be very serious. They can cause permanent brain damage, affecting your child for a lifetime.

TELL YOUR CHILD'S COACH ABOUT ANY PREVIOUS CONCUSSION. Coaches should know if your child had a previous concussion. Your child's coach may not know about a concussion your child received in another sport or activity unless you tell the coach.

> **If you think your teen has a concussion:**
> Don't assess it yourself. Take him/her out of play. Seek the advice of a health care professional.

It's better to miss one game than the whole season.

For more information, visit **www.cdc.gov/Concussion**.

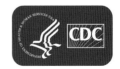

April 2013

Figure 8.3 CDC Heads Up concussion fact sheet.

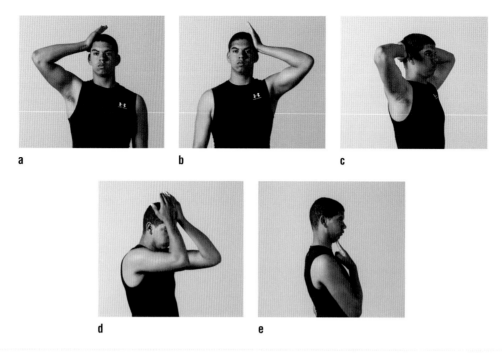

Figure 8.4 Isometric (no movement) neck strengthening exercises. (*a* and *b*) Lateral flexion, *(c)* extension, *(d)* forward flexion, and *(e)* chin retraction. For exercises a-d, place your hand or hands against your head and press against your hand as hard as possible without moving your head. For exercise e, tuck your chin in as far as possible and hold that position.

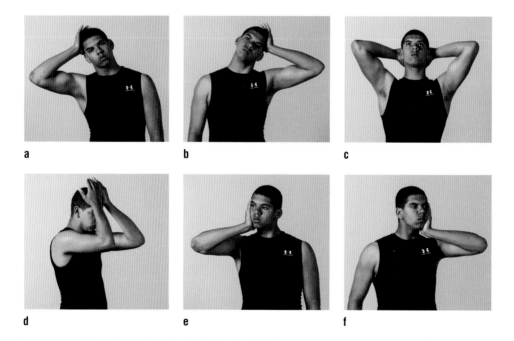

Figure 8.5 Isotonic (with movement) neck strengthening exercises. (*a* and *b*) Lateral flexion, *(c)* extension, *(d)* forward flexion, and *(e-f)* rotation. Move your head toward your shoulder, backward, and forward, and rotate to each side with self-resistance. Keep the chin tucked when performing each of these exercises.

SPINE INJURIES

A blow to the back, a swing of a club, or any sudden and forceful move can injure the spine or nerves. As discussed in chapter 3, the spine is a column of bones (vertebrae) that protect the spinal cord. The bones are held together by ligaments and muscles, and nerves branch out from between bones in the spinal column (see figure 3.6). Cartilage discs located between the vertebrae help absorb shock between the bones.

A direct blow, forceful twisting motion, compression, and forceful stretching beyond normal motion to any portion of the spine can cause a variety of spine injuries, including sprains, strains, contusions, fractures, and ruptured discs. Sprains, strains, and contusions are the most common sport-related back injuries. More severe spine and neck injuries like ruptured discs and vertebral fractures are less common. Table 8.3 lists the frequency of neck injuries in various high school sports. Injuries to the spinal cord, nerves, and cartilage can cause numbness and, in more severe injuries, paralysis—a temporary or permanent loss of function in certain body parts.

Table 8.3 Frequency of Neck Injuries by Sport

Sport	Percent of injuries in that sport
Girls' swimming and diving	4.5
Cheerleading	3.1
Wrestling	3.1

Data from Comstock, Collins, and McIlvain 2012.

It's not important to know the type of back or spine injury an athlete has suffered. Your first aid care will be dictated by the signs and symptoms described here. Always suspect a serious head or spine injury in an unconscious athlete. Never move the athlete during the evaluation unless you are unable to check for breathing or you need to move the athlete away from a dangerous area.

If the athlete is wearing a helmet, leave it on! Removing it can cause further harm. If you suspect a serious spine injury, immediately stabilize the head and spine.

Athlete With a Possible Spine Injury

Causes
- Direct blow
- Compression
- Torsion or twisting

If you suspect a back or spine injury, look for these red flag symptoms and signs:

Ask if Experiencing Symptoms
- Pain over or near the spine
- Numbness or tingling in the feet or hands (ask the athlete to name the finger or toe that you are touching)

Check for Signs
- Responsiveness (if unresponsive or not fully alert, assume a head or neck injury)
- Inadequate breathing
- Profuse bleeding
- Blood or fluid leaking from the mouth, nose, or ears
- Spine deformity (if another trained rescuer can check without moving the athlete)
- Paralysis (ask athlete to move fingers or toes)

✚ FIRST AID

If any red flags are present, assume the athlete has a spine injury and administer appropriate first aid.

1. Send for emergency medical assistance.
2. Check for breathing without moving the athlete. If the athlete is not breathing, have someone hold the head and neck still while you perform CPR.
3. If the athlete is breathing, stabilize the head and neck until EMS takes over. Leave an athlete's helmet on when stabilizing the head and neck. You don't want to jar the head or neck unnecessarily. This is especially true if the athlete is also wearing shoulder pads. If the athlete's breathing is normal, continue to monitor and perform CPR if necessary.
4. Control any profuse bleeding but avoid applying excess pressure over a head wound.
5. Monitor and treat for shock if necessary.
6. Let EMS immobilize any other possible fractures or unstable injuries.

Playing Status
- The athlete cannot return to activity until examined and released by a physician.

Prevention
There are many ways to prevent nerve and spine injuries:

- Incorporate neck strengthening exercises into your preseason and in-season conditioning programs (see figures 8.4 and 8.5).
- Prevent players from using their helmets as a point of contact when tackling or checking.
- Recommend that all football players who have had neck injuries wear neck rolls (figure 8.6).
- Prohibit diving into water less than 6 feet deep.
- Require spotters for gymnasts or cheerleaders practicing skills or routines.

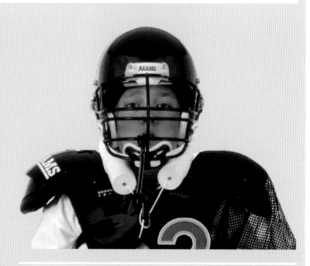

Figure 8.6 Neck rolls help prevent football players' heads from suddenly snapping to the side.
© Adams USA.

NERVE INJURIES

During sports, sometimes a nerve can get pinched, stretched, or bruised. This can occur close to the spinal column or near a joint where a nerve is located (for example, the nerve along the inside of the elbow, often called the funny bone). In this chapter we limit the discussion of nerve injuries to one that occurs near the cervical spine. It is called a burner or stinger and is a common nerve injury suffered by athletes, especially those in contact sports.

Burner or Stinger

A burner or stinger occurs when a group of nerves (brachial plexus) coming out of the neck and running to the shoulder are overstretched.

Cause

- The head is flexed or extended and forced quickly to one side and tilted down, as shown in figure 8.7.

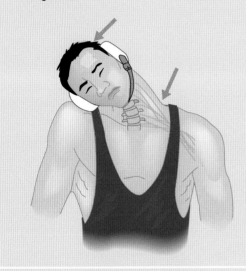

Figure 8.7   Mechanism of a burner injury.

Ask if Experiencing Symptoms

- Tingling or burning in the neck, shoulder, or arm
- Electrical shock sensation in the neck or shoulder
- Arm feeling dead or heavy

Check for Signs

- Arm or hand numbness on one side (ask the athlete to name the finger that you are touching)
- Arm or hand weakness on one side (have the athlete squeeze your fingers with each hand; any significant difference in the strength of the injured arm compared to the uninjured arm means that the nerve has been stretched and possibly injured)

✚ FIRST AID

If sensation and strength do not return within 5 minutes, or there is tenderness or deformity of the spine, do the following:

1. Send for emergency medical assistance.
2. Stabilize the head and spine.
3. Monitor breathing and provide CPR if needed.
4. Monitor and treat for shock as needed.
5. Stabilize any other unstable injuries.

If the sensation and strength return within a few minutes, call the athlete's parents or guardians and have them take the athlete to their physician.

(continued)

Burner or Stinger *(continued)*

Playing Status

It's best to err on the side of caution and have athletes exhibiting signs and symptoms of a nerve injury evaluated and released by a physician before returning to activity. This is especially true with burners since they can become a recurring problem and lead to long-term nerve damage.

Prevention

There are a number of ways to prevent nerve and spine injuries:

- Incorporate neck strengthening exercises into your preseason and in-season conditioning programs (see figures 8.4 and 8.5).
- Prevent players from using their helmets as a point of contact when tackling or checking.
- Recommend that all football players who have had neck injuries wear neck rolls (figure 8.6).
- Prohibit diving into water less than 6 feet deep.
- Require spotters for gymnasts or cheerleaders practicing skills or routines.

Chapter 8 *REPLAY*

☐ If an injury is the result of a direct blow, sudden or forceful movement to the head, spinal compression, or spinal torsion or twisting, check for head or spine injuries. You must evaluate these injuries quickly and treat them correctly to reduce further complications. (p. 104)

☐ What are some signs and symptoms of a head injury? (pp. 104, 107)

☐ When is it acceptable for an athlete with a mild traumatic brain injury to return to activity? (p. 105)

☐ What are some signs and symptoms of a spine injury? (p. 110)

☐ Describe the injury mechanism for a burner or stinger. (p. 111)

☐ When is it acceptable for an athlete with a burner or stinger to return to activity? (p. 112)

☐ What can be done to help prevent neck burners or stingers? (p. 112)

REFERENCES

Centers for Disease Control and Prevention. 2013. *Heads up: Concussion in high school sports: A fact sheet for parents.* www.cdc.gov/concussion/pdf/Parents_Fact_Sheet-a.pdf.

Comstock, R.D., C.L. Collins, J.D. Corlette, and E.N. Fletcher. 2013. Summary report: National high school sports-related injury surveillance study, 2011-2012 school year. Retrieved June 21, 2013 from www.nationwidechildrens.org/cirp-rio-study-reports.

Comstock, R.D., C.L. Collins, and N.M. McIlvain, 2012. Convenience sample summary report. National high school sports-related injury sur-veillance study, 2010-2011 school year. Retrieved June 21, 2013 from www.nationwidechildrens.org/cirp-rio-study-reports.

Comstock, R.D., C.L. Collins, and N.M. McIlvain. 2011. Convenience summary report. National high school sports-related injury surveillance study, 2009-2010 school year. Retrieved June 6, 2013 from www.nationwidechildrens.org/cirp-rio-study-reports.

Marar, M., N.M McIlvain, S.K Fields, and R.D. Yard. 2012. Epidemiology of concussions among United States high school athletes in 20 sports. *The American Journal of Sports Medicine* 40: 747-755.

Internal Organ Injuries

IN THIS CHAPTER, YOU WILL LEARN:

- ▸ How to recognize when an athlete has an internal injury, such as a ruptured spleen, bruised kidney, or testicular trauma.
- ▸ How to discern whether an athlete is in an early or an advanced, life-threatening stage of an internal organ injury.
- ▸ How to care for the injured athlete while waiting for emergency medical assistance.
- ▸ What to monitor if an athlete is exhibiting minor signs of an internal injury.
- ▸ What information to give the parents of an athlete who has incurred an internal organ injury.

INJURIES IN THIS CHAPTER

The body is often subjected to tremendous forces in sport. With 90-mile-per-hour pitches careening off a batter's flanks, and the shoulder pads of 230-pound linebackers slamming into a quarterback's numbers, it's a wonder that delicate internal organs aren't injured more often. Fortunately, the body has built-in armor—the ribs and pelvis—to help deflect some of the blows to the body's organs. In the rare instances when one of an athlete's internal organs is injured, prompt recognition and emergency medical care are critical. These injuries may initially appear minor, but can quickly progress into life-threatening conditions. So it's essential that medical personnel handle internal organ injuries.

You can help minimize complications of these injuries by learning how to

1. recognize the signs and symptoms of spleen, kidney, and testicular injuries;

2. monitor the athlete until medical help arrives; and

3. educate the athlete and parents about the signs and symptoms of internal injuries.

It often takes a few hours for a serious internal injury to appear. Therefore, it is essential that an injured athlete be monitored in case the athlete's condition worsens. You should inform the athlete's parents or guardian about the injury and provide information on what serious signs and symptoms to look for that may indicate that the athlete's condition has become life threatening. You may want to give them copies of the first aid protocols (see pages 273 to 275 in appendix A).

The most common internal injuries in sports are

- ruptured spleen,
- bruised kidney, and
- testicular trauma.

Collapsed lung is also considered an internal injury. It is included in chapter 7 as a respiratory emergency.

See page 273 in appendix A for an overview of first aid protocol for spleen injuries.

Page 274 in appendix A gives an overview of first aid protocol for a bruised kidney.

For an overview of first aid protocol for testicular trauma, see page 275 in appendix A.

→ Playing It Safe...
With Suspected Internal Injuries

- Do not give an athlete with suspected internal injuries food or water. If any of the digestive organs are injured, food or fluid intake can potentially leak out into the abdominal cavity, increasing the risk of infection. If an internal injury requires surgery, food or fluid intake can increase the likelihood of vomiting and potential aspiration during general anesthesia.

- Do not allow an athlete with possible internal injuries to leave a game or practice without being monitored by a responsible adult.

- If an athlete suffers an apparently minor blow in the area of an internal organ, before you allow the athlete to go home, inform both the athlete and the parents of the signs and symptoms of a serious internal injury.

Ruptured Spleen

Life-threatening contusion injury to the spleen, which is an organ that acts as a reservoir of red blood cells.

Cause
- A direct blow to the left side of the body, underneath the stomach and lower ribs (figure 9.1). The blow injures the spleen tissue and can cause profuse internal bleeding.

Ask if Experiencing Symptoms
Early Stage
- Pain in the left upper abdominal area

Advanced (Life-Threatening) Stage

- Pain progresses to the left shoulder or neck (figure 9.2)
- Feels faint
- Dizziness

Check for Signs

Early Stage

- Tenderness over left upper abdominal area
- Abrasion or bruise over injured area

Advanced (Life-Threatening) Stage

- Pale skin
- Rapid pulse
- Vomiting
- Rigid abdominal muscles
- Low blood pressure
- Shortness of breath

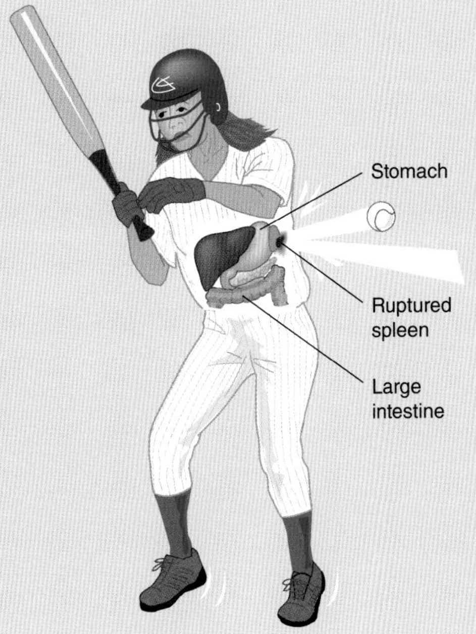

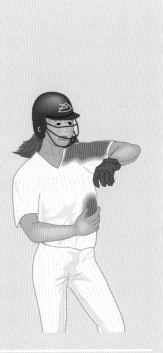

Stomach

Ruptured spleen

Large intestine

Figure 9.1 Location of a spleen injury.

Figure 9.2 A spleen injury can result in referred pain at the left shoulder and neck area.

⊕ FIRST AID

1. Send for emergency medical assistance if the initial signs and symptoms progress to the advanced stages.
2. Monitor breathing and provide CPR if needed (if CPR is needed, send for emergency medical assistance).
3. Treat for shock if necessary and send for emergency medical assistance if it occurs.
4. Treat other injuries, such as possible rib fractures.
5. If signs and symptoms do not progress to the advanced stages, but tenderness over the upper abdominal area persists for more than 15 minutes, call the athlete's parents or guardian to take the athlete to a physician.

Playing Status

- If sent to a physician or required emergency medical personnel, the athlete cannot return to activity until examined and released by a physician.
- If the athlete returns to participation before a spleen injury fully heals, another direct blow could cause profuse bleeding. This is true even if an athlete's signs and symptoms do not progress to the advanced stages.

Prevention

- Require athletes to wear appropriate protective padding in contact sports.
- Do not allow athletes who have mononucleosis to participate until examined and released by a physician. Mono can cause the spleen to enlarge and be at risk of contusion injuries.

Bruised Kidney

Contusion to the kidney (figure 9.3).

Cause

- Direct blow to either side of the midback

Ask if Experiencing Symptoms

Early Stage

- Pain at the site of the blow

Advanced (Life-Threatening) Stage

- Pain moves to the low back, outside thighs, or front pelvic area (figure 9.4)
- Feels faint
- Dizziness

Check for Signs

Early Stage

- Bruise or abrasion
- Tenderness over the injured area

Advanced Stage

- Abdominal swelling
- Increased heart rate
- Frequent and burning urination
- Cloudy or bloody urine
- Vomiting
- Rigid back muscles over the injury site
- Skin cool to touch
- Pale skin

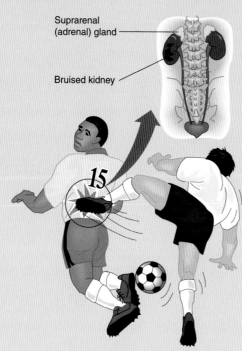

Suprarenal (adrenal) gland

Bruised kidney

Figure 9.3 Location of a kidney injury.

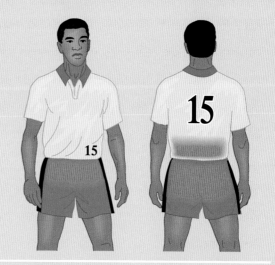

Figure 9.4 A kidney injury can result in referred pain at the low back, outside thighs, or front pelvic area.

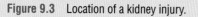

FIRST AID

1. Send for emergency medical assistance if the initial signs and symptoms progress to the advanced steps.
2. Monitor breathing and provide CPR if needed (if CPR is needed, send for emergency medical assistance).
3. Monitor and treat for shock (if necessary) and send for emergency medical assistance if it occurs.
4. Treat other injuries as needed.
5. If signs and symptoms do not progress to the advanced stages, but pain over the bruised area persists for more than 15 minutes, call the athlete's parents or guardian to take the athlete to a physician.

Playing Status

- If sent to a physician or required emergency medical personnel, the athlete cannot return to activity until examined and released by a physician. A mildly bruised kidney can worsen over time and become life threatening.

Prevention

- Require athletes to wear appropriate protective padding such as kidney pads or a flak jacket in contact sports.

Testicular Trauma

Contusion or trauma to the testicles. In severe injuries, the testicles can rupture or the testicular cord can be twisted (cutting off blood flow to the testicles, which can cause sterility).

Cause

- A direct blow to the groin area

Ask if Experiencing Symptoms

- Pain
- Nausea

Check for Signs

For All Cases

- Have athlete perform a self-exam, looking for swelling, discoloration, and deformity
- Spasm of testicles

Advanced Stage

- Testicles draw upward
- Bloody or cloudy urine
- Vomiting

⊕ FIRST AID

1. Assist the athlete into a position that feels the most comfortable.
2. Encourage the athlete to take slow, deep breaths.
3. Apply ice to the area for 15 minutes.
4. Send the athlete to a physician if the pain does not stop after 20 minutes, if the testicles draw upward, if the athlete has bloody or cloudy urine, or if the testicles exhibit swelling, discoloration, or tenderness more than an hour after the injury occurred (Koester 2000).
5. If the athlete recovers within a few minutes or if the testicles exhibit swelling, discoloration, or tenderness more than an hour after the injury occurred (Koester 2000), notify the athlete's parents and explain how to identify signs and symptoms of a more severe injury (bloody or cloudy urine; testicles drawing upward; or testicles exhibit swelling, discoloration, or tenderness).

Playing Status

- The athlete cannot return to activity until the pain subsides or until examined and released by a physician.

Prevention

- Require athletes to wear athletic supporters and protective cups (in contact sports).

Chapter 9 *REPLAY*

☐ What are the symptoms and signs of a ruptured spleen? (pp. 114-115)

☐ Why should an athlete with a possible internal organ injury not be given food or fluid? (p. 114)

☐ What are the advanced symptoms and signs of a potentially life-threatening kidney injury? (p. 116)

☐ What are the signs and symptoms of a serious testicular injury? (p. 117)

REFERENCES

Koester, M.C. 2000. Initial evaluation and management of acute scrotal pain. *Journal of Athletic Training* 35(1):76-79.

CHAPTER 10

Sudden Illnesses

IN THIS CHAPTER, YOU WILL LEARN:

▶ How to recognize when an athlete is suffering from a diabetic emergency and how to provide first aid care.

▶ How to recognize the signs and symptoms of grand mal and petit mal seizures.

▶ How to recognize adverse reactions to drugs and supplements.

▶ How to prevent and provide first aid care for fainting.

▶ How to recognize the signs and symptoms of influenza.

▶ How to recognize the signs and symptoms of gastroenteritis.

▶ How to prevent influenza and gastroenteritis from spreading among your athletes.

INJURIES AND REACTIONS IN THIS CHAPTER

A botched dismount, wild pitch, dropped baton, or net serve can suddenly change the course of a competition. Likewise, an acute illness can suddenly change an athlete's ability to perform.

An immediate onset of illness can happen to anyone. But all too often, athletes continue to play while sick and attempt to hide their illness from the coach. So ask your athletes to report, and be alert to, common illnesses such as the flu. It's also essential that you are aware of athletes who have specific medical conditions such as diabetes and epilepsy. This chapter will help you to recognize and provide first aid care for diabetic emergencies, seizures, drug overdose or reaction, adverse supplement reactions, fainting, influenza, and gastroenteritis.

DIABETES

Diabetes is a condition that affects the body's ability to properly produce and regulate insulin. Insulin is produced in the pancreas and controls the uptake of glucose (sugar) by body tissues. Glucose is the primary energy source for tissues, especially the brain and kidneys. Without proper insulin lev-

els, the tissues can receive either too much glucose (hyperglycemia) or not enough (hypoglycemia).

In type 1 diabetes, the body does not produce insulin. This type often begins during childhood. Type 2 diabetes prevents the body from properly using insulin. It is more common than type 1 diabetes and is becoming increasingly prevalent among children.

Individuals with serious diabetic problems may need to take insulin injections or use an insulin pump, which delivers insulin in small amounts via a small tube inserted just under the skin. People with type 2 diabetes often take insulin pills. Because exercise and diet can affect the amount of insulin the body needs, diabetic athletes should be closely monitored for signs of diabetic illness. An athlete who is having problems regulating diabetes will be prone to either an insulin reaction or ketoacidosis, both of which can become life threatening. This section explains appropriate first aid measures for these diabetes-related conditions.

Page 276 in appendix A summarizes first aid techniques for an insulin reaction.

For a summary of first aid techniques for ketoacidosis, see page 277 in appendix A.

Insulin Reaction

Condition in which an athlete's glucose (sugar) levels drop below normal levels (hypoglycemia).

Cause

- High insulin levels, which may result from medications taken to control blood glucose levels.

Ask if Experiencing Symptoms

Mild

- Hunger

Check for Signs

Mild

- Irritability
- Slight weakness

Moderate

- Dilated pupils
- Trembling
- Sweating
- Strong, rapid pulse

Severe

- Confusion
- Convulsions
- Unresponsiveness

Mild to Moderate

1. Remove the athlete from all activity.
2. Give the athlete sugar, candy, pop, or fruit juice.
3. Send for emergency medical assistance if the athlete does not recover within a few minutes or signs progress to severe.
4. Monitor breathing and provide CPR if needed.
5. Inform the athlete's parents or guardian.

Severe

1. Send for emergency medical assistance.
2. Place an unresponsive athlete in recovery position (if uninjured) or HAINES position (if injured) to allow vomit or fluids to drain from the mouth.
3. Monitor breathing and provide CPR if needed.

Playing Status

Mild to Moderate

- Rest the athlete from all activity for the remainder of the day.
- The athlete cannot return to activity until insulin level is stabilized.

Severe

- The athlete cannot return to activity until examined and released by a physician.

Prevention

- During practice and competitions, carefully monitor athletes who have diabetes. This may include the use of predetermined hand signals by the athletes when they are not feeling well.
- Suggest that athletes who have diabetes bring fruit juice or candy to practice and games.
- Do not allow an athlete with uncontrolled diabetes to participate.

Ketoacidosis

Condition caused by a severe or prolonged insulin deficiency that can result in a high blood glucose (sugar) level (hyperglycemia). The body tries to compensate by eliminating excess sugar through urine. This causes increased urination and therefore dehydration and electrolyte (chemical) imbalance.

Causes

- Low insulin levels may result from stress, certain medications, too much food, or not enough exercise

Ask if Experiencing Symptoms

Early Stage

- Excessive thirst
- Dry mouth
- Nausea

Advanced Stage

- Headaches
- Abdominal pain

Check for Signs

Early Stage

- Sweet, fruity-smelling breath
- Excessive urination

Advanced Stage

- Dry, red, and warm skin
- Weak, rapid pulse
- Heavy breathing
- Vomiting

(continued)

Ketoacidosis   *(continued)*

✚ FIRST AID

Early Stage

1. Remove the athlete from all activity.
2. Recommend that the athlete check blood glucose levels (if the athlete has a monitor) and take insulin if appropriate.
3. Send for emergency medical assistance if the athlete does not recover within a few minutes or signs progress to severe.
4. Monitor breathing and provide CPR as needed.
5. Inform the athlete's parents or guardian.

Advanced Stage

1. Send for emergency medical assistance.
2. Place an unresponsive athlete in recovery position (if uninjured) or HAINES position (if injured) to allow vomit or fluids to drain from the mouth.
3. Monitor breathing and provide CPR if needed.

Playing Status

Early Stage

- Rest the athlete from all activity for the remainder of the day.
- The athlete cannot return to activity until insulin and blood sugar levels are stabilized.

Advanced Stage

- The athlete cannot return to activity until examined and released by a physician.

Prevention

- Provide athletes who have diabetes with frequent fluid breaks during practice and competitions.
- Do not allow an athlete with uncontrolled diabetes to participate.

SEIZURES

Because seizures can be caused by a wide variety of problems, it's important to look for other health problems when evaluating an athlete who has just suffered a seizure. Epilepsy is a primary cause of most seizures, but there are many other causes as well.

Page 278 in appendix A outlines the first aid protocol for petit and grand mal seizures.

Seizure

Episode of abnormal electrical activity within the brain. It can lead to sudden changes in an athlete's alertness, behavior, and muscle control.

Causes

- Epilepsy
- Head injuries
- Brain infection or tumor
- Drug abuse
- Respiratory arrest
- High fever
- Heatstroke
- Hypoglycemia
- Drug reactions
- Medication discontinuation

Check for Signs

Minor/Petit Mal Seizures

- Dazed or inattentive manner
- Confusion

- Loss of coordination
- Possibly loss of speech
- Repetitive blinking or other small movements
- Typically, these seizures are brief, lasting only seconds. However, some people may have many bouts in a day.

Major/Grand Mal Seizures (Typical Sequence)

- Eyes are generally open
- Body appears stiff or rigid
- Muscles contract violently in spasms or convulsions that usually stop in one to two minutes
- May temporarily stop breathing or appear to not be breathing, and progress to deep breathing after the seizure
- Bluish skin or lips
- Unresponsiveness, followed by gradual return to responsiveness
- Uncontrolled urination during the seizure
- Temporary confusion after the seizure

FIRST AID

Minor/Petit Mal Seizures

1. Monitor for possible progression into grand mal seizure.
2. Rest the athlete from activity.
3. Inform athlete's parents or guardian.

Grand Mal Seizures

1. Clear all objects away from the athlete. (Protect the athlete's head with a pillow or other soft material, if available.)
2. Do not restrain the athlete.
3. Do not try to place anything in the athlete's mouth or try to pry the teeth apart.
4. After the convulsions stop, check breathing and provide CPR if needed.
5. Check for other possible injuries or illnesses if the athlete is not an epileptic.
6. If the athlete has no suspected head, spine, or other injuries, place the athlete in the recovery position. If the athlete has injuries other than head or spine injuries, place the athlete in the HAINES position. This will allow fluids to drain from the mouth.
7. Treat for shock if necessary and send for emergency medical assistance if it occurs.
8. Call the parents or guardian if the athlete is known to have epilepsy and recovers within a few minutes.
9. If the athlete is suffering from an injury or illness, is experiencing seizure for the first time, has a prolonged epileptic seizure (more than 5 minutes), has prolonged confusion or unresponsiveness (more than 10-15 minutes), has difficulty breathing, or is not an epileptic, you should send for emergency medical assistance.
10. Encourage the athlete to rest.

Playing Status

- Rest the athlete for the remainder of the day.
- If the seizure is caused by an injury or illness, or is a first-time occurrence, the athlete must be examined and released by a physician before returning to activity.

Prevention

- Do not allow athletes with acute illnesses to participate until the illness subsides.

➔ Playing It Safe...
With Seizures

When an athlete has a seizure, do not
- restrain the athlete,
- try to place anything in the athlete's mouth, or
- try to pry the teeth apart.

SUBSTANCE ABUSE

Substance abuse is another possible cause of sudden illness in an athlete. An athlete may overdose on a substance or suffer an adverse reaction to it. There are several categories of drugs commonly used by athletes.

Depressants—These include alcohol, narcotics (morphine, heroin, and codeine), barbiturates (phenobarbital), GHB ("liquid ecstasy," "soap," "easy lay," and "Georgia home boy"), Rohypnol ("rophies," "roofies," "roach," and "rope"), and ketamine ("special K" or "vitamin K"). These drugs depress the central nervous system, so athletes may abuse them to achieve a relaxed,

calm feeling. Athletes may also use GHB as a synthetic steroid for bodybuilding.

Stimulants—Cocaine (crack and powdered) and amphetamines are the most common. These drugs stimulate the nervous system and make athletes feel quicker and more alert.

Combination drugs—MDMA (known as ecstasy, Adam, XTC, hug, beans, and love drug) includes both stimulant and hallucinogenic properties.

You should be able to recognize the signs and symptoms of possible overdose of or adverse reactions to these drugs. Moreover, you should educate and counsel your athletes so you won't have to take the following first aid measures.

Depressant Overdose or Reaction

Dangerous and possibly life-threatening reaction from using a depressant or taking an excessive amount of a depressant.

Ask if Experiencing Symptoms
- Relaxed feeling
- Fatigue
- Depression (ketamine)

Check for Signs
- Pale, cold, and clammy skin
- Constricted pupils that may not respond to light
- Rapid and weak pulse

- Possible unresponsiveness
- Shallow breathing that may stop
- Coma (GHB)
- Seizures (GHB)
- Anterograde amnesia—decreased ability to remember events experienced while taking the drug (Rohypnol and ketamine)
- Hallucinations (ketamine)
- Delirium (ketamine)
- Impaired motor function (ketamine)

⊕ FIRST AID

1. Rest the athlete from all activity.
2. Send for emergency medical assistance if the athlete exhibits breathing problems or altered responsiveness.
3. Monitor breathing and provide CPR if needed.
4. Place an unresponsive athlete in recovery position (if uninjured) or HAINES position (if injured) to allow fluids or vomit to drain from the mouth.
5. Treat for shock if necessary and send for emergency medical assistance if it occurs.
6. If the athlete recovers quickly, speak to the parents or guardian, and send the athlete to a physician.

Playing Status
- The athlete cannot return to activity until examined and released by a physician.

Prevention
- Provide drug abuse education.

- Monitor athletes who exhibit behaviors characteristic of depressant abuse: lethargy, inattentiveness, mood changes, fatigue, and slowed reactions.

Stimulant Overdose or Reaction

Dangerous and possibly life-threatening reaction from using a stimulant or taking an excessive amount of a stimulant.

Ask if Experiencing Symptoms
- Lack of fatigue
- Irritability
- Feeling of hyperstimulation
- Sense of mental clarity
- Restlessness
- Anxiety

Check for Signs
- Dilated pupils
- Increased body temperature
- Rapid pulse
- Hallucinations
- Paranoia (high doses of cocaine)
- Cardiac arrest (extreme cases)
- Confusion
- Mood changes

✚ FIRST AID

1. Rest the athlete from all activity.
2. Send for emergency medical assistance if the symptoms don't improve or if the athlete has breathing difficulties.
3. Monitor breathing and provide CPR if needed.
4. Place an unresponsive athlete in recovery position (if uninjured) or HAINES position (if injured) to allow fluids or vomit to drain from the mouth.
5. Treat for shock if necessary and send for emergency medical assistance if it occurs.
6. If the athlete recovers quickly, speak to the parents and send the athlete to a physician.

Playing Status
- The athlete cannot return to activity until examined and released by a physician.

Prevention
- Provide drug abuse education.
- Monitor any athletes who exhibit behaviors characteristic of stimulant abuse: hyperactivity or extreme fatigue, mood changes, dramatic changes in performance, and aggressiveness.

Ecstasy Overdose or Reaction

Dangerous and possibly life-threatening response from using ecstasy or taking an excessive amount of ecstasy.

Ask if Experiencing Symptoms
- Depression
- Anxiety
- Nausea
- Feeling faint
- Blurred vision

Check for Signs
- Muscle tension
- Involuntary teeth clenching
- Insomnia
- Paranoia
- Chills
- Sweating
- Increased heart rate
- Confusion

(continued)

Ecstasy Overdose or Reaction   *(continued)*

✚ FIRST AID

1. Rest the athlete from all activity.
2. Send for emergency medical assistance if the symptoms don't improve or if the athlete has breathing difficulties.
3. Monitor breathing and provide CPR if needed.
4. Place an unresponsive athlete in recovery position (if uninjured) or HAINES position (if injured) to allow fluids or vomit to drain from the mouth.
5. Treat for shock if necessary and send for emergency medical assistance if it occurs.
6. If the athlete recovers quickly, speak to the parents and send the athlete to a physician.

Playing Status

- The athlete cannot return to activity until examined and released by a physician.

Prevention

- Provide drug abuse education.
- Monitor any athletes who exhibit behaviors characteristic of ecstasy abuse: anxiety, confusion, involuntary teeth clenching, and insomnia.

SUPPLEMENT REACTIONS

Touted to enhance performance by boosting strength, decreasing fatigue, and improving endurance, supplements are becoming increasingly popular among athletes. However, since nutritional substances are not regulated by the Food and Drug Administration (FDA), they may contain substances that are not listed on the label. This can be especially problematic for athletes who have severe allergies to certain substances, such as bee pollen (a common supplement). A supplement commonly used by athletes is creatine.

Creatine

Creatine is a substance made from amino acids (the building blocks of protein). It is primarily found in the muscles, where it is used to help release the energy needed for short bouts of exercise or physical activity. Although creatine is synthesized in the body and also found in foods (primarily lean meat and fish), it has become very popular as a manufactured supplement. Creatine supplements are widely used by athletes in an effort to improve their performance in brief, high-intensity exercise or sports activity. Taken at certain dosages, creatine has been found to enhance intense, brief exercise performance in weightlifting, sprint cycling and jumping.

Creatine use among high school athletes has been reported to be anywhere between 5.6 to 16.7 percent (Castillo and Comstock 2007). This may be problematic, since the long-term effects and effects on growth of creatine use by adolescents is unknown. Also little research has been done to determine appropriate doses for adolescents. In addition, supplements are not subjected to the same rigorous restrictions placed upon over-the-counter and prescription medications; they are not regulated for content or purity. So it's best to play it safe and protect your athletes by prohibiting the use of performance-enhancing supplements such as creatine.

Some athletes have adverse effects from taking creatine. Here are some signs and symptoms to watch for.

Creatine Reaction

Creatine use may cause gastrointestinal distress, muscle cramps, weight gain, or dehydration.

Ask if Experiencing Symptoms

- Nausea
- Stomach discomfort (gas)
- Loss of appetite

Check for Signs

- Weight gain (due to water retention in the muscles)
- Muscle cramps
- Dehydration
- Diarrhea

✚ FIRST AID

1. Rest the athlete from activity until signs and symptoms subside.
2. Monitor the athlete for signs and symptoms of a more serious condition such as an abdominal injury (chapter 9) or heat illness (chapter 11) and provide appropriate first aid as needed.

Playing Status

- If the athlete exhibits signs of dehydration (see chapter 11), do not allow him or her to return to activity until adequately rehydrated.

Prevention

- Provide sport supplement education to athletes and their parents.
- Monitor athletes who exhibit signs and symptoms consistent with the side effects of creatine: weight gain, nausea, muscle cramps, dehydration and abdominal discomfort.

Anabolic Steroids

Anabolic steroids are manufactured substances derived from the male reproductive hormone testosterone. While these substances can be used for medical purposes, their use is legal only with a prescription. Steroids can increase muscle size, lean muscle mass, and muscle strength, so athletes use them illegally to enhance their athletic performance and appearance. Studies of steroid use by middle school and high school students have found use to vary from 2.5 percent to as much as 11 percent. Use by athletes, especially football players, has been found to be higher than for nonathletes (Castillo and Comstock 2007).

Despite their ability to enhance performance, anabolic steroids cause serious health effects. They can lead to high blood pressure, increased cholesterol, cardiovascular disease, liver damage and infertility (males). If used by adolescents, steroids may prematurely stop growth and result in shorter stature.

Anabolic Steroid Abuse

Ask if Experiencing Symptoms
- Mood swings
- Aching joints
- Nervousness

Check for Signs
Males
- Baldness
- Increased breast size
- Decreased testicular size

Females
- Increased facial hair

- Deepened voice
- Reduced breast size
- Menstrual cycle changes

Both Genders
- Yellowish skin (sign of jaundice)
- Swollen feet or ankles (signs of cardiovascular disease)
- Bad breath
- Trembling
- Increased acne

FIRST AID

1. Monitor the athlete for symptoms or signs of more serious illnesses or injuries and refer to a physician if necessary.

2. Speak to the athlete and his or her parents about the suspected steroid use.
3. Require the athlete to see a physician.

Playing Status
- The athlete cannot return to activity until examined and released by a physician.

Prevention
- Provide steroid abuse education to athletes and parents. For some helpful resources visit www.drugabuse.gov/drugs-abuse/steroids-anabolic and www.drugabuse.gov/Drugpages/PSAGamePlan.html.

- Monitor athletes who exhibit symptoms or signs of steroid use.

If you suspect any of your athletes are using steroids, talk with them about some of the drawbacks of steroid use and the fact that their use is illegal for non-medical purposes.

OTHER ACUTE ILLNESSES

Insect sting allergies, fainting, influenza, and gastroenteritis are other possible sudden illnesses that you may have to face. Anaphylactic shock may occur in athletes who are allergic to certain insect stings. This was covered in chapter 7. Fainting in athletes is most often caused by illness or dehydration. Influenza and some cases of gastroenteritis can happen at any time and quickly spread to other athletes. Each of these acute illnesses requires quick and accurate assessment and first aid intervention.

Fainting

Temporary unresponsiveness not caused by a head injury. Can be classified as a mild form of shock.

Cause

- Usually brought on by extreme fatigue, dehydration, low blood pressure, or illness

Ask if Experiencing Symptoms

- Nausea
- Weakness
- Headache
- Fatigue
- Dizziness

Check for Signs

- Pale, cool, clammy skin
- Possibly shallow and rapid breathing
- Possible loss of responsiveness

⊕ FIRST AID

If Athlete Is Responsive

1. Instruct the athlete to either sit (on a chair or bench) with head between knees, as shown in figure 10.1, or lie down.

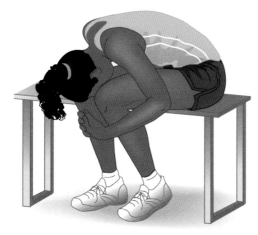

Figure 10.1 Position to prevent fainting.

2. Monitor and treat for shock if necessary and send for emergency medical assistance if it occurs.
3. If the athlete does not recover within a few minutes, send for emergency medical assistance.

If Athlete Is Unresponsive

1. Monitor breathing and provide CPR if needed.
2. Send for emergency medical assistance if the athlete does not recover within a few minutes.
3. Place athlete in recovery position (if uninjured) or HAINES position (if injured), not on back, to allow fluids to drain from the mouth.
4. Monitor and treat for shock if necessary and send for emergency medical assistance if it occurs.

Playing Status

- Rest the athlete for the remainder of the day.
- Inform the athlete's parents or guardian.
- The athlete must be examined and released by a physician if suffering from an illness.

Prevention

- If an athlete feels dizzy, seat the athlete with the head between the knees, as shown in figure 10.1.

Gastroenteritis

Sudden infection or toxin exposure affecting the stomach and intestines. This includes conditions commonly referred to as the stomach flu or food poisoning.

Cause

- Direct contact with bacteria, viruses, and certain parasites or germs that cause gastroenteritis. These can be spread through inhalation, personal contact, contact with contaminated surfaces, consumption of contaminated food or fluids, and handling of contaminated pets or animals.

Ask if Experiencing Symptoms

- Nausea
- Headache
- Abdominal pain
- Muscle aches
- Weakness
- Chills

Check for Signs

- Diarrhea
- Stomach cramps
- Vomiting
- Low-grade fever (99 degrees Fahrenheit)
- Dehydration (dry and parched lips, dry skin, extreme thirst, no urination in six hours)

⊕ FIRST AID

1. Rest the athlete from all activity.
2. Suggest the athlete avoid solid foods.
3. Encourage the athlete to consume only ice chips until vomiting stops, and then to drink clear fluids.
4. Immediately send the athlete to a physician if any of the following are present:
   a. Severe abdominal pain, particularly in the right lower abdomen
   b. Forceful vomiting
   c. Fever greater than 101 degrees
   d. Bloody stool or vomit
   e. Signs and symptoms lasting more than 48 hours
   f. Signs of dehydration
   g. Possibility of food poisoning

Playing Status

- The athlete cannot return to activity until signs and symptoms have been gone for 48 hours or until examined and released by a physician.

Prevention

- Prevent direct contact of an infected athlete with other athletes.
- Prevent indirect contact with an infected athlete via shared water bottles, towels, eating utensils, and so on.
- Make sure athletes wash their hands after using the bathroom.

Influenza

Infectious viral illness affecting the respiratory system (nose, throat, and lungs).

Cause

- Respiration of the virus or direct contact with the virus

Ask if Experiencing Symptoms

- Muscle or joint achiness
- Headache
- Fatigue

Check for Signs

- Fever
- Dry cough
- Nasal congestion
- Sore throat
- Runny nose
- Watery eyes

⊕ FIRST AID

1. Rest the athlete from all activity.

2. Encourage the athlete to drink liquids.

Playing Status

- The athlete cannot return to activity until signs and symptoms have been gone for 48 hours or until examined and released by a physician.

Prevention

- Prevent direct contact of an infected athlete with other athletes.
- Prevent indirect contact with an infected athlete via shared water bottles, towels, eating utensils, and so on.

Chapter 10 *REPLAY*

☐ Exercise and diet can affect the amount of insulin that the body needs. Thus, diabetic athletes need to be closely monitored for signs of diabetic illness. (p. 120)

☐ What causes an insulin reaction? (p. 120)

☐ What quick first aid care can you provide to help minimize an insulin reaction? (p. 121)

☐ Explain the cause of ketoacidosis. (p. 121)

☐ Discuss the difference between insulin reaction and diabetic ketoacidosis. (pp. 120-122)

☐ What first aid care can you provide for early stage ketoacidosis? (p. 122)

☐ What happens in the brain during a seizure? (p. 122)

☐ List some common causes of seizures. (p. 122)

☐ What are the signs and symptoms of a minor/petit mal seizure? (pp. 122-123)

☐ What are the signs and symptoms of a major/grand mal seizure? (p. 123)

☐ What are some substances that depress the central nervous system? (p. 124)

☐ What are the signs and symptoms of an overdose or adverse reaction to depressants? (p. 124)

☐ What are some substances that stimulate the central nervous system? (p. 124-125)

☐ What are the signs and symptoms of an overdose or adverse reaction to stimulants? (p. 125)

☐ Can you describe the first aid techniques for an overdose or adverse reaction to depressants and stimulants? (pp. 124-125)

☐ Describe the first aid care for fainting. (p. 129)

☐ What causes gastroenteritis? (p. 130)

☐ What are the signs and symptoms of gastroenteritis? (p. 130)

☐ What are the signs and symptoms of influenza (the flu)? (p. 131)

☐ What can you do to help prevent the spread of the flu and gastroenteritis among your athletes? (p. 131)

REFERENCES

Castillo, E.M. and R.D. Comstock. 2007. Prevalence of use of performance-enhancing substances among United States adolescents. *Pediatric Clinics of North America.* 54(4): 663-675.

Evans, N.A. and A. B. Parkinson. Special Q & A: Steroid use and the young athlete. *ACSM Fit Society Page,* Fall 2005, pp. 5-6. www. ladiesworkoutexpress.com/wellness/docs/fitsoc_fall05.pdf. Accessed 8/1/2007.

Lattavo, A., Kopperud, A., and P.D. Rogers. (2007). Creatine and Other Supplements. Pediatric Clinics of North America. 54: 735–760.

National Institute on Drug Abuse. *NIDA InfoFacts: Steroids (Anabolic-Androgenic).* www.nida.nih. gov/Infofacts/Steroids.html.

U.S. Department of Health and Human Services and SAMHA's National Clearinghouse for Alcohol & Drug Information – Publications. *Tips for teens: The truth about steroids.* http://ncadi. samhsa.gov/govpubs/phd726/.

RESOURCES

www.nida.nih.gov (National Institute on Drug Abuse)

www.playclean.org (Promoting anti-doping policies and preventing youth drug use through sport)

www.theantidrug.com (Parents Against Drugs)

www.joinaad.org (Athletes Against Drugs)

www.usantidoping.org (U.S. Anti-Doping Agency)

www.gssiweb.com (Gatorade Sports Science Institute)

Weather-Related Problems

IN THIS CHAPTER, YOU WILL LEARN:

- ▸ How to prevent heat-, cold-, and lightning-related injuries and illnesses.
- ▸ How to identify the symptoms and signs of heat cramps.
- ▸ How to identify and differentiate between the symptoms and signs of heat exhaustion and heatstroke.
- ▸ How to identify the symptoms and signs of first-, second-, and third-degree frostbite and mild to severe hypothermia.
- ▸ What first aid care to provide for heat cramps, heat exhaustion, heatstroke, frostbite, hypothermia, and lightning injuries.

INJURIES AND ILLNESSES IN THIS CHAPTER

Searing lightning, sweltering heat, and numbing cold are an accepted part of outdoor sport seasons. Even so, it's important to not overlook the serious illnesses and injuries that can result from these conditions. Lightning, heatstroke, and hypothermia can be life threatening, and frostbite can lead to disfiguration. Fortunately, almost all of these conditions can be prevented. You play a key role in preventing heat-related illnesses, cold-related illnesses, and lightning injuries as well as in identifying them quickly and providing appropriate first aid care.

TEMPERATURE REGULATION

Before learning the sport first aid specifics for temperature-related illnesses, it's essential to first understand how body temperature is regulated. There are several ways through which the body's temperature changes—metabolism, convection, conduction, radiation, and evaporation. Figure 11.1 helps illustrate each of these.

Metabolism

As the body's cells work and use energy (metabolism), heat is produced. So, when athletes are active, their body temperatures rise due to an increase in metabolic rate.

Convection

In convection, heat is lost or gained via air (wind) circulating around the body. If the air temperature is warmer than the body, the body will gain heat. If the air temperature is cooler, the body will lose heat.

Conduction

Another way the body loses or gains heat is by coming in contact with warmer or colder objects. This is called conduction. For example, sitting in a warm whirlpool will cause an athlete's body temperature to rise. Or, an athlete can lose body heat by sitting on a cold, metal bench.

Radiation

Radiation occurs when heat is gained through contact with electromagnetic waves, such as from

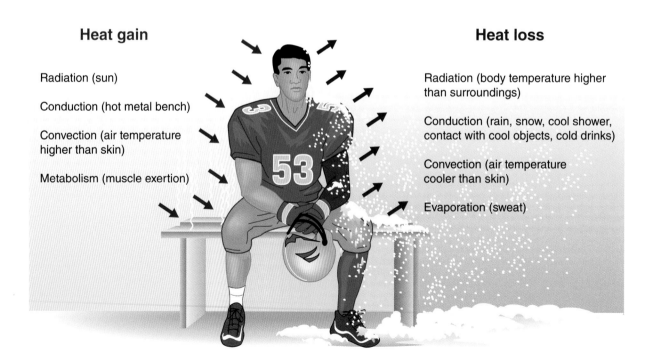

Heat gain

Radiation (sun)

Conduction (hot metal bench)

Convection (air temperature higher than skin)

Metabolism (muscle exertion)

Heat loss

Radiation (body temperature higher than surroundings)

Conduction (rain, snow, cool shower, contact with cool objects, cold drinks)

Convection (air temperature cooler than skin)

Evaporation (sweat)

Figure 11.1 Methods of body temperature change.

the sun. The degree of cloudiness and the angle of the sun can influence the sun's radiative effects. Heat can be lost through radiation from the body to the environment whenever the environmental temperature is less than body temperature.

Evaporation

Sweating is the body's built-in mechanism for cooling itself. However, it's only effective if the sweat actually evaporates from the skin. Humidity, or the amount of moisture already in the air, directly influences how much sweat will evaporate. The more humid the environment, the less sweat will evaporate, and the more difficult it is for the body to lose heat. Equipment and type of clothing can also affect sweat evaporation. For example, a helmet will prevent heat from the head from being dissipated through radiation, evaporation, and convection.

With this understanding of body temperature regulation, let's look at what can happen when body temperature goes awry. First we'll look at exertional heat-related illnesses, and then we will turn our attention to cold-related illnesses.

EXERTIONAL HEAT-RELATED ILLNESSES

After suffering heat exhaustion and leaving practice early the day before, perhaps he felt he couldn't afford to take it easy during drills and conditioning, even though it was another day of stifling heat. So, he pushed himself through practice. It was hard; he vomited several times. Finally it was time to head inside to the long-awaited air conditioning. There he developed symptoms of heatstroke, including weakness and rapid breathing. Although he was immediately evaluated and treated by athletic trainers, and transported to a hospital, Korey Stringer, offensive tackle for the Minnesota Vikings, was unresponsive at the time of arrival. His body temperature had soared to over 108 degrees, resulting in multiorgan system failure and, finally, death.

In 1997, within the span of one month, three college wrestlers died trying to make weight. A February 20, 1998, issue of the *Morbidity and Mortality Weekly Report*, published by the Centers for Disease Control and Prevention,

concluded that all three victims wore vapor-impermeable suits and exercised vigorously in hot environments. "These conditions promoted dehydration and heat-related illness," stated the report, which noted that the body temperature of one of the wrestlers was 108 degrees at the time of death.

Heat-related fatalities and illnesses are not unique to professional and collegiate sports. There were 15 heat-related deaths in high school sports in the United States from 1995 through July 2002, according to the National Federation for State High School Associations. Fortunately, heat-related illnesses are very preventable.

Prevention of Exertional Heat-Related Illnesses

The key to prevention is balancing all the factors that influence body temperature so that the body temperature stays within a safe range. Here's how:

• *Monitor weather conditions and adjust practices accordingly.* Table 11.1 shows the specific air temperature and humidity percentages that can be hazardous. Keep in mind, however that football exertional heat-related deaths have occurred at temperatures as low as 82 degrees with a relative humidity index at only 40 percent. If heat and humidity are equal to or higher than these conditions, make sure athletes are acclimated to the weather and are wearing light practice clothing. Schedule practices for early morning and evening to avoid the heat of the day.

• *Acclimate athletes to exercising in high heat and humidity.* If you are located in a warm-weather climate or have practices during the summer, athletes need time (approximately 7 to 10 days) to adjust to high heat and humidity. During this time, hold short practices at low to moderate activity levels and provide fluid and rest breaks every 15 to 20 minutes. The National Athletic Trainers' Association 2009 Consensus Statement offers more specific guidelines for acclimating high school athletes to hot environmental conditions. Table 11.2 summarizes the organization's recommendations.

• *Switch to light clothing and less equipment.* Athletes stay cooler if they wear shorts, white

Table 11.1 Warm-Weather Precautions

Temperature (98°F)	Humidity	Precautions
80-90	<70%	Monitor athletes prone to heat illness
80-90	>70%	5-minute rest after 30 minutes of practice
90-100	<70%	5-minute rest after 30 minutes of practice
90-100	>70%	Short practices in evenings or early morning

Table 11.2 Heat Acclimatization Recommendations

Week	Day(s)	Equipment	Practice length	Practice frequency	Practice activities	Walk-through
1	1	Helmets only	3 hours per day	Once per day	Warm-up, stretching, cool-down, walk-through (during 2-a-days), conditioning, and weightlifting are all considered practice activities. None of these should be tacked on to extend the activity beyond the recommended practice hours.	1 permitted per day in addition to practice, but athletes must have a 3-hour recovery period between walk-through and practice.
	2					
	3	Helmets and shoulder pads				
	4					
	5					
	6	Full equipment	No more than 5 hours per day for double-practice days No single practice lasting more than 3 hours	Alternate a double-practice day with a single-practice day or double-practice day with a recovery day.		1 permitted only on single-practice days but must be separated from the practice by a 3-hour recovery period.
	7					
2	8					
	9					
	10					
	11					
	12					
	13					
	14					

Note: Any athlete who misses a practice for any reason must still complete a full 14-day progression. Therefore, the athlete must pick up where he or she left off before the missed practice(s).

Adapted from D.J. Casa and D. Csillan, 2009, "Preseason heat-acclimatization guidelines for secondary school athletics," *Journal of Athletic Training.* 44 (3): 332–333.

T-shirts, and less equipment (especially helmets and pads). Equipment blocks the ability of sweat to evaporate. It's especially important for athletes to wear light clothing and minimal equipment while they are acclimating to the heat.

- *Identify and monitor athletes who are prone to heat illness.* Athletes who have previously suffered a heat illness and those with the sickle cell trait are particularly prone to exertional heat illness and should be continuously monitored during activity. Dehydrated, overweight, heavily muscled, or deconditioned athletes are at risk, as well as athletes taking certain medications (antihistamines, decongestants, some asthma medications, certain supplements, and attention-deficit/hyperactivity disorder medications). Closely monitor these athletes and make sure they drink plenty of fluids. Rest dehydrated athletes until they have become rehydrated (see next bullet for more information on adequate hydration).

The signs and symptoms of dehydration include

- thirst,
- flushed skin,
- fatigue,
- muscle cramps,
- apathy,
- dry lips and mouth,
- dark colored urine (should be clear or light yellow), and
- feeling weak.

- *Strictly enforce adequate hydration.* Athletes can lose a great deal of water through sweat. If this fluid is not replaced, the body will have less water to cool itself and will become dehydrated. Dehydration not only increases athletes' risk for heat illness, it also decreases their performance. In fact, athletic performance may worsen after only 2 percent of the body weight is lost through sweat. For example, dehydrated athletes may experience

- decreased muscle strength,
- increased fatigue,
- decreased mental function (e.g., concentration), and
- decreased endurance.

Sports Drinks Versus Water

If athletes are

- engaged in any vigorous or high-intensity activity,
- practicing or competing for more than one hour,
- competing or practicing more than once per day, or
- dehydrated,

then sports drinks (with 6 to 7 percent carbohydrate solution and sodium content) are preferred because they

- stimulate thirst,
- promote fluid retention,
- replenish carbohydrates utilized for energy,
- help to reduce muscle cramping, and
- appeal to athletes (because of the flavor), which causes them to drink more.

Don't rely on athletes to drink enough fluids on their own. Most won't actually feel thirsty until they've lost 3 percent or more of their body weight in sweat (water). By that time their performance will have started to decrease and their risk of exertional heat illness will have increased. Also, they may not drink enough fluid to replenish the water lost through sweat.

For proper hydration, the National Athletic Trainers' Association (Casa et al. 2000) recommends

- 17 to 20 fluid ounces of fluid at least 2 hours before workouts, practice, or competition;
- another 7 to 10 fluid ounces of water or sports drink 10 to 15 minutes before workouts, practice, or competition;
- as a general guideline, 7 to 10 fluid ounces of cool (50 to 59 degrees Fahrenheit) water or sports drink every 10 to 20 minutes during workouts, practice, or competition; and

- after workouts, practices, and competitions, 24 fluid ounces of water or sports drink for every pound of fluid lost through sweat (Manore et al. 2000).

To determine the amount of weight lost through sweat, weigh athletes in their underwear before and after practices and competitions that take place in high heat and humidity.

- *Replenish electrolytes lost through sweat.* During activities lasting longer than 45 to 50 minutes, substantial amounts of electrolytes such as sodium (salt) and potassium are lost in sweat. They are used in muscle contraction, fluid balance, and other body functions, and therefore must be replaced. In addition, sodium plays a role in activating the body's thirst mechanism, so it can stimulate athletes to drink (keep hydrated). The best way for athletes to replace these nutrients is by drinking a sports beverage (containing sodium) and eating a normal diet. Athletes can also replace sodium by lightly salting their food, so salt tablets are not recommended. Just a small amount of potassium is lost in sweat. Oranges and bananas are good sources of potassium.

- *Prohibit the use of sweatboxes, vinyl suits, diuretics, or other artificial means of quick weight reduction.* The NFHS Wrestling Rules Committee has already prohibited these methods.

Identifying and Treating Exertional Heat Illnesses

During physical activity, the body can produce 10 to 20 times the amount of heat that it produces at rest (metabolism). Approximately 75 percent of this heat must be eliminated. If the air temperature is less than the body temperature, radiation, conduction, and convection can help dissipate 65 to 75 percent of this heat. However, if the air temperature is near the body temperature, these modes of heat loss are less effective, and the body has to rely more on perspiration. High humidity reduces the amount of sweat evaporation, and thus leaves exercising athletes at risk of exertional heat illness.

The following sections will cover three types of exertional heat illness:

- Heat cramps
- Heat exhaustion
- Heatstroke

Each has different signs and symptoms, as well as different first aid interventions. Heatstroke is life threatening, whereas heat exhaustion and heat cramps typically are not. Therefore, it is important that you learn to evaluate the signs and symptoms and learn to apply the first aid techniques that are appropriate for each illness.

For a summary of first aid care for heat cramps, heat exhaustion, and heatstroke, see pages 279 to 281 in appendix A.

Heat Cramps

Sudden muscle spasms (commonly occur in the quadriceps, hamstrings, or calves).

Causes

- Dehydration
- Electrolyte (sodium and potassium) loss
- Decreased blood flow to the muscles
- Fatigue

Ask if Experiencing Symptoms

- Pain
- Fatigue

Check for Signs

- Severe muscle spasms, often in the quadriceps, hamstrings, or calves

⊕ FIRST AID

1. Rest the athlete.
2. Assist the athlete with stretching the affected muscle.
3. Give the athlete a sports beverage (containing sodium) to drink.
4. If the spasms do not stop with stretching or after a few minutes of rest, look for other possible causes.
5. If spasms continue or other injuries are found, inform parents or guardians and send athlete to a physician.

Playing Status

- The athlete can return to activity once the spasms stop and the athlete can run, jump, and cut without limping or pain.
- You should monitor the athlete for worsening signs and symptoms, or any signs of dehydration, and send the athlete to a physician if such occurs.
- If referred to a physician, the athlete cannot return to activity until examined and released.

Prevention

- Ensure that athletes stay well hydrated.
- Rest an athlete who is showing signs of dehydration.
- Educate parents and athletes about dehydration and heat illnesses. Visit www.nata.org/sites/default/files/Heat-Illness-Parent-Coach-Guide.pdf for an informative handout.

Heat Exhaustion

Shocklike condition caused by dehydration.

Cause

- Dehydration, which occurs when the body's water and electrolyte supplies are depleted through sweating

Ask if Experiencing Symptoms

- Headache
- Nausea
- Dizziness
- Chills
- Fatigue
- Thirst

Check for Signs

- Pale, cool, and clammy skin
- Rapid, weak pulse
- Loss of coordination
- Dilated pupils
- Profuse sweating

(continued)

✚ FIRST AID

1. Quickly move the athlete to a cool, shaded area. Allow athlete to rest on his or her back with feet elevated.

2. Take a rectal temperature. If it is approaching 104 degrees, skip to first aid step 9.

3. Apply ice or cold, wet towels to the athlete's neck, back, or stomach to help cool the body.

4. Give the athlete cool water or sports beverage to drink (if responsive and able to ingest fluid).

5. Monitor breathing and provide CPR if needed.

6. Monitor and treat for shock as needed and send for emergency medical assistance if it occurs.

7. Send for emergency medical assistance if the athlete does not recover, the athlete's condition worsens, or the athlete becomes unresponsive.

8. If the athlete recovers, call the parents or guardian to take the athlete home.

9. If the athlete is exhibiting signs or symptoms of life-threatening heat illness, vomiting, altered responsiveness, disorientation, staggering, fainting, belligerence, and so on, then do the following:

   a. Immediately remove excess clothing and equipment and immerse athlete in cold water (wading pool or tub).

   b. Send for emergency medical assistance.

   c. Monitor breathing and provide CPR if needed.

Playing Status

- An athlete must absolutely not return to activity on the same day that the athlete suffered heat exhaustion. If the athlete is sent to a physician or does not quickly recover, do not allow the athlete to return to activity until released by a physician.

- The athlete cannot return to activity until the weight lost through sweat is regained.

Prevention

- Ensure that athletes stay well hydrated.

- Rest an athlete who is showing signs of dehydration.

- Educate parents and athletes about dehydration and heat illnesses. Visit www.nata.org/sites/default/files/Heat-Illness-Parent-Coach-Guide.pdf for an informative handout.

Heatstroke

Life-threatening condition in which the body temperature rises dangerously high.

Cause

- A malfunction in the brain's temperature control center, caused by severe dehydration, fever, or inadequate balance of the body's temperature regulation

Ask if Experiencing Symptoms

- Feels extremely hot
- Nausea
- Irritability
- Fatigue

Check for Signs

- Hot and flushed or red skin
- Very high body temperature—rectal temperature 104 degrees or more
- Rapid pulse
- Rapid breathing
- Constricted pupils
- Vomiting
- Diarrhea
- Confusion
- Possible seizures
- Possible unresponsiveness
- Possible respiratory or cardiac arrest

🔴➕ FIRST AID

1. Send for emergency medical assistance.
2. Immediately remove excess clothing and equipment and immerse athlete in cold water (wading pool or tub).
3. Position the athlete in a semireclining position. If unresponsive, raise the athlete's head or roll him on his side as necessary to allow fluids and vomit to drain from the mouth.

4. Monitor breathing and provide CPR if needed.
5. Monitor and treat for shock as needed (**do not** cover the athlete with blankets).
6. Give the athlete cool water or sports beverage to drink (if responsive and able to ingest fluid).

Playing Status

- The athlete cannot return to activity until examined and released by a physician, and then should return to activity gradually.

Prevention

- Ensure that athletes stay well hydrated.
- Rest an athlete who is showing signs of dehydration.

- After an athlete suffers from heat exhaustion, do not allow the athlete to return to practice or competition until the athlete has fully rehydrated.
- Educate parents and athletes about dehydration and heat illnesses. Visit www.nata.org/sites/default/files/Heat-Illness-Parent-Coach-Guide.pdf for an informative handout.

COLD-RELATED ILLNESSES

As with heat illnesses, cold-related illnesses are caused by an imbalance in the factors that affect the body temperature. Exposure to cold weather and cold equipment causes the body temperature to drop below normal. To counteract this, the body tries to gain or conserve heat by shivering (increases metabolism) and reducing blood flow to the skin and extremities (to conserve heat and blood flow to the brain, heart, and lungs). This can result in frostbite or hypothermia.

Prevention of Cold-Related Illnesses

The body best withstands cold temperatures when it is prepared to handle them. Following are guidelines to reduce the risk of cold-related illnesses.

- *Make sure athletes wear appropriate protective clothing.* Athletes should dress in layers to allow sweat to evaporate and to protect against the cold. Wool, Gore-Tex™, and Lycra™ are excellent materials to wear. Also, be sure the head and neck are covered to prevent excessive heat loss. Mittens are preferable to gloves because they allow the fingers to warm each other.

- *Keep athletes active to maintain body heat.* Athletes who must stand along the sidelines should keep moving to help produce body heat. Jumping up and down and jogging in place are good sideline exercises.

- *Monitor the windchill (figure 11.2) and adjust exposure to the cold accordingly.* The combination of wind, cold temperatures, and wet conditions increases athletes' risk of hypothermia.

- *Monitor athletes who are at risk of cold-related illness.* Thin yet highly conditioned athletes may be prone to cold-related illness because they have less fat to help insulate their bodies. Dehydrated athletes are also at risk.

Temperature (°F)

Wind (mph)	40	35	30	25	20	15	10	5	0	-5	-10	-15	-20	-25	-30	-35	-40	-45
Calm																		
5	36	31	25	19	13	7	1	-5	-11	-16	-22	-28	-34	-40	-46	-52	-57	-63
10	34	27	21	15	9	3	-4	-10	-16	-22	-28	-35	-41	-47	-53	-59	-66	-72
15	32	25	19	13	6	0	-7	-13	-19	-26	-32	-39	-45	-51	-58	-64	-71	-77
20	30	24	17	11	4	-2	-9	-15	-22	-29	-35	-42	-48	-55	-61	-68	-74	-81
25	29	23	16	9	3	-4	-11	-17	-24	-31	-37	-44	-51	-58	-64	-71	-78	-84
30	28	22	15	8	1	-5	-12	-19	-26	-33	-39	-46	-53	-60	-67	-73	-80	-87
35	28	21	14	7	0	-7	-14	-21	-27	-34	-41	-48	-55	-62	-69	-76	-82	-89
40	27	20	13	6	-1	-8	-15	-22	-29	-36	-43	-50	-57	-64	-71	-78	-84	-91
45	26	19	12	5	-2	-9	-16	-23	-30	-37	-44	-51	-58	-65	-72	-79	-86	-93
50	26	19	12	4	-3	-10	-17	-24	-31	-38	-45	-52	-60	-67	-74	-81	-88	-95
55	25	18	11	4	-3	-11	-18	-25	-32	-39	-46	-54	-61	-68	-75	-82	-89	-97
60	25	17	10	3	-4	-11	-19	-26	-33	-40	-48	-55	-62	-69	-76	-84	-91	-98

Frostbite times ■ 30 minutes ■ 10 minutes ■ 5 minutes

$$\text{Wind Chill (°F)} = 35.74 + 0.6215T - 35.75(V^{0.16}) + 0.4275T(V^{0.16})$$

Where T = Air Temperature (°F); V = Wind Speed (mph) *Effective 11/01/01*

Figure 11.2 National Weather Service Wind Chill Temperature Index.

- *Stress adequate hydration.* For proper hydration, the National Athletic Trainers' Association recommends (Casa et al. 2000)

  - 17 to 20 fluid ounces of fluid at least 2 hours before workouts, practice, or competition;

  - another 7 to 10 fluid ounces of water or sports drink 10 to 15 minutes before workouts, practice, or competition;

  - as a general guideline for when profuse sweating is expected, 7 to 10 fluid ounces of water or sports drink every 10 to 20 minutes during workouts, practice, or competition; and

- after workouts, practices, and competitions 24 fluid ounces of water or sports drink for every pound of water lost through sweat (Manore et al. 2000).

Identifying and Treating Cold-Related Illnesses

Frostbite and hypothermia occur in varying degrees of severity, advancing from mild to severe. Each stage has specific signs and symptoms that will dictate the first aid that you administer.

For first aid protocols for frostbite and hypothermia, see pages 282 and 283 in appendix A.

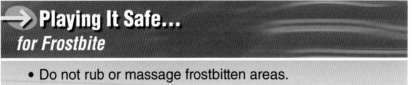

⇒ Playing It Safe...
for Frostbite

- Do not rub or massage frostbitten areas.
- Do not apply ice to frostbitten areas.
- Do not allow frostbitten tissue to refreeze.

Doing any of these things can worsen an athlete's condition.

Frostbite

A condition in which tissues freeze and blood vessels constrict.

Superficial frostbite involves localized freezing of the skin and the superficial tissues below it. The nose, ears, toes, and fingers are especially prone to superficial frostbite. Deep frostbite begins superficially but advances to deep tissues such as muscles and tendons.

Cause

- Exposure of body parts to cold, causing tissues to freeze and blood vessels to constrict

Ask if Experiencing Symptoms

- Painful, itchy, burning, or tingling areas that may become numb as the frostbite worsens. These symptoms may recur when the affected areas are rewarmed.

Check for Signs

First-Degree Frostbite (Superficial)

- Red or flushed skin that may turn white or gray

Second-Degree Frostbite

- Firm, white, and waxy skin
- Blisters and purple tint to skin may appear when the area is rewarmed

Third-Degree Frostbite (Deep)

- Blisters
- Bluish skin
- Frostbitten area feels very cold and stiff

✚ FIRST AID

First- and Second-Degree Frostbite

1. Move the athlete to a warm area.
2. Remove wet and cold clothing.
3. Monitor and treat for shock if necessary and call for emergency medical assistance if it occurs.
4. Rewarm the area by soaking it in clean, warm water (100 to 105 degrees Fahrenheit). Do not rewarm if the area might refreeze or the athlete is close to a medical facility.
5. Call the athlete's parents or guardian to take the athlete to a physician.

Third-Degree Frostbite

1. Send for emergency medical assistance.
2. Move the athlete to a warm area.
3. Remove wet and cold clothing.
4. Monitor breathing and provide CPR if needed.
5. Monitor and treat for shock if necessary.

Playing Status

- The athlete cannot return to activity until examined and released by a physician.

Hypothermia

Condition in which the body temperature drops below 95 degrees.

Causes

- Prolonged exposure to a wet, windy, and cold environment
- Extreme fatigue, such as that suffered after competition in a marathon or triathlon
- Dehydration

Ask if Experiencing Symptoms

When the body temperature drops below 95 degrees,

- Irritability
- Drowsiness
- Lethargy

Check for Signs

From 90 to 95 Degrees (Mild to Moderate Hypothermia)

- Loss of coordination
- Loss of sensation
- Shivering
- Pale and hard skin
- Numbness
- Irritability
- Mild confusion

- Depression
- Withdrawn behavior
- Slow, irregular pulse
- Slowed breathing
- Sluggish movements
- Inability to walk
- Difficulty speaking

From 86 to 90 Degrees (Severe Hypothermia)

- Hallucinations
- Dilated pupils
- Decreasing pulse rate
- Decreasing breathing rate
- Confusion
- Partial responsiveness
- Shivering stops
- Muscle rigidity
- Exposed skin blue and puffy

85 Degrees and Below (Also Severe Hypothermia)

- Unresponsiveness
- Respiratory arrest
- Erratic to no pulse

⊕ FIRST AID

Mild to Moderate Hypothermia

1. Move the athlete to a warm area.
2. Send for emergency medical assistance.
3. Gently remove cold and wet clothes.
4. Wrap the athlete in blankets.
5. Monitor and treat for shock as needed.

Severe Hypothermia

1. Send for emergency medical assistance.
2. Cover the athlete with blankets.
3. Handle the athlete very carefully. Excessive movements or jarring may cause cold blood to recirculate from the limbs to the heart and cause it to stop.
4. Monitor breathing and provide CPR if needed.
5. Monitor and treat for shock as needed.

Playing Status

- The athlete cannot return to activity until examined and released by a physician.

LIGHTNING-RELATED INJURIES

According to the National Weather Service, individuals in recreation and sporting activities comprise a third of all lightning injuries in the United States. Common sites for these injuries include athletic fields, golf courses, and swimming pools. Metal bats, fences, benches and bleachers; trees, and water are good conductors of lightning. Athletes, staff, and spectators are vulnerable to lightning while around these objects. Since lightning tends to strike taller objects, standing in an open playing field increases the risk of a lightning injury. Seeking shelter under a tree is also risky because lightning can travel through the tree to nearby objects. To minimize the risk of lightning injuries, review the safety guidelines in chapter 2 and develop a lightning safety policy.

Lightning Injury

Lightning can cause a gamut of injuries, from burns to fractures to cardiac arrest.

Cause
- Indirect or direct hit by lightning

Ask if Experiencing Symptoms
If responsive,
  - headache
  - dizziness

Check for Signs
- Burns at point of entrance and exit
- If responsive—disorientation
- Unresponsiveness

✚ FIRST AID

1. Quickly move (being mindful of other injuries) the athlete to a safe area, away from lightning.
2. Send for emergency medical assistance.
3. Monitor breathing and provide CPR if needed.
4. Monitor and treat for shock as needed.
5. Remove smoldering clothing, shoes, and belt to prevent burns.
6. If breathing is present and no fractures are suspected, place an unresponsive or incoherent athlete in recovery position (see chapter 4) to allow fluids and vomit to drain from the mouth.

Playing Status
- The athlete cannot return to activity until examined and released by a physician.

Prevention
- Develop a lightning injury prevention plan (see chapter 2).

- Stop activities when thunder occurs, even without lightning, or use the 30 to 30 rule (Walsh et al. 2000) for suspending recreational or sporting activities: If thunder occurs within 30 seconds of distant lightning, seek shelter. Do not leave the shelter until 30 minutes after the last lightning strike or clap of thunder.

Chapter 11 *REPLAY*

- ☐ Describe the five methods through which the body gains or loses heat. (pp. 134-135)
- ☐ Is an athlete who has a previous history of either a cold- or a heat-related illness prone to suffering the same condition again? (p. 137)
- ☐ What are the three common types of heat illness? (p. 138)
- ☐ What are the signs and symptoms of heat exhaustion? (p. 139)
- ☐ What are the signs and symptoms of heatstroke? (p. 140)
- ☐ What are the first aid steps for heatstroke? (p. 141)
- ☐ What steps can be taken to prevent heat illnesses? (pp. 135-138)
- ☐ What steps can be taken to prevent cold-related illnesses? (pp. 141-142)
- ☐ Explain what happens to a body part when it is affected by the different degrees of frostbite. (p. 143)
- ☐ What are the first aid steps for frostbite? (p. 143)
- ☐ Define hypothermia. (p. 144)
- ☐ What are the first aid steps for hypothermia? (p. 144)
- ☐ What types of injuries can result from a lightning strike? (p. 145)

REFERENCES

Casa, D.E., L.E. Armstrong, S.K. Hillman, S.J. Montain, R.V. Reiff, B.S.E. Rich, W.O. Roberts, and J.A. Stone. 2000. National Athletic Trainers' Association position statement: Fluid replacement for athletes. *Journal of Athletic Training* 35(2): 212-224.

Casa, D.E. and D. Csillan. 2009. Preseason heat-acclimatization guidelines for secondary school athletics. *Journal of Athletic Training* 44(3):332-3.

Centers for Disease Control and Prevention. 1998. Hyperthermia and dehydration-related deaths associated with intentional rapid weight loss–North Carolina, Wisconsin, and Michigan, November-December 1997. *Morbidity and Mortality Weekly Report* 47(6):105-108.

Manore, M.M., S.I. Barr, and G.E. Butterfield. 2000. Nutrition and athletic performance: Position of the American Dietetic Association, Dietitians of Canada, and the American College of Sports Medicine. *Journal of the American Dietetic Association* 100:1543-1556.

Walsh, K.M., B. Bennett, M.A. Cooper, R.L. Holle, R. Kithil, and R.E. Lopez. 2000. National Athletic Trainers' Association position statement: Lightning safety for athletics and recreation. *Journal of Athletic Training* 35(4):471-477.

CHAPTER 12

Upper Body Musculoskeletal Injuries

IN THIS CHAPTER, YOU WILL LEARN:

▸ How to recognize upper body musculoskeletal injuries.

▸ What first aid care to provide for each of these types of injuries.

▸ How to prevent upper body musculoskeletal injuries.

▸ What conditions are required before an injured athlete can return to play.

INJURIES IN THIS CHAPTER

(continued)

Sports that involve throwing, swinging, lifting, catching, pushing, or pulling place a lot of demand upon the upper body, shoulders, arms, wrists, and hands. For example, during the acceleration phase in throwing, the shoulder joint reaches an angular velocity of more than 7000 degrees per second (Fleisig, Dillman, and Andrew 1994). And in gymnastics, the elbow experiences approximately two times the body weight in compression force while doing a handspring (Koh, Grabiner, and Weiker 1992).

It's no wonder that upper body injuries are common in some sports. This chapter will help you identify and provide first aid care for these types of injuries.

First aid decisions for musculoskeletal injuries often depend on the severity of the injury—mild (Grade I), moderate (Grade II), and severe (Grade III). You may want to review the definitions and illustrations of Grade I, II, and III strains and sprains on pages 39 through 41. In addition, many of the first aid protocols in this chapter include icing and immobilizing (splinting) the injured part. You can find guidelines for ice application on page 76 and for splinting on pages 70 to 73.

SHOULDER

Acute shoulder injuries—those that occur suddenly—commonly occur in football and wrestling, whereas chronic shoulder injuries—those that develop gradually—typically occur in volleyball, swimming, baseball, and softball. For example, in a study conducted by Comstock, Collins, and Yard (2008), shoulder or arm injuries were the number one injury (19.6 percent) among high school baseball players and accounted for 19.3 percent of all injuries sustained by high school wrestlers. Table 12.1 illustrates the incidence of shoulder and arm injuries in several sports.

Page 284 in appendix A summarizes first aid care for shoulder fractures and sprains, and page 285 summarizes first aid care for shoulder strains.

Table 12.1 Frequency of Shoulder and Upper Arm Injury Out of All Reported Body Regions Injured

Sport	Percentage
Baseball	19.6
Wrestling	19.3
Ice Hockey	14.1 (male and female)
Lacrosse	12.3 (male and female)
Football	12.1
Softball	10.9

Data from Comstock, Collins, and Yard 2008, and Yard and Comstock 2006.

Clavicle Fracture

Crack or break in clavicle.

Cause
- Direct blow to the front or side of the shoulder

Ask if Experiencing Symptoms
- Pain in front of the shoulder along the collarbone
- Pain when raising the arm
- Grating sensation

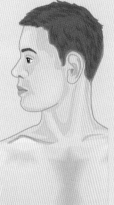

Check for Signs
- Deformity (figure 12.1)
- Swelling
- Point tenderness

Figure 12.1 Fractured collarbone.

FIRST AID

1. Immobilize the arm with a sling and secure the arm to the body with an elastic wrap (figure 12.2).
2. Send for emergency medical assistance if bones are grossly displaced or protruding through the skin, or if the athlete is suffering from shock.
3. Apply ice to the injury and send the athlete to a physician (if not suffering from shock).

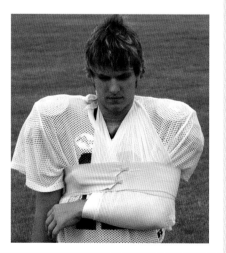

Figure 12.2 Sling and wrap immobilization for a broken collarbone.

(continued)

Playing Status

- The athlete cannot return to activity until examined and released by a physician; the shoulder is pain free; and the athlete has full strength, flexibility, and range of motion in the shoulder.

Prevention

- Require athletes to wear properly fitted shoulder pads if part of standard equipment.

Acromioclavicular (AC) Joint Sprain (Shoulder Separation)

Stretch or tear of the ligaments that connect the clavicle to the shoulder blade—the acromioclavicular joint (figure 12.3).

Causes

- Direct blow to the top or side of the shoulder
- Fall on outstretched arm

Ask if Experiencing Symptoms

Grade I

- Mild pain along the outer edge of the clavicle (collarbone)
- Mild pain with raising the arm overhead
- Mild pain with reaching the arm across the body

Grades II and III

- Moderate to severe pain along the outer edge of the clavicle (collarbone)
- Moderate to severe pain with raising the arm overhead
- Moderate to severe pain with reaching the arm across the body

Check for Signs

Grade I

- Slight elevation of the end of the clavicle

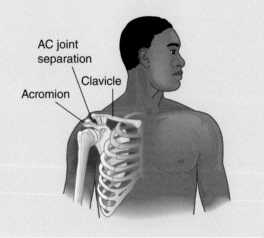

AC joint separation

Clavicle

Acromion

Figure 12.3   AC joint sprain.

- Mild point tenderness over outer edge of the clavicle

Grades II and III

- Moderate to severe elevation of the outer edge of the clavicle
- Moderate to severe point tenderness over outer edge of the clavicle

⊕ FIRST AID

Grade I

1. Rest the athlete from painful activities.
2. Apply ice.
3. Refer the athlete to a physician if symptoms and signs worsen (occur more often, especially with daily activities) or do not subside within a few days.

Grades II and III

1. Immobilize the arm with a sling and secure the arm to the body with an elastic wrap (see figure 12.2).
2. Monitor and treat for shock as needed and send for emergency medical assistance if it occurs.
3. Apply ice and send the athlete to a physician (if shock does not occur).

Playing Status

Grade I

- The athlete can return to activity if signs and symptoms subside; the shoulder is pain free; and the athlete has full strength, flexibility, and range of motion in the shoulder.
- If sent to a physician, the athlete cannot return to activity until examined and released.
- When returning to activity, the athlete may benefit from wearing a special protective pad over the injury.

Grades II and III

- The athlete cannot return to activity until examined and released by a physician; the shoulder is pain free; and the athlete has full strength, flexibility, and range of motion in the shoulder.
- When returning to activity, the athlete may benefit from wearing a special protective pad over the injury.

Prevention

- Require athletes to wear properly fitted shoulder pads if part of standard equipment.

Sternoclavicular (SC) Sprain (Shoulder Separation)

Stretch or tear of the ligaments that connect the clavicle to the sternum (breastbone) as shown in figure 12.4.

Causes

- Falling on an outstretched hand
- Direct blow that pushes the clavicle forward or backward

Ask if Experiencing Symptoms

Grade I

- Mild pain at the attachment of the clavicle to the sternum
- Mild pain when moving arm across chest, reaching arm backward while raised to shoulder level, and when shrugging shoulders

Grades II and III

- Dizziness (If the clavicle is pushed backward at the SC joint, it can potentially damage major blood vessels to the brain.)
- Moderate to severe pain at the attachment of the collarbone to the breastbone
- Moderate to severe pain when moving arm across chest, reaching arm backward while raised to shoulder level, and when shrugging shoulders

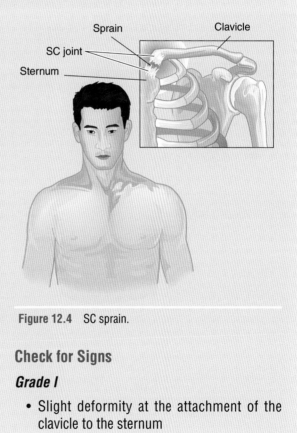

Figure 12.4 SC sprain.

Check for Signs

Grade I

- Slight deformity at the attachment of the clavicle to the sternum

(continued)

Grades II and III

- Moderate to severe deformity at the attachment of the clavicle to the sternum

- Possible unresponsiveness (if clavicle is displaced backward toward neck)
- Respiratory or cardiac arrest (if clavicle is displaced backward toward neck)

✚ FIRST AID

Grade I

For forward displacement of clavicle, do the following:

1. Rest the athlete from painful activities.
2. Apply ice.
3. Refer the athlete to a physician if symptoms and signs worsen (occur more often, especially with daily activities) or do not subside within a few days.

For backward displacement of clavicle, do the following:

1. Rest the athlete from all activities.
2. Apply ice to the injury and send the athlete to a physician.

Grades II and III

For forward displacement of clavicle, do the following:

1. Immobilize the arm with a sling and secure the arm to the body with an elastic wrap (see figure 12.2).
2. Monitor and treat for shock as needed and send for emergency medical assistance if it occurs.
3. Apply ice and send the athlete to a physician (if shock does not occur).

For backward displacement of clavicle, do the following:

1. Send for emergency medical assistance.
2. Monitor breathing and provide CPR if needed.
3. Monitor and treat for shock if needed.
4. Keep athlete from moving the arm.

Playing Status

- The athlete cannot return to activity until examined and released by a physician; the shoulder is pain free; and the athlete has full strength, flexibility, and range of motion in the shoulder.

- When returning to contact sports, the athlete should wear a protective pad over the injury.

Prevention

- Require athletes to wear shoulder pads if part of standard equipment.

Shoulder Dislocation or Subluxation

In a dislocation, the humerus (upper arm bone) pops out of the shoulder socket. In a subluxation, the humerus pops out of the shoulder socket and then spontaneously shifts back into the socket.

Causes

- Backward blow to upper arm while it is raised to the side, as shown in figure 12.5
- Forceful contraction of the shoulder muscles
- Fall on outstretched arm

Ask if Experiencing Symptoms

- Intense pain where the upper arm bone connects to the shoulder blade
- Sense of looseness or giving away
- Tingling in arm or hand (caused by the displaced bone pinching nerves)
- Felt or heard a pop

Check for Signs

Subluxation

- Lack of sensation in the arm or hand (caused by the displaced bone pinching nerves)
- Bluish arm or hand (caused by the displaced bone disrupting blood supply)

Dislocation

- Inability to move the arm
- Shoulder appears flat instead of rounded
- Arm is held slightly out to the side of the body
- Lack of sensation in the arm or hand (caused by the displaced bone pinching nerves and arteries)
- Bluish arm or hand (caused by the displaced bone disrupting blood supply)

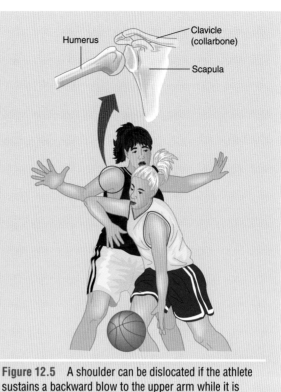

Figure 12.5 A shoulder can be dislocated if the athlete sustains a backward blow to the upper arm while it is raised to the side.

⊕ FIRST AID

Subluxation

1. Immobilize the arm with a sling and secure the arm to the body with an elastic wrap (see figure 12.2).
2. Monitor and treat for shock as needed and send for emergency medical assistance if it occurs.
3. Apply ice to the injury and send the athlete to a physician (if shock does not occur).

Dislocation

1. Send for emergency medical assistance.
2. If emergency medical assistance is delayed more than 20 minutes, stabilize the arm in the position in which you found it.
3. Do not try to put the humerus back into the socket.
4. Monitor and treat for shock as needed.
5. Apply ice.

Playing Status

- The athlete cannot return to activity until examined and released by a physician; the shoulder is pain free; and the athlete has full strength, flexibility, and range of motion in the shoulder.

Prevention

- Encourage athletes to perform preseason shoulder strengthening exercises.

Rotator Cuff Strain

Stretch or tear of the muscles used in throwing, swimming, and hitting motions and essential to holding the humerus in the socket (figure 12.6).

Causes

- Throwing sidearm
- Swinging a racquet or throwing with just the arm and not the body
- Weak and tight shoulder muscles

Ask if Experiencing Symptoms

All Grades

- Pain with swimming, throwing, spiking, serving, and forehand and backhand motions
- Pain with lifting arm overhead

Check for Signs

Grade I

- Mild tenderness over the front of the shoulder, just below the outer edge of the collarbone, along the shoulder blade, or the outside of the shoulder
- Muscle tightness

Grades II and III

- Indentation or lump where muscle or tendon is torn

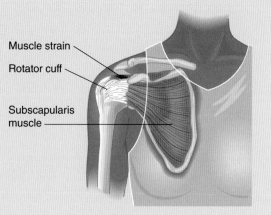

Figure 12.6 Rotator cuff strain.

- Inability to throw, spike, serve, or hit a forehand or backhand with a normal motion
- Moderate to severe tenderness over the front of the shoulder, just below the outer edge of the collarbone, along the shoulder blade, or the outside of the shoulder
- Arm weakness
- Swelling
- Muscle spasm

⊕ FIRST AID

Grade I

1. Rest the athlete from painful activities.
2. Apply ice.
3. Refer the athlete to a physician if symptoms and signs worsen (occur more often, especially with daily activities) or do not subside within a few days.

Grades II and III

1. Immobilize the arm with a sling and secure the arm to the body with an elastic wrap (see figure 12.2).
2. Monitor and treat for shock as needed and send for emergency medical assistance if it occurs.
3. Apply ice and send the athlete to a physician (if shock does not occur).

Playing Status

Grade I

- The athlete can return to activity if signs and symptoms subside; the shoulder is pain free; and the athlete has full strength, flexibility, and range of motion in the shoulder.

- If sent to a physician, the athlete cannot return to activity until examined and released.

Grades II and III

- The athlete cannot return to activity until examined and released by a physician; the shoulder is pain free; and the athlete has full strength, flexibility, and range of motion in the shoulder.

Prevention

- Encourage athletes to perform preseason shoulder strengthening and stretching exercises.
- At the beginning of the season, instruct athletes to gradually begin throwing, starting with slow speed and short distance throws, and gradually increasing the speed and distance.
- Instruct athletes to throw from an overhead position and to use the body and legs as well as the arms.

Pectoral Muscle Strain

Stretch or tear of the muscles used in bringing arm across chest (figure 12.7).

Causes

- Throwing sidearm
- Swinging a racquet or throwing with the arm only
- Weak and inflexible chest and shoulder muscles
- Lifting weights that are too heavy or using incorrect technique such as lowering the elbows too far in the bench press

Ask if Experiencing Symptoms

- Pain with swimming, spiking, serving, sidearm throwing, forehand motions, push-ups, and bench and incline presses
- Pain with reaching arm across chest
- Pain when arm is stretched straight out to the side
- Pain over the front of the shoulder or chest, below the clavicle
- Slight muscle tightness

Check for Signs

Grade I

- Mild point tenderness

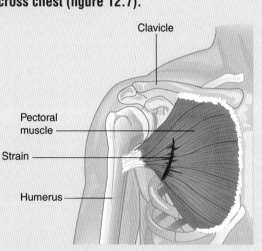

Figure 12.7 Pectoral muscle strain.

Grades II and III

- Indentation or lump where muscle or tendon is torn
- Inability to throw, spike, serve, or hit a forehand with a normal motion
- Arm weakness
- Moderate to severe point tenderness
- Swelling
- Muscle spasm

✚ FIRST AID

Grade I

1. Rest the athlete from painful activities.
2. Apply ice.

3. Refer the athlete to a physician if symptoms and signs worsen (occur more often, especially with daily activities) or do not subside within a few days.

(continued)

Grades II and III

1. Immobilize the arm with a sling and secure the arm to the body with an elastic wrap (see figure 12.2).

2. Monitor and treat for shock as needed and send for emergency medical assistance if it occurs.

3. Apply ice and send the athlete to a physician (if shock does not occur).

Playing Status

Grade I

- The athlete can return to activity if signs and symptoms subside; the shoulder is pain free; and the athlete has full strength, flexibility, and range of motion in the shoulder.

- If sent to a physician, the athlete cannot return to activity until examined and released.

Grades II and III

- The athlete cannot return to activity until examined and released by a physician; the shoulder is pain free; and the athlete has full strength, flexibility, and range of motion in the shoulder.

Prevention

- Encourage athletes to perform preseason shoulder strengthening and stretching exercises.

- At the beginning of the season, instruct athletes to gradually begin throwing, starting with slow speed and short distance throws, and gradually increasing the speed and distance.

- Instruct athletes to throw from an overhead position and to use the body and legs as well as the arms.

Deltoid Strain

Stretch or tear of the muscles around the front, back, and side of the shoulder (figure 12.8).

Causes

- Weak and inflexible shoulder muscles
- Throwing sidearm

Ask if Experiencing Symptoms

- Pain with throwing, spiking, serving, and swimming
- Pain when raising arm forward, to the side, or backward
- Slight muscle tightness

Check for Signs

Grade I

- Mild point tenderness over the front, side, or back of the shoulder below the clavicle or spine of the scapula

Grades II and III

- Indentation or lump where muscle or tendon is torn
- Inability to throw, spike, or serve with a normal motion

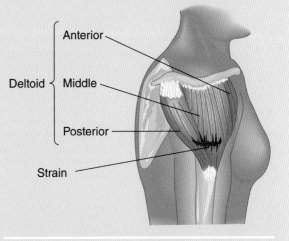

Figure 12.8   Deltoid muscle strain.

- Moderate to severe point tenderness over the front, side, or back of the shoulder below the clavicle or spine of the scapula
- Arm weakness
- Swelling
- Muscle spasm

156

Grade I

1. Rest the athlete from painful activities.
2. Apply ice.
3. Refer the athlete to a physician if symptoms and signs worsen (occur more often, especially with daily activities) or do not subside within a few days.

Grades II and III

1. Immobilize the arm with a sling and secure the arm to the body with an elastic wrap (see figure 12.2).
2. Monitor and treat for shock as needed and send for emergency medical assistance if it occurs.
3. Apply ice to the injury and send the athlete to a physician (if shock does not occur).

Playing Status

Grade I

- The athlete can return to activity if signs and symptoms subside; the shoulder is pain free; and the athlete has full strength, flexibility, and range of motion in the shoulder.
- If sent to a physician, the athlete cannot return to activity until examined and released.

Grades II and III

- The athlete cannot return to activity until examined and released by a physician; the shoulder is pain free; and the athlete has full strength, flexibility, and range of motion in the shoulder.

Prevention

- Encourage athletes to perform preseason shoulder strengthening and stretching exercises.
- Instruct athletes to throw from an overhead position and to use the body and legs as well as the arms.

Upper Trapezius (Trap) Muscle Strain

Stretch or tear of the trapezius muscle. This muscle extends from the base of the skull to the outer tips of the shoulder and down to just above the low back.

Different portions of the muscle shrug the shoulders, extend the head backward, and squeeze the shoulder blades together (figure 12.9).

Causes

- Weak upper back or neck muscles
- Tight chest muscles
- Lifting weights that are too heavy or doing shoulder shrugs incorrectly

Ask if Experiencing Symptoms

Grade I

- Mild pain with shrugging the shoulders, extending the head backward, and squeezing the shoulder blades together
- Mild pain with stretching arm across chest
- Tightness in neck and upper and mid back

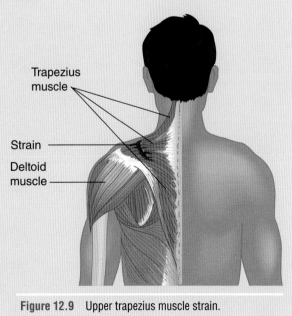

Figure 12.9 Upper trapezius muscle strain.

(continued)

Grades II and III

- Moderate to severe pain with shrugging the shoulders, extending the head backward, and squeezing the shoulder blades together
- Moderate to severe pain with stretching arm across chest

Check for Signs

Grade I

- Slight muscle tightness at the back of the neck, just above the shoulder blade, or down the upper and mid back
- Mild point tenderness at the neck, just above the shoulder blades, or down the upper and mid back

Grades II and III

- Indentation or lump where muscle or tendon is torn
- Inability to throw, spike, serve, or hit a forehand with a normal motion
- Moderate to severe point tenderness at the neck, just above the shoulder blades, or down the upper and mid back
- Weakness in extending upper arm backward or pushing head backward
- Swelling
- Muscle spasm

⊕ FIRST AID

Grade I

1. Rest the athlete from painful activities.
2. Apply ice.
3. Refer the athlete to a physician if symptoms and signs worsen (occur more often, especially with daily activities) or do not subside within a few days.

Grades II and III

1. Immobilize the arm with a sling and secure the arm to the body with an elastic wrap (see figure 12.2).
2. Monitor and treat for shock as needed and send for emergency medical assistance if it occurs.
3. Apply ice to the injury and send the athlete to a physician (if shock does not occur).

Playing Status

Grade I

- The athlete can return to activity if signs and symptoms subside; the shoulder is pain free; and the athlete has full strength, flexibility, and range of motion in the shoulder.
- If sent to a physician, the athlete cannot return to activity until examined and released.

Grades II and III

- The athlete cannot return to activity until examined and released by a physician; the neck, shoulder, or back is pain free; and the athlete has full strength, flexibility, and range of motion in the neck and shoulder.

Prevention

- Encourage athletes to perform preseason exercises that strengthen the neck and upper back and stretch the pectoral (pec or chest) and latissimus dorsi (lat) muscles.

Rhomboid Muscle Strain

Stretch or tear of the muscle between the scapula (shoulder blade) and spine (figure 12.10). These muscles pull the shoulder blades toward the spine.

Causes

- Weak upper back muscles and tight chest muscles

Ask if Experiencing Symptoms

Grade I

- Mild pain with shrugging the shoulders and squeezing the shoulder blades together
- Mild pain with stretching arm across chest
- Mild pain between the shoulder blades and spine
- Muscle tightness between the shoulder blade and spine

Grades II and III

- Moderate to severe pain with shrugging the shoulders and squeezing the shoulder blades together
- Moderate to severe pain with stretching arm across chest
- Moderate to severe pain between the shoulder blades and spine

Check for Signs

Grade I

- Mild muscle tightness between the shoulder blade and spine
- Mild point tenderness between the shoulder blade and spine

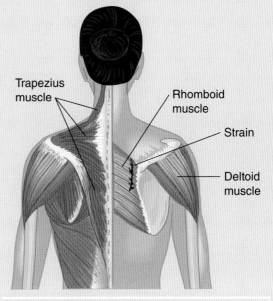

Figure 12.10 Rhomboid muscle strain.

Grades II and III

- Indentation or lump where muscle or tendon is torn
- Inability to swim or hit a backhand with a normal motion
- Moderate to severe point tenderness between the shoulder blade and spine
- Weakness in squeezing shoulder blades together and reaching upper arm backward (while raised out to the side at shoulder level)
- Swelling
- Muscle spasm

⊕ FIRST AID

Grade I

1. Rest the athlete from painful activities.
2. Apply ice.
3. Refer the athlete to a physician if symptoms and signs worsen (occur more often, especially with daily activities) or do not subside within a few days.

Grades II and III

1. Immobilize the arm with a sling and secure the arm to the body with an elastic wrap (see figure 12.2).
2. Monitor and treat for shock as needed and send for emergency medical assistance if it occurs.
3. Apply ice to the injury and send the athlete to a physician (if shock does not occur).

(continued)

Rhomboid Muscle Strain   *(continued)*

Playing Status

Grade I

- The athlete can return to activity if signs and symptoms subside; the shoulder is pain free; and the athlete has full strength, flexibility, and range of motion in the shoulder.
- If sent to a physician, the athlete cannot return to activity until examined and released.

Grades II and III

- The athlete cannot return to activity until examined and released by a physician; the muscle is pain free; and the athlete has full strength, flexibility, and range of motion in the shoulder.

Prevention

- Encourage athletes to perform preseason exercises that strengthen the upper back and stretch the pectoral (pec or chest) and latissimus dorsi (lat) muscles.

CHEST

In contact sports, the ribs are subjected to being jabbed by elbows; crunched by helmets; pelted by pucks, baseballs, or softballs; and crushed by the weight of other players. As a coach, you'll need to be able to tell the difference between a potentially life-threatening rib fracture and a simple contusion.

Rib Fracture or Contusion

Rib bruise or break (figure 12.11).

Cause

- Direct blow to rib cage

Ask if Experiencing Symptoms

Contusion

- Mild pain with breathing, coughing, sneezing, or laughing

Fracture

- Moderate to severe pain with breathing, coughing, sneezing, or laughing

Check for Signs

Contusion

- Swelling
- Bruising
- Mild point tenderness

Fracture

- Deformity
- Pain when rib cage is gently compressed on either side of injury

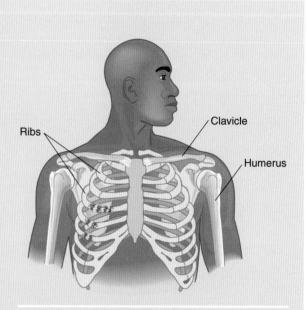

Figure 12.11   Rib fracture.

- Moderate to severe point tenderness over the site of the injury
- Swelling
- Breathing difficulties (if fractured rib punctures lung)

🛡️ FIRST AID

Contusion

1. Rest the athlete from all activities.
2. Apply ice and send the athlete to a physician.

Fracture

1. Rest the athlete from all activities.

2. If the athlete has breathing difficulties, an open chest wound, or a backward displaced (toward internal organs) rib, or the athlete is suffering from shock, call for emergency medical assistance.

3. If none of the above, apply ice and send the athlete to a physician.

Playing Status

- The athlete cannot return to activity until examined and released by a physician.
- If the athlete returns to contact sports, the injured area should be padded.

Prevention

- Require athletes to wear rib pads if appropriate for the sport (football and ice hockey).

UPPER ARM

The humerus (upper arm bone) and the muscles that span its length are subject to direct blow, torsion, and tension injuries in sports. Specifically, acute injuries to the upper arm include fractures and biceps and triceps strains. In addition, repetitive pushing, pulling, and lifting activities can irritate muscle tendons over time and lead to biceps or triceps tendinitis.

Acute Upper Arm Injuries

Humerus Fracture

Crack or break in the humerus (figure 12.12).

Causes
- Direct blow
- Torsion injury
- Compression injury

Ask if Experiencing Symptoms
- Severe pain

Check for Signs
- Deformity
- Swelling
- Severe point tenderness
- Inability to move arm
- Bluish skin on forearm, wrist, hand, or fingers (if fracture injures blood vessels)
- Loss of sensation and tingling in forearm, wrist, hand, or fingers (if fracture injures nerves)

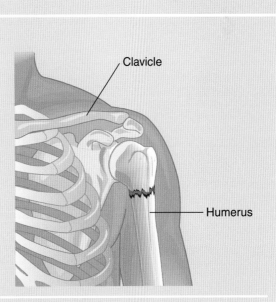

Figure 12.12 Humerus fracture.

(continued)

🞢 FIRST AID

1. Send for emergency medical assistance.
2. Monitor breathing and provide CPR as needed.
3. Monitor and treat for shock as needed.
4. Prevent the athlete from moving the arm.
5. Apply ice for 15 minutes.

Playing Status

- The athlete cannot return to activity until examined and released by a physician; the shoulder and elbow are pain free; and the athlete has full strength, flexibility, and range of motion in the shoulder and elbow.

Prevention

- Instruct athletes to tuck arm to side if falling.

Biceps Muscle Strain

Stretch or tear to biceps (figure 12.13).

Cause

- Sudden forceful contraction or stretch of the biceps muscle

Ask if Experiencing Symptoms

Grade I

- Mild pain along front of upper arm (figure 12.14)
- Mild pain with bending elbow
- Mild pain when elbow is straight and arm is extended back past body
- Tightness along front of upper arm
- Mild pain when raising upper arm forward

Grades II and III

- Moderate to severe pain along front of upper arm
- Moderate to severe pain with bending elbow
- Moderate to severe pain when elbow is straight and arm is extended back past body
- Moderate to severe pain when raising upper arm forward

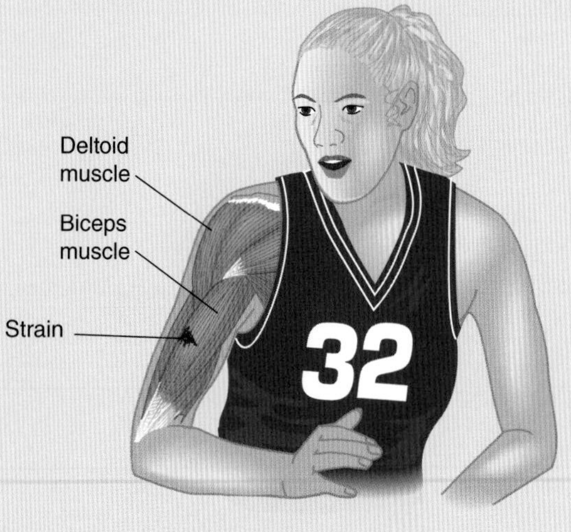

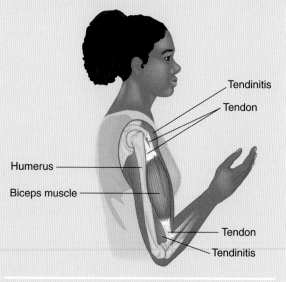

Figure 12.13   Biceps strain.

Deltoid muscle
Biceps muscle
Strain

Tendinitis
Tendon
Humerus
Biceps muscle
Tendon
Tendinitis

Figure 12.14   Areas of pain of biceps strain, biceps tendinitis, golfer's elbow, and growth plate stress fracture.

Check for Signs

Grade I

- Slight muscle tightness along front of upper arm
- Mild point tenderness

Grades II and III

- Indentation or lump where muscle or tendon is torn
- Inability to lift objects while bending elbow (arm curl)
- Inability to bend elbow or to fully straighten elbow
- Inability to raise upper arm forward
- Moderate to severe point tenderness
- Swelling
- Discoloration—occurs several days after a partial or complete tear of the muscle
- Muscle spasm

✚ FIRST AID

Grade I

1. Rest the athlete from painful activities.
2. Apply ice.
3. Refer the athlete to a physician if symptoms and signs worsen (occur more often, especially with daily activities) or do not subside within a few days.

Grades II and III

1. Immobilize the arm with a sling.
2. Monitor and treat for shock as needed and send for emergency medical assistance if it occurs.
3. Apply ice and send the athlete to a physician (if shock does not occur).

Playing Status

Grade I

- The athlete can return to activity if signs and symptoms subside; the biceps is pain free; and the athlete has full range of motion in the shoulder and elbow, and full strength and flexibility in the biceps.
- If sent to a physician, the athlete cannot return to activity until examined and released.

Grades II and III

- The athlete cannot return to activity until examined and released by a physician; the biceps is pain free; and the athlete has full range of motion in the shoulder and elbow, and full strength and flexibility in the biceps.

Prevention

- Encourage athletes to perform preseason upper arm strengthening and stretching exercises.

Triceps Muscle Strain

Stretch or tear of the triceps muscle. This muscle straightens the elbow and extends the upper arm backward (figure 12.15).

Causes

- Repeated forceful contraction or stretch of the triceps
- Weak or inflexible triceps

Ask if Experiencing Symptoms

Grade I

- Mild pain along back of upper arm
- Mild pain with extending upper arm backward past body

(continued)

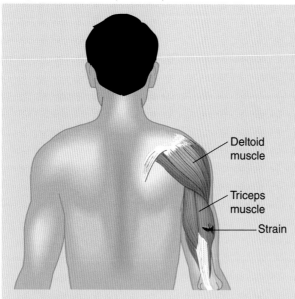

Figure 12.15 Triceps muscle strain.

- Mild pain with straightening the elbow against resistance (triceps extension)
- Mild pain when the elbow is bent and the upper arm is stretched forward and up toward head
- Tightness along back of upper arm

Grades II and III

- Moderate to severe pain along back of upper arm
- Moderate to severe pain with extending upper arm backward past body
- Moderate to severe pain with straightening the elbow against resistance (triceps extension)
- Moderate to severe pain when the elbow is bent and the upper arm is stretched forward and up toward head

Check for Signs

Grade I

- Slight muscle tightness along back of upper arm
- Mild point tenderness

Grades II and III

- Indentation or lump where muscle or tendon is torn
- Inability to fully straighten or bend elbow
- Moderate to severe point tenderness
- Swelling
- Discoloration—occurs several days after a partial or complete tear of the muscle
- Muscle spasm

⊕ FIRST AID

Grade I

1. Rest the athlete from painful activities.
2. Apply ice.
3. Refer the athlete to a physician if symptoms and signs worsen (occur more often, especially with daily activities) or do not subside within a few days.

Grades II and III

1. Immobilize the arm with a sling, if tolerated.
2. Monitor and treat for shock as needed and send for emergency medical assistance if it occurs.
3. Apply ice and send the athlete to a physician (if shock does not occur).

Playing Status

Grade I

- The athlete can return to activity if signs and symptoms subside; the triceps is pain free; and the athlete has full range of motion in the shoulder and elbow, and full strength and flexibility in the triceps.
- If sent to a physician, the athlete cannot return to activity until examined and released.

Grades II and III

- The athlete cannot return to activity until examined and released by a physician; the triceps is pain free; and the athlete has full range of motion in the shoulder and elbow, and full strength and flexibility in the triceps.

Prevention

- Encourage athletes to perform preseason upper arm strengthening and stretching exercises.

Chronic Upper Arm Injuries

Biceps Tendinitis

Irritation to biceps tendon (see figure 12.14).

Causes

- Repeated forceful contraction or stretch of the biceps
- Weak or inflexible biceps

Ask if Experiencing Symptoms

Mild

- Mild pain along front of upper arm near shoulder or elbow
- Mild pain with raising upper arm forward
- Mild pain when elbow is straight and arm is extended back past body

Moderate to Severe

- Moderate to severe pain along front of upper arm near shoulder or elbow
- Moderate to severe pain with raising upper arm forward
- Moderate to severe pain when elbow is straight and arm is extended back past body

Check for Signs

Mild

- Slight tenderness along front of upper arm near shoulder or elbow

Moderate to Severe

- Decreased ability or inability to lift objects while bending elbow and raising upper arm
- Swelling
- Moderate to severe point tenderness along front of upper arm near shoulder or elbow

✚ FIRST AID

Mild

1. Rest the athlete from painful activities.
2. Apply ice.
3. Refer the athlete to a physician if symptoms and signs worsen (occur more often, especially with daily activities) or do not subside within a few days.

Moderate to Severe

1. Rest the arm from all activities.
2. Apply ice to the injury and send the athlete to a physician.

Playing Status

Mild

- The athlete can return to activity if signs and symptoms subside; the tendon is pain free; and the athlete has full range of motion in the shoulder and elbow, and full strength and flexibility in the biceps.
- If sent to a physician, the athlete cannot return to activity until examined and released.

Moderate to Severe

- The athlete cannot return to activity until examined and released by a physician; the tendon is pain free; and the athlete has full range of motion in the shoulder and elbow, and full strength and flexibility in the biceps.

Prevention

- Encourage athletes to perform preseason upper arm strengthening and stretching exercises.

Triceps Tendinitis

Irritation to the triceps tendon (see figure 12.15).

Causes

- Repeated forceful contraction or stretch of the triceps
- Weak or inflexible triceps

Ask if Experiencing Symptoms

Mild

- Mild pain along back of the upper arm near shoulder or elbow
- Mild pain with straightening the elbow
- Mild pain when the elbow is bent and the upper arm is stretched forward and up toward head
- Mild pain when extending upper arm backward

Moderate to Severe

- Moderate to severe pain along back of the upper arm near shoulder or elbow
- Moderate to severe pain with straightening the elbow
- Moderate to severe pain when the elbow is bent and the upper arm is stretched forward and up toward head
- Moderate to severe pain when extending upper arm backward

Check for Signs

Mild

- Slight point tenderness along back of the elbow

Moderate to Severe

- Moderate to severe point tenderness along back of elbow
- Decreased ability or inability to straighten the elbow against resistance (triceps extension)
- Decreased ability or inability to extend the upper arm backward
- Swelling

⊕ FIRST AID

Mild

1. Rest the athlete from painful activities.
2. Apply ice.
3. Refer the athlete to a physician if symptoms and signs worsen (occur more often, especially with daily activities) or do not subside within a few days.

Moderate to Severe

1. Rest the arm from all activities.
2. Apply ice and send the athlete to a physician.

Playing Status

Mild

- The athlete can return to activity if signs and symptoms subside; the tendon is pain free; and the athlete has full range of motion in the elbow, and full strength and flexibility in the triceps.
- If sent to a physician, the athlete cannot return to activity until examined and released.

Moderate to Severe

- The athlete cannot return to activity until examined and released by a physician; the elbow and triceps are pain free; and the athlete has full range of motion in the elbow, and full strength and flexibility in the triceps.

Prevention

- Encourage athletes to perform preseason upper arm strengthening and stretching exercises.

ELBOW

The elbow is injured most often in tennis, baseball, softball, and wrestling. Tennis, baseball, and softball players are particularly susceptible to chronic injuries such as tennis elbow, whereas wrestlers and gymnasts are more prone to acute injuries such as dislocation. In a study of high school sports injuries, Comstock, Collins, and Yard (2008) reported that 9.6 percent of all injuries in wrestlers occurred at the elbow, and baseball players had a 6.7 percent elbow injury rate.

For the first aid care protocol for acute elbow injuries, see page 286 in appendix A.

For a summary of first aid care for chronic elbow injuries, see page 287 in appendix A.

Acute Elbow Injuries

Elbow Fracture

Break of any or all of the three elbow bones: bottom of the humerus (upper arm; figure 12.16), radius (forearm), and ulna (forearm).

Cause

- Direct blow

Ask if Experiencing Symptoms

- Numbness around the area or down the forearm and hand (if fracture injures nerves)
- Severe pain
- Grating sensation at the site of injury

Check for Signs

- Deformity

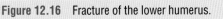

Figure 12.16   Fracture of the lower humerus.

Humerus
Blood vessel
Nerve
Ulna
Radius

- Swelling
- Severe point tenderness at the site of injury
- Inability to bend or straighten elbow
- Bluish skin on forearm, wrist, hand, or fingers (if fracture injures blood vessels)
- Loss of sensation and tingling in forearm, wrist, hand, or fingers (if fracture injures nerves)

⊕ FIRST AID

Send for emergency medical assistance if bones are grossly displaced (deformity) or sticking through the skin, if there are signs of nerve damage or disrupted circulation, or if the athlete is suffering from shock.

If none of the above, do the following:

1. Splint the arm in the position in which you found it.
2. Secure the arm to the body with an elastic wrap.
3. Monitor and treat for shock if necessary and send for emergency medical assistance if it occurs.
4. Apply ice (avoid the nerve that runs to the hand—see figure 12.17) and send the athlete to a physician.

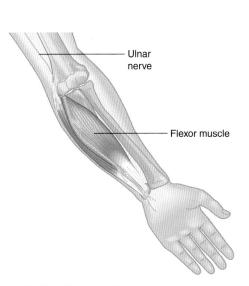

Ulnar nerve
Flexor muscle

Figure 12.17   When applying ice to the elbow area, keep the ice away from the inner elbow to avoid the ulnar nerve, which runs to the hand.

(continued)

Playing Status

- The athlete cannot return to activity until examined and released by a physician; the elbow is pain free; and the athlete has full strength, flexibility, and range of motion in the elbow.

Prevention

- Encourage athletes to wear protective elbow pads during high-impact sports such as football, ice hockey, lacrosse, and basketball.

Elbow Dislocation or Subluxation

In a dislocation, the bones of the elbow joint move out of place. In a subluxation, the bones of the elbow joint move out of place and then spontaneously shift back into position.

Causes

- Direct blow
- Falling on an outstretched hand
- Severe elbow sprain
- Elbow forcefully extended backward

Ask if Experiencing Symptoms

Subluxation

- Tingling down the forearm and hand (if subluxated bone pinches nerves)
- Felt or heard a pop
- Sense of looseness or giving away

Dislocation

- Intense pain
- Tingling down the forearm and hand (if dislocated bone pinches nerves)
- Felt or heard a pop
- Sense of looseness or giving away

Check for Signs

Subluxation

- Lack of sensation in hand (if subluxated bone pinches nerves)
- Extreme tenderness around the elbow
- Swelling

Dislocation

- Elbow in a slightly bent position
- Swelling or other deformity around the elbow area
- Inability to bend or straighten elbow
- Lack of sensation in hand (if dislocated bone pinches nerves)
- Extreme tenderness around the elbow

✚ FIRST AID

Subluxation

1. Rest the athlete from all activity.
2. Immobilize the arm with a sling and secure the arm to the body with an elastic wrap.
3. Monitor and treat for shock as needed, and send for emergency medical assistance if it occurs.
4. Apply ice (avoid the nerve that runs to the hand—see figure 12.17) and send the athlete to a physician.

Dislocation

1. Send for emergency medical assistance.
2. Monitor and treat for shock as needed.
3. Keep the athlete from moving the elbow.
4. Apply ice (avoid the nerve that runs to the hand—see figure 12.17).

Playing Status

- The athlete cannot return to activity until examined and released by a physician; the elbow is pain free; and the athlete has full range of motion in the elbow, and full strength and flexibility in the elbow, wrist, and hand.
- When returning to activity, the athlete may need to use protective taping or bracing.

Prevention

- Encourage athletes to perform preseason exercises that strengthen and stretch the biceps, triceps, and forearm muscles.

Ulnar Nerve Contusion

Bruise of the ulnar nerve on the back of the elbow joint (figure 12.18). Sometimes called "hitting the funny bone."

Cause

- Direct blow to the inside back of the elbow

Ask if Experiencing Symptoms

Mild

- Tingling down the forearm and hand (if injury bruises nerve) that lasts a few minutes
- Mild pain shooting from elbow down to forearm

Moderate to Severe

- Tingling down the forearm and hand (if injury bruises nerve) that lasts more than five minutes
- Moderate to severe pain shooting from elbow down to forearm

Check for Signs

Mild

- Mild point tenderness

Moderate to Severe

- Moderate to severe point tenderness

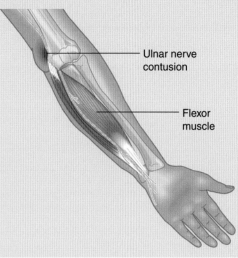

Figure 12.18   Ulnar nerve contusion.

- Loss of grip strength
- Swelling
- Discoloration
- Hand weakness
- Loss of sensation in ring and little fingers

⊕ FIRST AID

Mild

1. Rest the athlete from activity until numbness and tingling are gone, and until the athlete has full elbow range of motion and full hand strength.

Moderate to Severe

1. Rest the athlete from all activity.
2. Immobilize the arm with a sling, if tolerated.
3. Treat for shock if necessary and send for emergency medical assistance if such occurs.
4. Send the athlete to a physician.

Playing Status

Mild

- If numbness and tingling disappear within a few minutes and grip strength is equal to the other side, the athlete can return to activity.

Moderate to Severe

- The athlete cannot return to activity until examined and released by a physician; the elbow is pain free; and the athlete has full elbow range of motion and hand strength.

Prevention

- Encourage athletes to wear protective elbow pads during high-impact sports such as football, ice hockey, lacrosse, and basketball.

Elbow Sprain

Stretch or tear of the ligaments holding the elbow bones together (figure 12.19).

Cause

- Direct blow or torsion (twisting) injury that forces the elbow sideways or backward

Ask if Experiencing Symptoms

Grade I

- Mild pain along sides, back, or front of elbow
- Mild pain with bending and straightening elbow

Grades II and III

- Moderate to severe pain along sides, back, or front of elbow
- Moderate to severe pain with bending and straightening elbow
- Elbow feels loose or unstable

Check for Signs

Grade I

- Mild point tenderness over the sides, back, or front of elbow

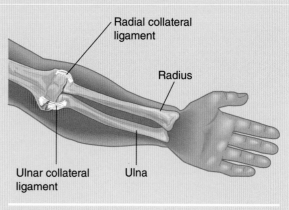

Figure 12.19 Elbow sprain.

Grades II and III

- Moderate to severe point tenderness over the sides, back, or front of elbow
- Inability to fully bend or straighten elbow
- Swelling

⊕ FIRST AID

Grade I

1. Rest the athlete from painful activities.
2. Apply ice.
3. Refer the athlete to a physician if symptoms and signs worsen (occur more often, especially with daily activities) or do not subside within a few days.

Grades II and III

1. Rest the arm from all activities.
2. Immobilize the arm with a sling, if tolerated.
3. Monitor and treat for shock if needed and send for emergency medical assistance if it occurs.
4. Apply ice (avoid the nerve that runs to the hand—see figure 12.17) and send the athlete to a physician.

Playing Status

Grade I

- The athlete can return to activity if pain subsides and the athlete has full range of motion in the elbow and full strength and flexibility in the elbow and wrist.
- If sent to a physician, the athlete cannot return to activity until examined and released.

Grades II and III

- The athlete cannot return to activity until examined and released by a physician; the elbow is pain free; and the athlete has full range of motion in the elbow, and full strength and flexibility in the elbow and wrist.

Prevention

- Encourage athletes to do preseason arm and forearm strengthening and flexibility training.

Chronic Elbow Injuries

Tennis Elbow

Chronic strain or inflammation where the wrist muscles attach to outside of the elbow joint (figure 12.20).

Causes

- Weak or inflexible wrist muscles
- Incorrect stroke technique (particularly backhand) in racquet sports—using the wrist for all the force of the swing instead of the shoulder and body
- Racquet strung too tight

Ask if Experiencing Symptoms

Mild

- Mild pain typically with backhand strokes in racquet sports
- Mild pain when gripping or making a fist
- Mild pain when lifting objects when the palm is facing down (figure 12.21)

Moderate to Severe

- Moderate to severe pain typically with backhand strokes in racquet sports
- Moderate to severe pain when gripping or making a fist
- Moderate to severe pain when lifting objects when the palm is facing down (figure 12.21)

Check for Signs

Mild

- Slight point tenderness over outside of elbow

Moderate to Severe

- Moderate to severe point tenderness over outside of elbow
- Inability to lift objects when the palm is facing down
- Swelling over outside of elbow

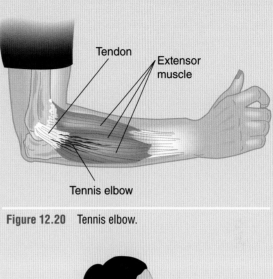

Figure 12.20   Tennis elbow.

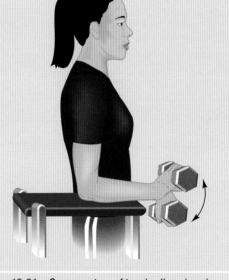

Figure 12.21   One symptom of tennis elbow is pain when lifting objects with the wrist when the palm is facing down.

(continued)

Tennis Elbow   *(continued)*

⊕ FIRST AID

Mild

1. Rest the arm from painful activities.
2. Apply ice.
3. Refer the athlete to a physician if symptoms and signs worsen (occur more often, especially with daily activities) or do not subside.

Moderate to Severe

1. Rest the arm from all activities.
2. Apply ice and send the athlete to a physician.

Playing Status

Mild

- The athlete can return to activity if signs and symptoms subside; the elbow is pain free; and the athlete has full strength, flexibility, and range of motion in the elbow and wrist.
- If sent to a physician, the athlete cannot return to activity until examined and released.

Moderate to Severe

- The athlete cannot return to activity until examined and released by a physician; the elbow is pain free; and the athlete has full strength, flexibility, and range of motion in the elbow and wrist.

Prevention

- Encourage athletes to do preseason upper arm and forearm strengthening and flexibility training.
- Instruct athletes to use the shoulder and body for power when performing a backhand stroke.

Golfer's Elbow

Chronic strain or inflammation where the wrist muscles attach to inside of the elbow joint (figure 12.22).

Causes

- Overuse of weak or inflexible wrist muscles
- Throwing sidearm
- Using only the forearm and wrist for power in forehand racquet stroke

Ask if Experiencing Symptoms

Mild

- Mild pain typically with forehand strokes in racquet sports
- Mild pain when gripping or making a fist
- Mild pain when lifting objects with the wrist when palm is facing up (figure 12.23)

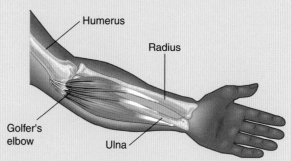

Figure 12.22   Golfer's elbow.

Moderate to Severe

- Moderate to severe pain typically with forehand strokes in racquet sports
- Moderate to severe pain when gripping or making a fist
- Moderate to severe pain when lifting objects with the wrist when palm is facing up (figure 12.23)

Check for Signs

Mild

- Slight point tenderness over inside of elbow

Moderate to Severe

- Moderate to severe point tenderness over inside of elbow
- Inability to lift objects when the palm is facing up
- Swelling over inside of elbow

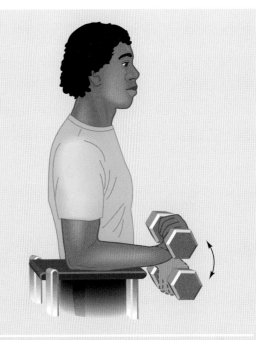

Figure 12.23 One symptom of golfer's elbow is pain when lifting objects with the wrist while the palm is facing up.

⊕ FIRST AID

Mild

1. Rest the arm from painful activities.
2. Apply ice (avoid the nerve that runs to the hand—see figure 12.17).
3. Refer the athlete to a physician if symptoms and signs worsen (occur more often, especially with daily activities) or do not subside.

Moderate to Severe

1. Rest the arm from all activities.
2. Apply ice (avoid the nerve that runs to the hand—see figure 12.17) and send the athlete to a physician.

Playing Status

Mild

- The athlete can return to activity if signs and symptoms subside; the elbow is pain free; and the athlete has full strength, flexibility, and range of motion in the elbow and wrist.
- If sent to a physician, the athlete cannot return to activity until examined and released.

Moderate to Severe

- The athlete cannot return to activity until examined and released by a physician; the elbow is pain free; and the athlete has full strength, flexibility, and range of motion in the elbow and wrist.

Prevention

- Encourage athletes to do preseason upper arm and forearm strengthening and flexibility training.
- Instruct athletes to use the shoulder and body for power when performing a forehand stroke.

Elbow Epiphyseal (Growth Plate) Stress Fracture

Break in the growth plate of the humerus (upper arm bone) at the elbow (figure 12.24; also see figure 12.14).

Cause

- Repetitive and forceful throwing weakens the growth plate until it breaks

Ask if Experiencing Symptoms

- Pain over the inside edge of the elbow that gradually worsens with activity
- Achiness when at rest

Check for Signs

- Swelling over the inside of elbow
- Point tenderness over the inside of elbow

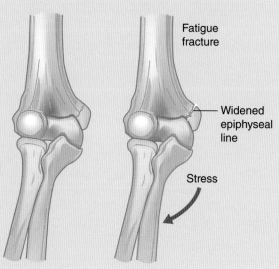

Figure 12.24   Elbow growth plate stress fracture.

⊕ FIRST AID

Mild

1. Rest the arm from all activities.
2. Apply ice (avoid the nerve that runs to the hand—see figure 12.17) and send the athlete to a physician.

Moderate to Severe

1. Rest the athlete from all activities.
2. Immobilize the arm with a sling (if tolerated).
3. Monitor and treat for shock as needed, and send for emergency medical assistance if it occurs.
4. Apply ice (avoid the nerve that runs to the hand—see figure 12.17) and send the athlete to a physician.

Playing Status

- The athlete cannot return to activity until examined and released by a physician.

Prevention

- Encourage athletes to do preseason upper arm and forearm strengthening and flexibility training.
- Follow league guidelines for limiting forceful throwing by growing athletes.

Elbow Bursitis

Irritation of the elbow bursa.

Causes

- Single blow or repetitive blows to the elbow
- Infection

Ask if Experiencing Symptoms

- Pain along the back of elbow

Check for Signs

- Gradual or sudden localized swelling on the back of elbow
- Noticeable bump on the back of the elbow
- Warmth over the area (indicates possible infection)

✚ FIRST AID

1. Rest the elbow from all activities.

2. Apply ice and send the athlete to a physician.

Playing Status

- The athlete cannot return to activity until examined and released by a physician; the elbow is pain free; and the athlete has full strength, flexibility, and range of motion in the elbow.
- When returning to activity, the athlete should wear a protective elbow pad.

Prevention

- Encourage athletes to wear protective elbow pads during high-impact sports such as football, ice hockey, lacrosse, wrestling, and basketball.

FOREARM, WRIST, AND HAND

Almost all of the sports injuries involving the forearm, wrist, and hand are acute. Forearm, wrist, and hand injuries are the most common of all injuries in softball (15 percent), baseball (11 percent), volleyball (10 percent), and wrestling (7.9 percent) (Comstock, Collins, and Yard 2008). Table 12.2 illustrates the occurrences of wrist and hand injuries in several sports. Following are the most common forearm, wrist, and hand problems in sports.

Page 288 in appendix A summarizes first aid care for common forearm, wrist, and hand injuries.

Table 12.2 Frequency of Hand and Wrist Injury Out of All Reported Body Regions Injured

Sport	Percentage
Field hockey	34.0 (male and female)
Lacrosse	22.9 (male and female)
Ice Hockey	15.8 (male and female)
Softball	15
Baseball	11.1
Volleyball	10
Football	9.2
Basketball – Boys	8.1
Wrestling	7.9
Basketball – Girls	7.8

Data from Comstock, Collins, and Yard 2008, and Yard and Comstock 2006.

Forearm Fracture

Break in the radius, ulna, or both (figure 12.25).

Causes

- Direct blow
- Falling on an outstretched hand

Ask if Experiencing Symptoms

- Pain

Check for Signs

- Swelling
- Deformity
- Severe point tenderness
- Inability to rotate or twist forearm to turn palm up or down
- Inability to bend or straighten wrist or elbow (depending on the site of the injury along the forearm)

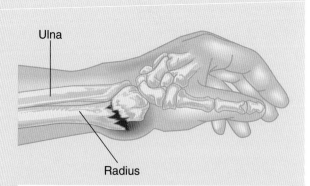

Figure 12.25 In a forearm fracture, the radius, ulna, or both forearm bones may be broken.

- Bluish skin on hand or fingers (if fracture injures blood vessels)
- Loss of sensation and tingling in hand and fingers (if fracture injures nerves)

⊕ FIRST AID

Send for emergency medical assistance if bones are grossly displaced or sticking through the skin, if there are signs of nerve damage or disrupted circulation, or if the athlete is suffering from shock.

If none of the above, do the following:

1. Splint the arm in the position in which you found it.

2. Monitor and treat for shock if necessary and send for emergency medical assistance if it occurs.
3. Apply ice (avoid the nerve that runs to the hand—figure 12.17) and send the athlete to a physician.

Playing Status

- The athlete cannot return to activity until examined and released by a physician; the forearm is pain free; and the athlete has full strength, flexibility, and range of motion in the elbow and wrist, and equal handgrip strength.

Prevention

- Encourage athletes to wear protective forearm pads in football and ice hockey.

Wrist Fracture

Break in one or more of the little wrist bones (figure 12.26).

Causes

- Direct blow
- Falling on an outstretched hand

Ask if Experiencing Symptoms

- Pain when rotating wrist
- Pain when bending wrist
- Pain when tilting wrist from side to side

Check for Signs

- Swelling
- Deformity
- Point tenderness
- Inability to rotate or twist forearm and wrist
- Inability to bend wrist

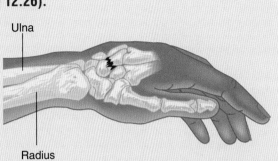

Figure 12.26   Fractured wrist bones.

- Bluish skin on hand and fingers (if fracture injures blood vessels)
- Loss of sensation and tingling in hand and fingers (if fracture injures nerves)

✚ FIRST AID

Send for emergency medical assistance if bones are grossly displaced or sticking through the skin, if there are signs of nerve damage or disrupted circulation, or if the athlete is suffering from shock.

If none of the above, do the following:

1. Splint the forearm and hand in the position in which you found them.
2. Apply a sling (if tolerated).
3. Monitor and treat for shock if necessary and send for emergency medical assistance if it occurs.
4. Apply ice and send the athlete to a physician.

Playing Status

- The athlete cannot return to activity until examined and released by a physician; the wrist is pain free; and the athlete has full range of motion in the wrist, and full strength and flexibility in the hand and forearm.

Prevention

- Instruct athletes to avoid falling on outstretched hand.

Wrist Sprain

Stretch or tear of the ligaments that hold the wrist bones together (figure 12.27).

Causes

- Torsion (twisting) injury
- Falling on an outstretched hand

Ask if Experiencing Symptoms

Grade I

- Mild pain along sides, back, or front of wrist
- Mild pain with bending wrist to extremes
- Mild pain with rotating palm up or down

Grades II and III

- Moderate to severe pain along sides, back, or front of wrist
- Moderate to severe pain with bending wrist to extremes
- Moderate to severe pain with rotating palm up or down
- Wrist feels loose or unstable

Check for Signs

Grade I

- Mild point tenderness over the sides, back, or front of wrist

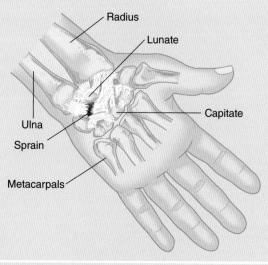

Figure 12.27 Wrist sprain.

Grades II and III

- Moderate to severe point tenderness over the sides, back, or front of wrist
- Decreased grip strength
- Swelling
- Deformity if sprain results in wrist bone shifting out of position

---

✚ FIRST AID

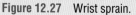

Grade I

1. Rest the athlete from painful activities.
2. Apply ice.
3. Refer the athlete to a physician if symptoms and signs worsen (occur more often, especially with daily activities) or do not subside within a few days.

Grades II and III

1. Rest the arm from all activities.
2. Splint the wrist and hand and secure to the body with a sling.
3. Monitor and treat for shock if needed and send for emergency medical assistance if it occurs.
4. Apply ice and send the athlete to a physician.

Playing Status

Grade I

- The athlete can return to activity if pain subsides and the athlete has full strength, flexibility, and range of motion in the wrist, and equal grip strength.

- If sent to a physician, the athlete cannot return to activity until examined and released.

Grades II and III

- The athlete cannot return to activity until examined and released by a physician; the wrist is pain free; and the athlete has full strength, flexibility, and range of motion in the wrist, and equal grip strength.

Prevention

- Encourage athletes to do preseason arm and forearm strengthening and flexibility training.

- Instruct athletes to avoid falling on outstretched hand.

Hand Fracture

Break in the bone(s) of the hand (figure 12.28).

Causes

- Direct blow
- Falling on an outstretched hand

Ask if Experiencing Symptoms

- Pain localized around the injured area
- Grating sensation
- Pain with gripping or making a fist

Check for Signs

- Point tenderness
- Swelling
- Deformity
- Loss of function
- Grip weakness

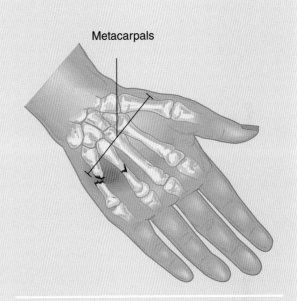

Metacarpals

Figure 12.28 In a hand fracture, one or more of the bones of the hand are broken.

⊕ FIRST AID

Send for emergency medical assistance if bones are grossly displaced or sticking through the skin, if there are signs of nerve damage or disrupted circulation, or if the athlete is suffering from shock.

If none of the above, do the following:

1. Immobilize the hand and fingers.

2. Secure the hand to the body by applying an arm sling.
3. Monitor and treat for shock as needed and send for emergency medical assistance if it occurs.
4. Apply ice and send the athlete to a physician.

Playing Status

- The athlete cannot return to activity until examined and released by a physician; the hand is pain free; and the athlete has full range of motion in the wrist, and full strength and flexibility in the wrist and hand.

Prevention

- Encourage athletes to wear protective hand pads in football, lacrosse, and ice hockey.

Finger Dislocation

In a dislocation, finger bones move out of position (figure 12.29).

Causes

- Direct blow to the end of the finger
- Forceful crushing or pinching of finger between two objects

Ask if Experiencing Symptoms

- Intense pain
- Tingling in finger (if dislocated bone pinches nerves)
- Felt or heard a pop
- Sense of looseness or giving away

Check for Signs

- Finger in a bent position
- Swelling
- Deformity
- Inability to bend or straighten finger

- Lack of sensation in finger (if dislocated bone pinches nerves)
- Extreme tenderness around finger joint

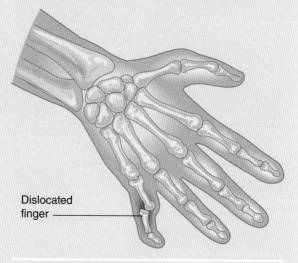

Dislocated finger

Figure 12.29 Finger dislocation.

⊕ FIRST AID

Send for emergency medical assistance if

1. the athlete is suffering from shock, or
2. there are signs of nerve damage or disrupted circulation.

If none of the above, do the following:

1. Immobilize the hand and finger (in position in which you found it).
2. Monitor and treat for shock as needed.
3. Apply ice and send the athlete to a physician.

Playing Status

- The athlete cannot return to activity until examined and released by a physician; the finger is pain free; and the athlete has full strength, flexibility, and range of motion in the wrist, hand, and finger.
- When returning to activity, the athlete may need protective taping for the finger. Buddy tape the finger to an adjacent finger toward the midline of the hand (figure 12.30).

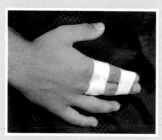

Figure 12.30 Protective taping for finger.

Prevention

- Encourage athletes to perform preseason wrist and hand muscle strengthening and stretching exercises.
- Recommend athletes tape previously injured fingers before practices and games.

180

Finger Sprain

Finger joint ligaments are stretched or torn (figure 12.31).

Cause

- Direct blow to the end of the finger
- Twisting or torsion of finger joint

Ask if Experiencing Symptoms

Grade I

- Mild pain when bending or straightening injured joint
- Mild pain along sides, back, or front of finger joint

Grades II and III

- Moderate to severe pain when bending or straightening injured joint
- Moderate to severe pain along sides, back, or front of finger joint
- Feeling of looseness or instability at the joint
- Grating sensation
- Heard or felt a pop

Check for Signs

Grade I

- Mild point tenderness over the sides, back, or front of finger joint

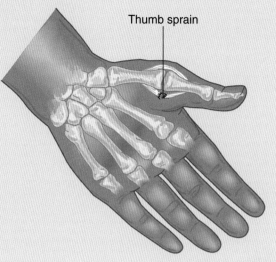

Figure 12.31   In a thumb sprain, the ligaments are torn (shown here) or stretched.

Grades II and III

- Moderate to severe point tenderness over the sides, back, or front of finger joint
- Inability to bend or straighten injured finger joint
- Decreased grip strength
- Swelling

⊕ FIRST AID

Grade I

1. Rest the athlete from painful activities.
2. Apply ice.
3. Refer the athlete to a physician if symptoms and signs worsen (occur more often, especially with daily activities) or do not subside within a few days.

Grades II and III

1. Rest the hand from all activities.
2. Splint the finger.
3. Monitor and treat for shock as needed and send for emergency medical assistance if it occurs.
4. Apply ice, instruct athlete to elevate the injury, and send the athlete to a physician.

Playing Status

Grade I

- The athlete can return to activity if pain subsides and the athlete has full strength and range of motion in the finger.

- If sent to a physician, the athlete cannot return to activity until examined and released.
- When the athlete returns to activity, protective taping should be applied to the finger (see figure 12.30). This is not applicable to thumb sprains.

(continued)

Grades II and III

- The athlete cannot return to activity until examined and released by a physician; the finger is pain free; and the athlete has full strength and range of motion in the finger.
- When returning to activity, the athlete may need protective taping (see figure 12.30).

Prevention

- Encourage athletes to do preseason forearm and hand strengthening exercises.
- Instruct athletes to avoid falling on outstretched hand.
- Recommend athletes tape previously injured fingers before practices and games.

Finger or Thumb Fracture

Break of one or more of the finger or thumb bones (figure 12.32).

Causes

- Direct blow to the end of the finger or thumb
- Forceful crushing or pinching of finger or thumb between two objects

Ask if Experiencing Symptoms

- Pain with bending or straightening the finger or thumb
- Pain when the end of the finger is tapped

Check for Signs

- Swelling
- Deformity
- Inability to bend or straighten finger

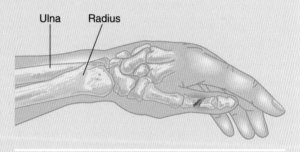

Figure 12.32 Thumb fracture.

⊕ FIRST AID

Send for emergency medical assistance if bones are sticking through the skin, if there are signs of nerve damage or disrupted circulation, or if the athlete is suffering from shock.

If none of the above, do the following:

1. Immobilize the hand and fingers.
2. Secure the hand to the body by applying an arm sling.
3. Monitor and treat for shock as needed and send for emergency medical assistance if it occurs.
4. Apply ice and send the athlete to a physician.

Playing Status

- The athlete cannot return to activity until examined and released by a physician; the finger is pain free; and the athlete has full strength, flexibility, and range of motion in the wrist, hand, and finger.
- When returning to activity, the athlete may need protective taping (see figure 12.30).

Prevention

- Recommend athletes tape previously injured fingers before practices and games.

Chapter 12 *REPLAY*

- ☐ What is a mechanism of injury for a clavicle fracture? (p. 149)
- ☐ Where is pain or tenderness felt for an AC joint sprain? (p. 150)
- ☐ Why is it potentially life threatening if the clavicle is pushed back in an SC joint sprain? (p. 151)
- ☐ What sport activities may cause pain for an athlete who has a rotator cuff strain? (p. 154)
- ☐ What shoulder motions would cause pain if an athlete has a pectoral muscle strain? (p. 155)
- ☐ Where is the deltoid muscle located? (p. 156)
- ☐ What are three actions of the trapezius muscle? (p. 157)
- ☐ What are two possible causes of a rhomboid muscle strain? (p. 159)
- ☐ How might you differentiate between a contused rib and a fractured rib? (p. 160)
- ☐ What sign might indicate that a humeral fracture has injured a nerve? (p. 161)
- ☐ What are two mechanisms of injury for a biceps strain? (p. 162)
- ☐ What are signs of a Grade II and III triceps strain? (pp. 163-164)
- ☐ A moderate to severe biceps tendinitis could cause inability or decreased ability to do what? (p. 165)
- ☐ When is it acceptable for an athlete with a moderate to severe triceps tendinitis to return to activity? (p. 166)
- ☐ If applying ice for a potential lower humerus fracture, what portion of the elbow should be avoided and why? (p. 167)
- ☐ Where is the ulnar nerve located? (p. 167)
- ☐ In what position is the elbow usually in after it is dislocated? (p. 168)
- ☐ What are the potential causes of an elbow sprain? (p. 170)
- ☐ Where is the pain typically felt with tennis elbow? (p. 171)
- ☐ When lifting an object, which hand position typically causes pain when an athlete has golfer's elbow? (pp. 172-173)
- ☐ Which part of the elbow is usually injured if an athlete has an elbow growth plate fracture resulting from throwing? (p. 174)
- ☐ What are the signs of elbow bursitis? (p. 175)
- ☐ In a forearm fracture, what conditions would necessitate sending for emergency medical assistance? (p. 176)
- ☐ How would you splint a suspected wrist fracture? (You may want to review page 72 in chapter 5.) (p. 177)
- ☐ What actions can be taken to help prevent a wrist sprain? (p. 179)
- ☐ In a hand fracture, what hand motions might cause pain? (p. 179)
- ☐ What are the signs of a dislocated finger? (p. 180)
- ☐ What are the signs of a finger sprain? (p. 181)
- ☐ How would you immobilize a finger or thumb fracture? (p. 182)

REFERENCES

Comstock, R.D., C.L. Collins, and E. E. Yard. National high school sports-related injury surveillance study, 2005-06 and 2006-07 school years (Personal communication, February 1, 2008).

Fleisig, G.S., C.J. Dillman, and J.R. Andrew. 1994. Biomechanics of the shoulder during throwing. In *The Athletic Shoulder,* edited by J.E. Andrews and K.E. Wilk. New York: Churchill Livingstone.

Koh, T.J., M.D. Grabiner, and G.G. Weiker. 1992. Technique and ground reaction forces in the back handspring. *American Journal of Sports Medicine* 20:61-66.

Yard, E.E. and R.D. Comstock. 2006. Injuries sustained by pediatric ice hockey, lacrosse, and field hockey athletes presenting to United States emergency departments. *Journal of Athletic Training,* 41(4): 441-449.

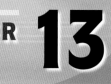

Lower Body Musculoskeletal Injuries

IN THIS CHAPTER, YOU WILL LEARN:

▸ How to recognize lower body musculoskeletal injuries.

▸ What first aid care to provide for each of these types of injuries.

▸ How to prevent lower body musculoskeletal injuries.

▸ What conditions are required before an injured athlete can return to play.

INJURIES IN THIS CHAPTER

(continued)

From the waist down, the lower body has to withstand some amazingly large forces. For example, when running, the hip absorbs a force that is seven times greater than the body's weight. And in basketball, landing from a layup or jump shot produces vertical forces from five to seven times the body's weight (Cavanaugh and Robinson 1989). These forces can take their toll on the back and abdominal muscles as well as the hips, thighs, knees, lower legs, ankles, feet, and toes. Your ability to quickly evaluate injuries to these areas and provide first aid care will help minimize the amount of time these injuries sideline your athletes.

This chapter will help you to recognize and provide first aid care for acute and chronic injuries to the lower body.

ABDOMEN AND BACK

Since the abdominal and back muscles help support the body during all movements, injuries to these areas can become very debilitating and chronic if not caught quickly and provided appropriate care.

Pages 289-290 in appendix A summarize first aid care for abdominal and low back injuries.

Abdominal Strain

Stretch or tear of abdominal muscle fibers.

Causes

- Sudden stretch or contraction of the abdominal muscles (figure 13.1)
- Weak or inflexible abdominal muscles

Ask if Experiencing Symptoms

Grade I

- Mild pain when abdominal muscles contracted
- Mild pain with rising to sitting position from lying down
- Mild pain with abdominal crunches

Grades II and III

- Moderate to severe pain when abdominal muscles contracted
- Moderate to severe pain with rising to sitting position from lying down
- Moderate to severe pain with abdominal crunches

Check for Signs

Grade I

- Mild tenderness

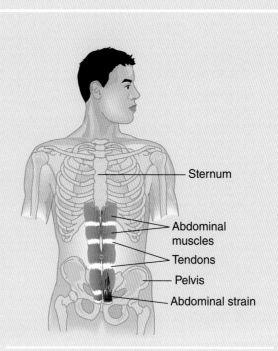

Figure 13.1 An abdominal strain.

Grades II and III

- Moderate to severe tenderness
- Lump or indentation where the muscle is torn
- Abdominal weakness
- Bruising (appears a day or two after initial injury)

✚ FIRST AID

Grade I

1. Rest the athlete from painful activities.
2. Apply ice.
3. Refer the athlete to a physician if symptoms and signs worsen (occur more often, especially with daily activities) or do not subside within a few days.

Grades II and III

1. Rest the athlete from all activities.
2. Monitor and treat for shock as needed and send for emergency medical assistance if it occurs.
3. Send for emergency medical assistance if
   a. the athlete has symptoms and signs of a constricted muscle hernia—bulge in the abdominal wall, accompanied by nausea or vomiting; or
   b. the injury was caused by a direct blow and the athlete has symptoms and signs of internal injury—shock, vomiting, bloody urine, or referred pain.
4. Apply ice to the injury and send the athlete to a physician (if emergency medical assistance is not sent for).

(continued)

Playing Status

Grade I

- The athlete can return to activity if signs and symptoms subside; the abdomen is pain free; and the athlete has full abdominal muscle flexibility and strength.
- If sent to a physician, the athlete cannot return to activity until examined and released.

Grades II and III

- The athlete cannot return to activity until examined and released by a physician; the abdomen is pain free; and the athlete has full abdominal and hip muscle flexibility and strength, and full trunk and hip range of motion.

Prevention

- Encourage athletes to do preseason exercises to strengthen and stretch the abdominal, lower back, and hip muscles.

Side Stitch

Cramping or spasm felt in either the right or left side. It's most often experienced by runners or athletes who lack cardiovascular endurance.

Cause

- Unknown

Ask if Experiencing Symptoms

- Sharp pain in the side during activity

- Pain usually disappears after the athlete rests

Check for Signs

- None

FIRST AID

1. Instruct the athlete to bend over and push fingertips into the painful side.
2. Have the athlete take a deep breath and blow it out through tight lips.
3. Instruct the athlete to stretch the muscles by placing the arm overhead and bending at the waist over to the opposite side.

Playing Status

- The athlete can return to activity once the pain subsides and breathing and heart rates are normal.
- If the pain does not subside, the athlete must be examined and released by a physician to rule out other problems.

Prevention

- Instruct athletes to perform an adequate aerobic or cardiovascular warm-up before activity.
- Instruct athletes to not eat within two hours before strenuous activity.

Low Back Strain

Stretch or tear of back muscle fibers.

Causes

- Sudden stretch or contraction of the low back muscles (figure 13.2)
- Weak abdominal muscles
- Tight low back muscles and hip muscles

Ask if Experiencing Symptoms

Grade I

- Mild pain when low back muscles contracted
- Mild pain with rising from lying down to sitting
- Mild pain when bending forward
- Mild pain when arching back
- Mild pain when twisting at the waist

Grades II and III

- Moderate to severe pain when low back muscles contracted
- Moderate to severe pain with rising from lying down to sitting
- Moderate to severe pain when bending forward
- Moderate to severe pain when arching back
- Moderate to severe pain when twisting at the waist

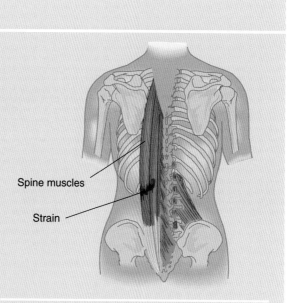

Spine muscles

Strain

Figure 13.2 Back strain.

Check for Signs

Grade I

- Mild tenderness over site of injury (toward either side from the spine)

Grades II and III

- Moderate to severe tenderness over site of injury (toward either side from the spine)
- Lump or indentation where the muscle is torn
- Back weakness
- Bruising (appears a day or two after initial injury)

✚ FIRST AID

Grade I

1. Rest the athlete from painful activities.
2. Apply ice.
3. Refer the athlete to a physician if symptoms and signs worsen (occur more often, especially with daily activities) or do not subside within a few days.

Grades II and III

1. Rest the athlete from all activities.
2. Monitor and treat for shock as needed and send for emergency medical assistance if it occurs.

3. Send for emergency medical assistance if
   a. the injury was caused by a direct blow and resulted in spine deformity or tenderness directly over the spine, or
   b. the athlete has signs and symptoms of nerve damage—sharp shooting pain, numbness or tingling down one leg, leg weakness, lower extremity paralysis, or incontinence.
4. Apply ice to the injury and send the athlete to a physician (if emergency medical assistance is not sent for).

(continued)

Low Back Strain   *(continued)*

Playing Status

Grade I

- The athlete can return to activity if signs and symptoms subside; the back is pain free; and the athlete has full range of motion in the trunk and hip, and full flexibility and strength in the back muscles.
- If sent to a physician, the athlete cannot return to activity until examined and released.

Grades II and III

- The athlete cannot return to activity until examined and released by a physician; the back is pain free; and the athlete has full range of motion in the trunk and hip, and full flexibility and strength in the back, hip, and abdominal muscles.

Prevention

- Encourage athletes to do preseason exercises to strengthen and stretch the lower back, abdominal, and hip muscles.

For a summary of first aid care for a low back strain, see page 290 in appendix A.

HIP AND THIGH

Now let's move down and examine the common acute and chronic injuries that can occur to the hips and thigh. Hip injuries can be extremely painful and debilitating. And thigh injuries, especially muscle strains and contusions, are common to most sports. During the early season, many athletes suffer strains to the quadriceps, hamstrings, and groin muscles of the thigh because they are out of shape, with weak, inflexible muscles.

In the high school sports studied by Comstock, Collins, and Yard (2008), soccer reported a high incidence of hip and leg injuries at 19.6 percent and 13.3 percent of all injuries in, respectively, male and female soccer athletes. Table 13.1 illustrates the occurrence of these injuries in other sports. The following section will help you to address the painful hip and prevalent thigh injuries your athletes might experience.

Pages 291 and 292 in appendix A will serve as a handy reference to help you properly care for your athletes' hip and thigh injuries.

Table 13.1   Frequency of Hip and Thigh Injuries Out of All Body Regions Injured

Sport	Percentage
Soccer – Boys	19.6
Soccer – Girls	13.3
Wrestling	10.5
Lacrosse – Boys	10.3
Football	10.1
Softball	9
Basketball – Boys	8.2
Basketball – Girls	8.2
Lacrosse – Girls	8.2

Data from Comstock, Collins, and Yard 2008, and Hinton et al. 2005.

Hip Dislocation and Subluxation

In a dislocation, the head of the thighbone pops out of the socket on the pelvis (figure 13.3). In a subluxation, the head of the thighbone pops out of the socket on the pelvis and spontaneously shifts back into the socket.

Cause

- 70 to 80 percent of all hip dislocations are caused by the head of the femur (thighbone) dislocating backward out of the socket. Typically, these occur when an athlete lands on a bent knee while the thigh is rotated inward and positioned close to the midline of the body.

An example is a running football player who is tackled and falls forward on a bent knee.

Ask if Experiencing Symptoms

- Severe pain in hip and thigh
- Tingling in leg and foot (if displaced bone pinches nerves)
- Sense of looseness or instability
- Felt or heard a pop
- Knee, lower leg, or even back pain

Check for Signs

Subluxation

- Lack of sensation in the leg, foot, or toes (if displaced bone pinches nerves)
- Bluish leg, foot, or toes (if displaced bone disrupts blood supply)
- Limping

Dislocation

- Inability to walk
- Inability to move thigh

- Injured leg may appear shorter (backward dislocation)
- Lack of sensation in the leg, foot, or toes (if displaced bone pinches nerves)
- Bluish leg, foot, or toes (if displaced bone disrupts blood supply)

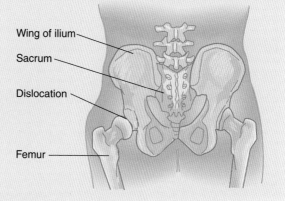

Wing of ilium

Sacrum

Dislocation

Femur

Figure 13.3   In most hip dislocations, the head of the thighbone slips backward out of its socket in the pelvis.

⊕ FIRST AID

Subluxation

1. Prevent the athlete from walking on the injured leg.
2. Monitor and treat for shock as needed and send for emergency medical assistance if it occurs.
3. Send for emergency medical assistance if the athlete has extreme pain, limited hip motion, or signs and symptoms of nerve damage or disrupted blood supply.

4. Apply ice to the injury and send the athlete to a physician.

Dislocation

1. Call for emergency medical assistance.
2. Prevent the athlete from moving entire leg.
3. Monitor and treat for shock as needed.
4. Apply ice.

Playing Status

- The athlete cannot return to activity until examined and released by a physician; the hip is pain free; and the athlete has full range of motion in the hip, and full strength and flexibility in the hip and thigh.

Prevention

- Encourage athletes to do preseason core and hip strengthening exercises.

Hip Contusion (Hip Pointer)

Bruise to the front, top of the hipbone (figure 13.4).

Cause

- Compression

Ask if Experiencing Symptoms

Mild

- Mild pain with raising thigh forward
- Mild pain with arching back

Moderate to Severe

- Moderate to severe pain with raising thigh forward
- Moderate to severe pain with arching back

Check for Signs

Mild

- Slight point tenderness over front of hip bone

Moderate to Severe

- Inability to raise the thigh forward
- Swelling

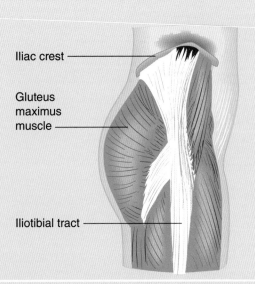

Figure 13.4   Hip contusion.

- Bruising (appears one to two days after initial injury)
- Moderate to severe point tenderness over front of hip bone
- Moderate to severe pain when walking
- Limping or inability to walk

✚ FIRST AID

Mild

1. Rest the athlete from painful activities.
2. Apply ice.
3. Refer the athlete to a physician if symptoms and signs worsen (occur more often, especially with daily activities) or do not subside within a few days.

Moderate to Severe

1. Rest the athlete from all activities.
2. Prevent the athlete from walking on the injured leg.
3. Monitor and treat for shock as needed and send for emergency medical assistance if it occurs.
4. Apply ice to the injury and send the athlete to a physician (if shock does not occur).

Playing Status

Mild

- The athlete can return to activity if signs and symptoms subside; the hip is pain free; and the athlete has full range of motion in the hip, and full strength and flexibility in the hip and thigh muscle.
- If sent to a physician, the athlete cannot return to activity until examined and released.
- When returning to activity, the athlete should wear a protective pad over the hip.

- The athlete cannot return to activity until examined and released by a physician; the hip is pain free; and the athlete has full range of motion in the hip, and full flexibility and strength in the hip and thigh muscle.

- When returning to activity, the athlete should wear a protective pad over the hip.

Prevention

- Encourage athletes to wear protective hip pads during football, volleyball, ice hockey, baseball, and softball.

Hip Flexor Strain

Stretch or tear of the muscles located high on the front of the thigh or pelvis (figure 13.5).

Causes

- Forceful contraction or stretch (tension injury) of the muscles
- Weak or inflexible hip and thigh muscles

Ask if Experiencing Symptoms

Grade I

- Mild pain high on the front of the thigh
- Mild pain when trying to raise thigh forward
- Mild pain when running

Grades II and III

- Moderate to severe pain high on the front of the thigh
- Moderate to severe pain when trying to raise thigh forward
- Moderate to severe pain when running
- Heard or felt a pop

Check for Signs

Grade I

- Mild tenderness over the front of the hip

Grades II and III

- Moderate to severe tenderness over the front of the hip

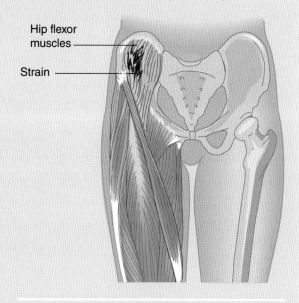

Figure 13.5 Hip flexor strain.

- Lump or indentation where the muscle is torn
- Hip and thigh weakness
- Bruising (appears a day or two after initial injury)
- Inability to raise thigh forward or up
- Swelling
- Limping

(continued)

FIRST AID

Grade I

1. Rest the athlete from painful activities.
2. Apply ice.
3. Refer the athlete to a physician if symptoms and signs worsen (occur more often, especially with daily activities) or do not subside within a few days.

Grades II and III

1. Rest the athlete from all activities.
2. Monitor and treat for shock as needed and send for emergency medical assistance if it occurs.
3. Send for emergency medical assistance if the muscle is completely torn (rolled up).
4. Prevent the athlete from walking on the injured leg.
5. Apply ice to the injury and send the athlete to a physician (if emergency medical assistance is not sent for).

Playing Status

Grade I

- The athlete can return to activity if signs and symptoms subside; the hip is pain free; and the athlete has full strength, flexibility, and range of motion in the hip.
- If sent to a physician, the athlete cannot return to activity until examined and released.
- When returning to activity, the athlete may benefit from wearing an elastic wrap to support the hip and thigh.
- When returning to activity, the athlete should stretch the upper hip and quadriceps muscles daily.

Grades II and III

- The athlete cannot return to activity until examined and released by a physician; the hip is pain free; and the athlete has full strength, flexibility, and range of motion in the hip.
- When returning to activity, the athlete may benefit from wearing an elastic wrap to support the hip and thigh.
- When returning to activity, the athlete should stretch the upper hip and quadriceps muscles daily.

Prevention

- Encourage athletes to do preseason core, hip, and thigh strengthening and stretching exercises.
- Instruct athletes to perform an adequate aerobic or cardiovascular warm-up before activity.

Inner Thigh Strain

Stretch or tear of the adductor (inner thigh) muscles (figure 13.6).

Causes

- Forceful contraction or stretch (tension injury) of the inner thigh muscles
- Weak or inflexible inner thigh muscles
- Twisting the upper body while the foot is planted

Ask if Experiencing Symptoms

Grade I

- Mild pain along inside of the thigh
- Mild pain when trying to move thigh inward toward other leg
- Mild pain when running
- Mild pain with cutting and pivoting maneuvers
- Mild pain when moving sideways

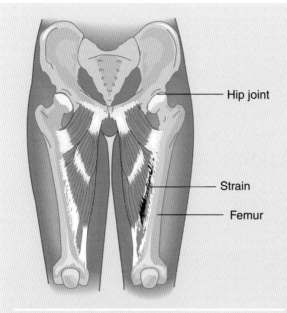

Figure 13.6 Inner thigh strain.

Grades II and III

- Moderate to severe pain along inside of the thigh
- Moderate to severe pain when trying to move thigh inward toward other leg

- Moderate to severe pain when running
- Moderate to severe pain with cutting and pivoting maneuvers
- Moderate to severe pain when moving sideways
- Heard or felt a pop

Check for Signs

Grade I

- Mild tenderness along the inner thigh

Grades II and III

- Moderate to severe tenderness over the inner thigh
- Lump or indentation where the muscle is torn
- Inner thigh weakness
- Bruising down inner thigh or knee (appears a day or two after initial injury)
- Inability to move the thigh inward toward the other thigh (such as kicking leg across body)
- Inability to stretch legs apart
- Swelling
- Limping

✚ FIRST AID

Grade I

1. Rest the athlete from painful activities.
2. Apply ice.
3. Refer the athlete to a physician if symptoms and signs worsen (occur more often, especially with daily activities) or do not subside within a few days.

Grades II and III

1. Rest the athlete from all activities.

2. Monitor and treat for shock as needed and send for emergency medical assistance if it occurs.
3. Send for emergency medical assistance if the muscle is completely torn (rolled up).
4. Prevent the athlete from walking on the injured leg.
5. Apply ice to the injury and send the athlete to a physician (if emergency medical assistance is not sent for).

Playing Status

Grade I

- The athlete can return to activity if signs and symptoms subside; the thigh is pain free; and the athlete has full range of motion in the hip, and full strength and flexibility in the hip and thigh.

- If sent to a physician, the athlete cannot return to activity until examined and released.
- When returning to activity, the athlete may benefit from wearing an elastic wrap or neoprene (rubberized) thigh sleeve to support the inner thigh.
- When returning to activity, the athlete should stretch the inner thigh muscles daily.

(continued)

Grades II and III

- The athlete cannot return to activity until examined and released by a physician; the thigh is pain free; and the athlete has full range of motion in the hip, and full flexibility and strength in the hip and thigh.
- When returning to activity, the athlete may benefit from wearing an elastic wrap or neoprene (rubberized) thigh sleeve to support the thigh.

- When returning to activity, the athlete should stretch the inner thigh muscles daily.

Prevention

- Encourage athletes to do preseason core, hip, and thigh strengthening and stretching exercises.
- Instruct athletes to perform an adequate aerobic or cardiovascular warm-up before activity.

Thigh Fracture

Break of the femur (thighbone).

Causes

- Compression
- Twisting or torsion injury

Ask if Experiencing Symptoms

- Heard or felt a pop or snap
- Grating feeling
- Pain at the site of the injury when gently squeezing the thigh above and then below the injury
- Severe pain with any movement

Check for Signs

- Deformity
- Inability to move thigh
- Lack of sensation in the leg, foot, or toes (if displaced bone pinches nerves)
- Bluish leg, foot, or toes (if displaced bone disrupts blood supply)
- Muscle spasm

⊕ FIRST AID

1. Send for emergency medical assistance.
2. Prevent the athlete from moving the hip and the entire leg.

3. Monitor and treat for shock as needed.
4. Apply ice for 15 minutes.

Playing Status

- The athlete cannot return to activity until examined and released by a physician; and the athlete has full range of motion in the hip and knee, and full strength and flexibility in the quadriceps and hamstring.

- When returning to contact sports, the athlete should wear a protective pad over the thigh.

Prevention

- Require athletes to wear protective thigh pads in football and ice hockey.

Thigh Contusion

Bruise to the soft tissues or bones of the thigh (figure 13.7).

Cause

- Compression

Ask if Experiencing Symptoms

Mild

- Mild pain with raising thigh forward or extending it backward (depending upon the site of the injury)
- Mild pain with running
- Mild pain when bending or straightening the knee

Moderate to Severe

- Moderate to severe pain with raising thigh forward or extending it backward (depending upon the site of the injury)
- Moderate to severe pain with running
- Moderate to severe pain when bending or straightening the knee

Check for Signs

Mild

- Slight point tenderness over site of the injury
- Mild pain with walking

Moderate to Severe

- Inability to raise the thigh forward or extend it backward (depending upon the site of the injury)

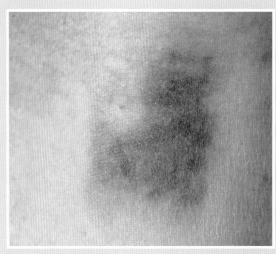

Figure 13.7 Thigh contusion.
© Custom Medical Stock Photo.

- Inability to bend or straighten the knee
- Swelling
- Bruising (appears one to two days after initial injury)
- Moderate to severe point tenderness over site of the injury
- Moderate to severe pain when walking
- Muscle spasm
- Decreased thigh strength
- Limping

⊕ FIRST AID

Mild

1. Rest the athlete from painful activities.
2. Apply ice for 15 minutes, then a compression wrap.
3. Refer the athlete to a physician if symptoms and signs worsen (occur more often, especially with daily activities) or do not subside within a few days.

Moderate to Severe

1. Rest the athlete from all activities.
2. Prevent the athlete from walking on the injured leg.
3. Monitor and treat for shock as needed and send for emergency medical assistance if it occurs.
4. Apply ice to the injury and send the athlete to a physician (if shock does not occur).

(continued)

Playing Status

Mild

- The athlete can return to activity if signs and symptoms subside; the thigh is pain free; and the athlete has full range of motion in the hip and knee, and full flexibility and strength in the thigh muscle.
- If sent to a physician, the athlete cannot return to activity until examined and released.
- When returning to contact sports, the athlete should wear a protective pad over the area, as repeated blows could cause calcification of the muscle tissue.

Moderate to Severe

- The athlete cannot return to activity until examined and released by a physician; the thigh is pain free; and the athlete has full range of motion in the hip and knee, and full flexibility and strength in the thigh muscle.
- When returning to activity, the athlete should wear a protective pad over the area, as repeated blows could cause calcification of the muscle tissue.

Prevention

- Require athletes to wear protective thigh pads in football and ice hockey.

Quadriceps Strain

Stretch or tear of the quadriceps muscles (figure 13.8).

Causes

- Forceful contraction or stretch of the quad muscles
- Weak or inflexible muscles

Ask if Experiencing Symptoms

Grade I

- Mild pain on the front of the thigh
- Mild pain when trying to raise thigh forward or straighten knee
- Mild pain when running
- Mild pain when extending the thigh backward while the knee is bent

Grades II and III

- Moderate to severe pain on the front of the thigh
- Moderate to severe pain when trying to raise thigh forward or straightening knee
- Moderate to severe pain when running
- Moderate to severe pain when extending the thigh backward while the knee is bent
- Heard or felt a pop
- Pain going up and down stairs

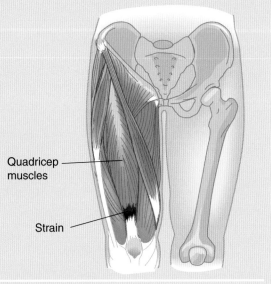

Quadricep muscles

Strain

Figure 13.8 Quadriceps strain.

Check for Signs

Grade I

- Mild tenderness over the front of the thigh

Grades II and III

- Moderate to severe tenderness over the front of the thigh
- Lump or indentation where the muscle is torn

- Bruising down thigh, knee, or lower leg (appears a day or two after initial injury)
- Decreased ability or inability to flex thigh forward or straighten the knee

- Swelling
- Limping

Grade I

1. Rest the athlete from painful activities.
2. Apply ice.
3. Refer the athlete to a physician if symptoms and signs worsen (occur more often, especially with daily activities) or do not subside within a few days.

Grades II and III

1. Rest the athlete from all activities.
2. Monitor and treat for shock as needed and send for emergency medical assistance if it occurs.
3. Send for emergency medical assistance if the muscle is completely torn (rolled up).
4. Prevent the athlete from walking on the injured leg.
5. Apply ice to the injury and send the athlete to a physician (if emergency medical assistance is not sent for).

Playing Status

Grade I

- The athlete can return to activity if signs and symptoms subside; the thigh is pain free; and the athlete has full range of motion in the hip and knee, and full strength and flexibility in the quadriceps.
- If sent to a physician, the athlete cannot return to activity until examined and released.
- When returning to activity, the athlete may benefit from wearing an elastic wrap or neoprene (rubberized) thigh sleeve to support the thigh.
- When returning to activity, the athlete should stretch the quadriceps daily.

Grades II and III

- The athlete cannot return to activity until examined and released by a physician; the thigh is pain free; and the athlete has full range of motion in the hip and knee, and full strength and flexibility in the quadriceps.
- When returning to activity, the athlete may benefit from wearing an elastic wrap or neoprene (rubberized) thigh sleeve to support the thigh.
- When returning to activity, the athlete should stretch the quadriceps daily.

Prevention

- Encourage athletes to do preseason exercises that strengthen and stretch the core, knee, hip, and thigh.
- Instruct athletes to perform an adequate aerobic or cardiovascular warm-up before activity.

Hamstring Strain

Stretch or tear of the hamstring muscles (figure 13.9).

Causes

- Forceful contraction or stretch (tension injury) of the hamstring muscles
- Weak or inflexible hamstrings

Ask if Experiencing Symptoms

Grade I

- Mild pain on the back of the thigh
- Mild pain when trying to extend thigh backward or bend knee

(continued)

- Mild pain when running
- Mild pain when flexing the thigh forward while straightening the knee

Grades II and III

- Moderate to severe pain on the back of the thigh
- Moderate to severe pain when trying to extend thigh backward or bend knee
- Moderate to severe pain when walking
- Moderate to severe pain when flexing the thigh forward while straightening the knee
- Heard or felt a pop

Check for Signs

Grade I

- Mild tenderness over back of the thigh

Grades II and III

- Moderate to severe tenderness over back of the thigh
- Lump or indentation where the muscle is torn

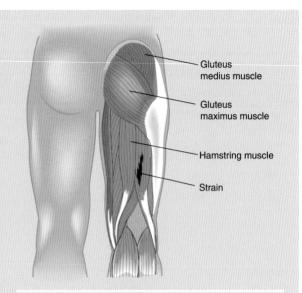

Figure 13.9 Hamstring strain.

- Bruising down back of thigh, knee, or lower leg (appears a day or two after initial injury)
- Decreased ability or inability to extend thigh backward or bend the knee
- Swelling
- Limping

⊕ FIRST AID

Grade I

1. Rest the athlete from painful activities.
2. Apply ice.
3. Refer the athlete to a physician if symptoms and signs worsen (occur more often, especially with daily activities) or do not subside within a few days.

Grades II and III

1. Rest the athlete from all activities.

2. Monitor and treat for shock as needed and send for emergency medical assistance if it occurs.
3. Send for emergency medical assistance if the muscle is completely torn (rolled up).
4. Prevent the athlete from walking on the injured leg.
5. Apply ice to the injury and send the athlete to a physician (if emergency medical assistance is not sent for).

Playing Status

Grade I

- The athlete can return to activity if signs and symptoms subside; the thigh is pain free; and the athlete has full range of motion in the hip and knee, and full strength and flexibility in the hamstring.

- If sent to a physician, the athlete cannot return to activity until examined and released.
- When returning to activity, the athlete may benefit from wearing an elastic wrap or neoprene (rubberized) thigh sleeve to support the thigh.
- When returning to activity, the athlete should stretch the hamstring muscles daily.

Grades II and III

- The athlete cannot return to activity until examined and released by a physician; the thigh is pain free; and the athlete has full range of motion in the hip and knee, and full strength and flexibility in the hamstring.
- When returning to activity, the athlete may benefit from wearing an elastic wrap or neoprene (rubberized) thigh sleeve to support the thigh.

- When returning to activity, the athlete should stretch the hamstring muscles daily.

Prevention

- Encourage athletes to do preseason exercises that strengthen and stretch the core, thigh, hip, and knee.
- Instruct athletes to perform an adequate aerobic or cardiovascular warm-up before activity.

KNEE

The knee is probably the second most commonly injured area in all of sport. In high school sports, girls suffer a proportionally higher rate of knee injuries than boys (Comstock, Collins, and Yard 2008). Girls' soccer and lacrosse players experienced the highest rates at 21.8 percent and 21.4 percent, respectively. Table 13.2 highlights the occurrence of knee injuries in other sports. Figure 13.10 shows the areas of pain of common knee injuries.

Refer to pages 293 and 294 in appendix A if you have any questions about the proper care for common knee injuries in sports.

Table 13.2 Frequency of Knee Injuries Out of All Body Regions Injured

Sport	Percentage
Soccer – Girls	21.8
Lacrosse – Girls	21.4
Basketball – Girls	18.4
Lacrosse – Boys	15.5
Football	15.4
Soccer - Boys	15.4
Wrestling	14.4
Softball – Girls	11.9
Volleyball – Girls	11.0
Baseball	7.7

Data from Comstock, Collins, and Yard 2008, and Hinton et al. 2005.

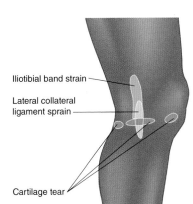

Figure 13.10a Outside of leg areas of pain for lateral collateral ligament sprain, cartilage tear, and iliotibial band strain.
© Breslich & Foss.

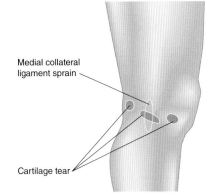

Figure 13.10b Inside of leg areas of pain for a cartilage tear and medial collateral ligament sprain.
© Breslich & Foss.

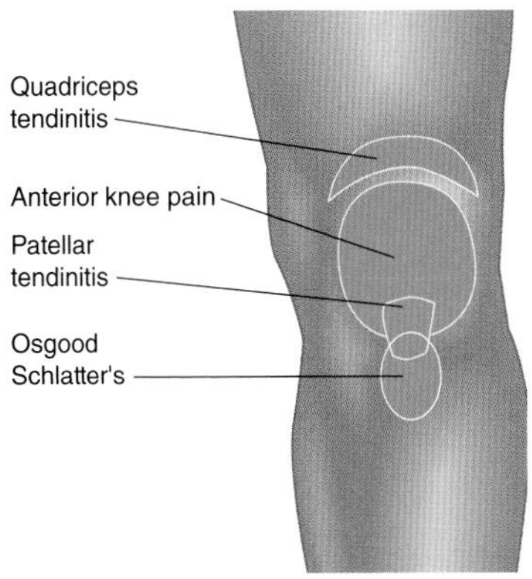

Figure 13.10c Front of knee areas of pain for Osgood Schlatter's, quadriceps tendinitis, anterior knee pain, and patellar tendinitis.
© Breslich & Foss.

Acute Knee Injuries

Knee Sprain

Stretch or tear of the ligaments that hold the knee bones in place (figure 13.11, a-d; also see figure 13.10, a and b for areas of pain).

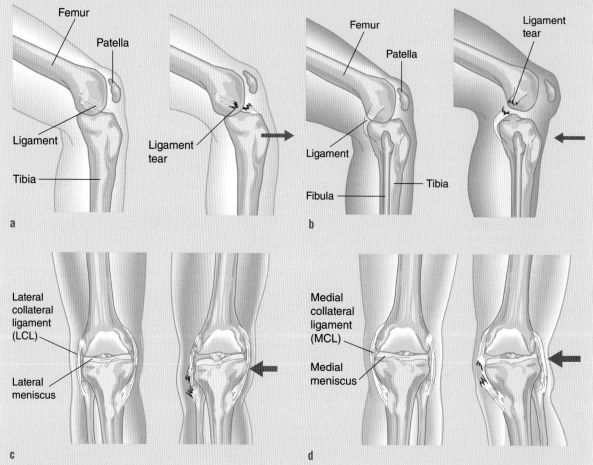

Figure 13.11 Knee sprains of the *(a)* anterior cruciate ligament (ACL), *(b)* posterior cruciate ligament (PCL), *(c)* lateral collateral ligament (LCL), and *(d)* medial collateral ligament (MCL).

Causes
- Compression to either the front, side, or back of the knee
- Twisting or torsion injury
- Hyperextension or hyperflexion of the knee
- Weak thigh muscles

Ask if Experiencing Symptoms

Grade I
- Mild pain straightening or bending knee (see figure 13.10, a and b)

Grades II and III
- Moderate to severe pain straightening or bending knee (see figure 13.10, a and b for possible areas of pain)
- Feeling of looseness or instability
- Heard or felt a pop

Check for Signs

Grade I
- Slight point tenderness

Grades II and III
- Moderate to severe point tenderness
- Swelling
- Limping

Grade I

1. Rest the athlete from painful activities.

2. Apply ice.

3. Refer the athlete to a physician if symptoms and signs worsen (occur more often, especially with daily activities such as walking) or do not subside within a few days.

Grades II and III

1. Rest the athlete from all activities.

2. Prevent the athlete from walking on the injured leg.

3. Monitor and treat for shock as needed and send for emergency medical assistance if it occurs.

4. Send for emergency medical assistance if any of the following are present:

   a. Symptoms and signs of nerve injury (tingling or numbness in lower leg, foot, or toes)

   b. Symptoms and signs of disrupted blood supply (bluish foot, toes, or toenails)

5. Apply ice to the injury and send the athlete to a physician (if emergency medical assistance is not sent for).

Playing Status

Grade I

- The athlete can return to activity if signs and symptoms subside; the knee is pain free; and the athlete has full range of motion in the knee, and full strength and flexibility in the quadriceps, hamstring, and calf.

- If sent to a physician, the athlete cannot return to activity until examined and released.

Grades II and III

- The athlete cannot return to activity until examined and released by a physician; the knee is pain free; and the athlete has full range of motion in the knee, and full strength and flexibility in the quadriceps, hamstring, and calf.

Prevention

- Encourage athletes to do preseason exercises that strengthen and stretch the hip, quadriceps, hamstring, and calf.

Dislocated or Subluxated Patella (Kneecap)

In a dislocation, the patella slips out of the groove on the femur (figure 13.12). In a subluxation, the patella slips out of the groove on the femur and then spontaneously shifts back into the groove.

Causes

- Compression to the inside of the kneecap
- Forceful contraction of the outside quadriceps muscles
- Twisting or torsion
- Weak inside quadriceps muscle

Ask if Experiencing Symptoms

Subluxation

- Pain with bending or straightening knee
- Feeling of kneecap "going out of place"
- Pain felt along the inside of the knee

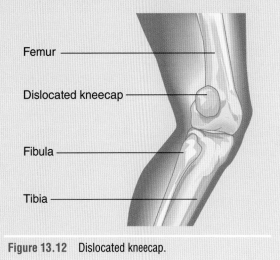

Figure 13.12 Dislocated kneecap.

(continued)

- Heard or felt a pop
- Grating sensation

- Swelling
- Limping

Dislocation

- Feeling of kneecap "going out of place"
- Pain felt along the inside of the knee
- Heard or felt a pop

Dislocation

- Obvious deformity—patella displaced to the outside of the knee
- Swelling
- Inability to bend or straighten knee
- Severe point tenderness along the inside of the kneecap or patella

Check for Signs

Subluxation

- Point tenderness along the inside of the knee

✚ FIRST AID

Subluxation

1. Rest the athlete from all activity.
2. Prevent the athlete from walking on the injured leg.
3. Monitor and treat for shock as needed, and send for emergency medical assistance if it occurs.
4. Apply ice to the injury and send the athlete to a physician.

Dislocation

1. Send for emergency medical assistance.
2. Do not try to put the patella back into place.
3. Monitor and treat for shock as needed.
4. Prevent the athlete from moving the leg.
5. Apply ice (if tolerated by the athlete).

Playing Status

- The athlete cannot return to activity until examined and released by a physician; the knee is pain free; and the athlete has full range of motion in the knee, and full strength and flexibility in the quadriceps, hamstring, and calf.

Prevention

- Encourage athletes to do preseason exercises that strengthen and stretch the quadriceps, hamstring, and calf.

Cartilage Tear

Tear of the cartilage on top of the tibia (figure 13.13; also see figure 13.10b for areas of pain).

Causes

- Compression
- Twisting or torsion injury, especially while knee is bent and foot is planted
- Knee is bent to an extreme while foot is planted

Ask if Experiencing Symptoms

- Feeling that knee "locks" or "won't move"
- Feeling of the knee "giving out"
- Feeling of looseness or instability
- Pain at the injury site, especially along the joint line between the femur and tibia (see figure 13.10a and b)
- Felt or heard a pop

Check for Signs

- Decreased ability or inability to completely bend or straighten the knee
- Delayed swelling (cartilage injury alone) or immediate swelling (cartilage injury and ligament sprain)
- Knee is "locked" (can't bend or straighten)
- Walking with knee bent or foot pointed
- Limping

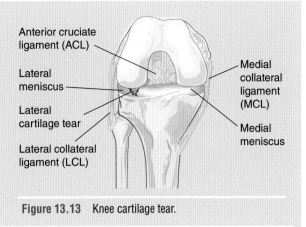

Figure 13.13   Knee cartilage tear.

✚ FIRST AID

1. Rest the athlete from activity.
2. Prevent the athlete from walking on the injured leg.
3. Monitor and treat for shock as needed and send for emergency medical assistance if it occurs.
4. Apply ice and send the athlete to a physician.

Playing Status

- The athlete cannot return to activity until examined and released by a physician; the knee is pain free; and the athlete has full range of motion in the knee, and full strength and flexibility in the quadriceps, hamstring, and calf.

Prevention

- Encourage athletes to do preseason exercises that strengthen and stretch the hip muscle, quadriceps, hamstring, and calf.

Chronic Knee Injuries

Patellar Tendinitis

Inflammation of the tendon that attaches the kneecap to the lower leg bone (see figure 13.14 for anatomy and figure 13.10c for area of pain).

Causes

- Forceful contraction of the quadriceps muscles
- Weak quad muscles and inflexible quadriceps, hamstring, and calf muscles

Ask if Experiencing Symptoms

Mild

- Mild pain from the bottom of the patella to the top of the tibia (see figure 13.10c)
- Mild pain with running and jumping activities
- Mild pain when forcefully straightening the knee

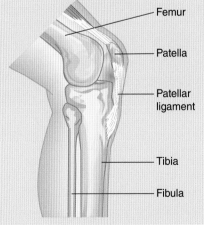

Figure 13.14   Patellar tendinitis is an inflammation of the tendon that attaches the kneecap to the tibia.

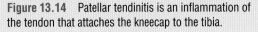

(continued)

Moderate to Severe

- Moderate to severe pain from the bottom of the patella to the top of the tibia (see figure 13.10c)
- Moderate to severe pain with running and jumping activities
- Moderate to severe pain when forcefully straightening the knee

Check for Signs

Mild

- Slight point tenderness between the patella and upper tibia

Moderate to Severe

- Decreased ability or inability to forcefully straighten the knee, especially when jumping, lifting weights, and running
- Thickening of the patellar tendon
- Moderate to severe point tenderness between the patella and upper tibia
- Localized swelling
- Limping

✚ FIRST AID

Mild

1. Rest the athlete from painful activities.
2. Apply ice.
3. Refer the athlete to a physician if symptoms and signs worsen (occur more often, especially with daily activities) or do not subside within a few days.

Moderate to Severe

1. Rest the athlete from all activities.
2. Monitor and treat for shock as needed and send for emergency medical assistance if it occurs.
3. Prevent the athlete from walking on the injured leg.
4. Apply ice to the injury and send the athlete to a physician (if shock does not occur).

Playing Status

Mild

- The athlete can return to activity if signs and symptoms subside; the knee is pain free; and the athlete has full knee range of motion, quadriceps strength, and quadriceps, hamstring, and calf flexibility.
- If sent to a physician, the athlete cannot return to activity until examined and released.
- When returning to activity, the athlete may benefit from wearing a rubberized neoprene knee sleeve to keep the tendon warm during activity.
- When returning to activity, the athlete should stretch the hamstring, quadriceps, and calf muscles daily.

Moderate to Severe

- The athlete cannot return to activity until examined and released by a physician; the knee is pain free; and the athlete has full knee range of motion, quadriceps strength, and quadriceps, hamstring, and calf flexibility.
- When returning to activity, the athlete may benefit from wearing a rubberized neoprene knee sleeve to keep the tendon warm during activity.
- When returning to activity, the athlete should stretch the hamstring, quadriceps, and calf muscles daily.

Prevention

- Encourage athletes to do preseason exercises that strengthen the core, gluteals, and quadriceps and stretch the quadriceps, hamstring, and calf.
- Instruct athletes to perform an adequate aerobic or cardiovascular warm-up before activity.

Anterior Knee Pain

Irritation between the patella and femur (see figure 13.10c). Typically occurs over time.

Causes

- Compression to the top of the patella
- Inability of the patella to properly track in the groove in the femur
- Repeated episodes of patellar dislocation and subluxation
- Weak quadriceps and gluteal (buttocks) muscles or inflexible quadriceps, hamstring, and calf muscles

Ask if Experiencing Symptoms

Mild

- Mild pain with running, jumping, or using stairs
- Mild pain behind the patella (see figure 13.10c)
- Grating feeling behind the patella
- Mild achiness while sitting for extended periods

Moderate to Severe

- Moderate to severe pain with running, jumping, or using stairs
- Moderate to severe pain behind the patella (see figure 13.10c)
- Grating feeling behind the patella
- Moderate to severe achiness while sitting for extended periods

Check for Signs

Mild

- Mild point tenderness underneath the patella

Moderate to Severe

- Moderate to severe point tenderness underneath the patella
- Decreased ability or inability to forcefully straighten the knee, especially when jumping, lifting weights, and running
- Limping

FIRST AID

Mild

1. Rest the athlete from painful activities.
2. Apply ice.
3. Refer the athlete to a physician if symptoms and signs worsen (occur more often, especially with daily activities) or do not subside within a few days.

Moderate to Severe

1. Rest the athlete from all activities.
2. Monitor and treat for shock as needed and send for emergency medical assistance if it occurs.
3. Prevent the athlete from walking on the injured leg.
4. Apply ice to the injury and send the athlete to a physician (if shock does not occur).

Playing Status

Mild

- The athlete can return to activity if signs and symptoms subside; the knee is pain free; and the athlete has full knee range of motion, quadriceps strength, and quadriceps, hamstring, and calf flexibility.

- If sent to a physician, the athlete cannot return to activity until examined and released.
- When returning to activity, the athlete should stretch the hamstring, quadriceps, and calf muscles daily.

Moderate to Severe

- The athlete cannot return to activity until examined and released by a physician; the

(continued)

knee is pain free; and the athlete has full knee range of motion, quadriceps strength, and quadriceps, hamstring, and calf flexibility.

- When returning to activity, the athlete should stretch the hamstring, quadriceps, and calf muscles daily.

Prevention

- Encourage athletes to do preseason exercises that strengthen the core, gluteals, and quadriceps and stretch the quadriceps, hamstring, and calf.
- Instruct athletes to perform an adequate aerobic or cardiovascular warm-up before activity.

Iliotibial Band Strain

Stretch or irritation of the connective tissue along the outside of the thigh (see figure 13.10a). Typically occurs over time.

Causes

- Forceful stretch of the connective tissue that attaches to the outside of the knee
- Weak or inflexible thigh muscles
- Running the same direction on a track or running on the sloped edge of a road
- Weak or inflexible hip muscles

Ask if Experiencing Symptoms

Mild

- Mild pain along the outside of the knee (see figure 13.10a)
- Mild pain with running, jumping, biking, or using stairs

Moderate to Severe

- Moderate to severe pain along the outside of the knee (see figure 13.10a)
- Moderate to severe pain with running, jumping, biking, or using stairs

Check for Signs

Mild

- Slight point tenderness along outside of knee

Moderate to Severe

- Moderate to severe point tenderness along outside of knee
- Swelling
- Limping

⊕ FIRST AID

Mild

1. Rest the athlete from painful activities.
2. Apply ice.
3. Refer the athlete to a physician if symptoms and signs worsen (occur more often, especially with daily activities) or do not subside within a few days.

Moderate to Severe

1. Rest the athlete from all activities.
2. Monitor and treat for shock as needed and send for emergency medical assistance if it occurs.
3. Prevent the athlete from walking on the injured leg.
4. Apply ice to the injury and send the athlete to a physician (if shock does not occur).

Playing Status

Mild

- The athlete can return to activity if the knee is pain free and the athlete has full knee range of motion, gluteal strength, and iliotibial band, quadriceps, and hamstring flexibility.
- If sent to a physician, the athlete cannot return to activity until examined and released.
- When returning to activity, the athlete should stretch the hamstrings and quadriceps daily.
- When returning to activity, the athlete may benefit from wearing a rubberized neoprene knee sleeve to keep the iliotibial band warm during activity.

Moderate to Severe

- The athlete cannot return to activity until examined and released by a physician; the knee is pain free; and the athlete has full knee range of motion, gluteal strength, and iliotibial band, quadriceps, and hamstring flexibility.
- When returning to activity, the athlete should stretch the hamstrings and quadriceps daily.
- When returning to activity, the athlete may benefit from wearing a rubberized neoprene knee sleeve to keep the iliotibial band warm during activity.

Prevention

- Encourage athletes to do preseason exercises that strengthen the core and the hip (gluteal) and stretch the iliotibial band, quadriceps, hamstring, and calf.
- Instruct athletes to perform an adequate aerobic or cardiovascular warm-up before activity.
- Instruct athletes to avoid running the same direction on a track or running on a sloped edge of a road.

LOWER LEG, ANKLE, AND FOOT

Ankle injuries are probably the most common injuries in sports. In the study by Comstock, Collins, and Yard (2008), basketball ankle injuries accounted for 38.3 percent of boys' injuries and 32.5 percent of girls'. And in high school volleyball, the ankle was the site of 46 percent of all injuries. Ankle injury occurrence in other sports can be found in table 13.3. Table 13.4 lists the occurrence of lower leg and foot injuries by sport.

Let's take a look at varies acute and chronic lower leg, ankle, and foot injuries.

Table 13.3 Frequency of Ankle Injuries Out of All Body Regions Injured

Sport	Percentage
Volleyball – Girls	46
Basketball – Boys	38.3
Basketball – Girls	32.5
Lacrosse – Girls	25.1
Soccer – Girls	24.7
Soccer – Boys	22.1
Softball – Girls	17.7
Lacrosse – Boys	16.1
Football	14.5

Data from Comstock, Collins, and Yard 2008, and Hinton et al. 2005.

Table 13.4 Frequency of Lower Leg and Foot Injuries Out of All Body Regions Injured

Sport	Percentage
Soccer – Boys	14.8
Soccer – Girls	13.8
Lacrosse – Girls	9.5
Basketball – Boys	8.5
Basketball – Girls	8.3
Lacrosse – Boys	8.0
Football	7.2
Volleyball – Girls	5.9

Data from Comstock, Collins, and Yard 2008, and Hinton et al. 2005.

Acute Lower Leg and Ankle Injuries

Calf Strain

Stretch or tear of the calf muscles (figure 13.15).

Causes

- Forceful contraction of the calf muscles
- Forced stretch (tension injury) of the calf muscles (moving toes up toward knee)
- Weak or inflexible calf muscles
- Explosive jumping or sprinting

Ask if Experiencing Symptoms

Grade I

- Mild calf pain
- Mild pain when pointing foot down
- Mild pain when foot is stretched up toward shin
- Mild pain when jumping and running

Grades II and III

- Moderate to severe calf pain
- Moderate to severe pain when pointing foot down
- Moderate to severe pain when foot is stretched up toward shin
- Moderate to severe pain when jumping and running

Check for Signs

Grade I

- Slight point tenderness

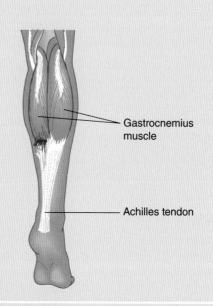

Figure 13.15 Calf strain—a stretch or tear (shown here) of the calf muscle.

Grades II and III

- Moderate to severe point tenderness
- Swelling
- Indentation or lump where muscle is torn
- Decreased ability or inability to point the foot
- Decreased ability or inability to jump or run
- Bruising down back of lower leg, ankle, or foot (appears a day or two after initial injury)
- Limping

✚ FIRST AID

Grade I

1. Rest the athlete from painful activities.
2. Apply ice.
3. Refer the athlete to a physician if symptoms and signs worsen (occur more often, especially with daily activities) or do not subside within a few days.

Grades II and III

1. Rest the athlete from all activities.

2. Monitor and treat for shock as needed and send for emergency medical assistance if it occurs.
3. Send for emergency medical assistance if the muscle is completely torn (rolled up).
4. Prevent the athlete from walking on the injured leg.
5. Apply ice to the injury and send the athlete to a physician (if emergency medical assistance is not sent for).

Playing Status

Grade I

- The athlete can return to activity if the calf is pain free and the athlete has full range of motion in the knee and ankle, and full strength and flexibility in the calf.
- If sent to a physician, the athlete cannot return to activity until examined and released.
- When returning to activity, the athlete should stretch the calf and Achilles tendon daily.
- When returning to activity, the athlete may benefit by wearing an elastic wrap or neoprene calf sleeve to support the calf.

Grades II and III

- The athlete cannot return to activity until examined and released by a physician; the calf is pain free; and the athlete has full range of motion in the knee and ankle, and full strength and flexibility in the calf.
- When returning to activity, the athlete should stretch the calf and Achilles tendon daily.
- When returning to activity, the athlete may benefit by wearing an elastic wrap or neoprene calf sleeve to support the calf.

Prevention

- Encourage athletes to do preseason exercises that strengthen the calf and stretch the calf and Achilles tendon.
- Instruct athletes to perform an adequate aerobic or cardiovascular warm-up before activity.

Lower Leg Fracture

Break in one or both of the lower leg bones (tibia and fibula).

Causes

- Direct blow
- Compression injury (such as landing from an apparatus)
- Twisting or torsion (see figure 3.23)

Ask if Experiencing Symptoms

- Pain
- Numbness or tingling in lower leg or foot if fracture injures nerves
- Grating sensation
- Heard or felt a pop or snap
- Severe pain with any movement

Check for Signs

- Deformity
- Lack of sensation in the lower leg, foot, or toes (if displaced bone injures nerves)
- Bluish lower leg, foot, or toes (if displaced bone injures blood supply)
- Possible inability to bend or straighten knee, if the fracture is near the knee
- Possible inability to flex foot up or down, if the fracture is near the ankle
- Swelling
- Pain at the site of the fracture of tibia and fibula when gently squeezed above and then below the injured area
- Inability to walk on injured leg

✚ FIRST AID

1. Send for emergency medical assistance.
2. Prevent athlete from moving the entire leg.
3. Monitor and treat for shock as needed.

(continued)

Playing Status

- The athlete cannot return to activity until examined and released by a physician and has full knee and ankle range of motion, and full quadriceps, hamstring, and lower leg muscle strength and flexibility.

- Recommend the athlete wear a protective pad over site of the injury when the athlete returns to activity.

Prevention

- Require athletes to wear protective padding when appropriate for sport, such as soccer, baseball, or softball.

Ankle Sprain

Stretch or tear of the ligaments holding the ankle bones together.

In an inversion sprain, the foot rolls in and damages the outside ankle ligaments and sometimes the inside ligaments (figure 13.16 and figure 13.17). This is the most common type, occurring in about 80 percent of ankle sprains. In an eversion sprain, the foot rolls out and damages the inside ankle ligaments and sometimes the outside ligaments.

Causes

- Compression
- Twisting or torsion

Ask if Experiencing Symptoms

Grade I

- Mild pain around the inside or outside ankle bones

- Mild pain when flexing the foot up or pointing it down

Grades II and III

- Moderate to severe pain around the inside or outside ankle bones
- Moderate to severe pain when flexing the foot up or pointing it down
- Feeling of looseness or instability
- Heard or felt a pop

Check for Signs

Grade I

- Slight point tenderness just below the outside or inside ankle bones (tibia and fibula)

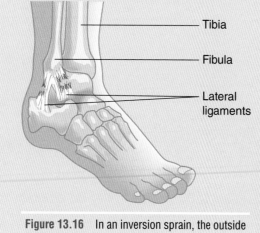

Figure 13.16 In an inversion sprain, the outside ankle ligaments are damaged.

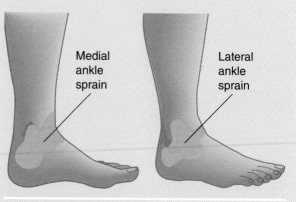

Figure 13.17 Ankle sprain areas of pain.
© Breslich & Foss.

Grades II and III

- Moderate to severe point tenderness just below the outside or inside ankle bones (tibia and fibula)

- Swelling
- Inability to bear weight or limps when walking

Grade I

1. Rest the athlete from painful activities.
2. Apply ice for 15 minutes, then apply a compression wrap.
3. Refer the athlete to a physician if symptoms and signs worsen (occur more often, especially with daily activities such as walking) or do not subside within a few days.

Grades II and III

1. Rest the athlete from all activities that require use of the leg.
2. Prevent the athlete from walking on the injured leg.
3. Monitor and treat for shock as needed and send for emergency medical assistance if it occurs.

4. Send for emergency medical assistance if any of the following are present:
   a. Signs of fracture—obvious deformity or pain at the site of the injury when tibia and fibula are gently squeezed above or below the injury, or pain along the midline of the lower third of the tibia or fibula
   b. Symptoms and signs of nerve compression (tingling and numbness)
   c. Symptoms and signs of disrupted blood supply (bluish toes and toenails)
5. Apply ice to the injury and send the athlete to a physician (if emergency medical assistance is not sent for).

Playing Status

Grade I

- The athlete can return to activity if signs and symptoms subside; the ankle is pain free; and the athlete has full ankle range of motion, lower leg strength, and calf and Achilles tendon flexibility.
- If sent to a physician, the athlete cannot return to activity until examined and released.
- When returning to activity, the athlete should wear a protective brace.

Grades II and III

- The athlete cannot return to activity until examined and released by a physician; the ankle is pain free; and the athlete has full ankle range of motion, lower leg strength, and calf and Achilles tendon flexibility.
- When returning to activity, the athlete should wear a protective brace.

Prevention

- Encourage athletes to do preseason lower leg strengthening exercises and calf and Achilles tendon stretching and balance training.

Heel Contusion

Bruise to the bone or soft tissues of the heel (figure 13.18).

Causes

- Wearing shoes with little heel cushioning
- Exercising on hard surfaces such as concrete
- Landing flat on the foot
- Compression

Ask if Experiencing Symptoms

Mild

- Mild pain under the heel
- Mild pain when jumping and running

Moderate to Severe

- Moderate to severe pain under the heel
- Pain with walking
- Moderate to severe pain when jumping and running

Check for Signs

Mild

- Slight point tenderness under the heel

Moderate to Severe

- Decreased ability or inability to land or walk on heel

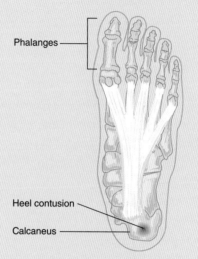

Figure 13.18 Bottom of foot: heel contusion.

- Moderate to severe point tenderness under the heel
- Swelling on the bottom of foot
- Decreased ability or inability to jump or run
- Bruising (appears a day or two after initial injury)
- Limping

⊕ FIRST AID

Mild

1. Rest the athlete from painful activities.
2. Apply ice.
3. Refer the athlete to a physician if symptoms and signs worsen (occur more often, especially with daily activities) or do not subside within a few days.

Moderate to Severe

1. Rest the athlete from all activities.
2. Monitor and treat for shock as needed and send for emergency medical assistance if it occurs.
3. Send for emergency medical assistance if any of the following are present:
   a. Signs of fracture—obvious deformity or pain when heel is gently tapped above or below the injury
   b. Symptoms and signs of nerve compression (tingling or numbness in foot or toes)
   c. Symptoms and signs of disrupted blood supply (bluish foot or toes)
4. Prevent the athlete from walking on the injured foot.
5. Apply ice to the injury and send the athlete to a physician (if emergency medical assistance is not sent for).

Playing Status

Mild

- The athlete can return to activity if the heel and foot are pain free and the athlete has full range of motion in the ankle and foot, and full flexibility in the calf and Achilles tendon.
- If sent to a physician, the athlete cannot return to activity until examined and released.
- When returning to activity, the athlete should stretch the calf and Achilles tendon daily.
- When returning to activity, the athlete should wear a shock-absorbing heel pad or cushion in both shoes.

Moderate to Severe

- The athlete cannot return to activity until examined and released by a physician; the heel and foot are pain free; and the athlete has full ankle range of motion, and full calf and Achilles tendon flexibility.
- When returning to activity, the athlete should stretch the calf and Achilles tendon daily.
- When returning to activity, the athlete should wear a shock-absorbing heel pad or cushion in both shoes.

Prevention

- Encourage athletes to wear shoes with plenty of heel cushioning.

Turf Toe

Hyperextension of the great toe (figure 13.19).

Cause

- Forced extension (pushing off) of big toe

Ask if Experiencing Symptoms

Grade I

- Mild pain underneath big toe
- Mild pain when bending or extending the big toe
- Mild pain when walking, running, or jumping, particularly when "toeing off"

Grades II and III

- Moderate to severe pain underneath big toe
- Moderate to severe pain when bending or extending the big toe
- Moderate to severe pain with walking, running, or jumping, particularly when "toeing off"

Check for Signs

Grade I

- Slight point tenderness over the joint between the big toe and foot

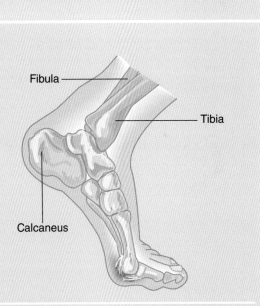

Figure 13.19 Turf toe occurs when the great toe is hyperextended.

Grades II and III

- Decreased ability or inability to land on ball of foot or walk on toes
- Moderate to severe point tenderness over joint between the big toe and foot
- Swelling
- Decreased ability or inability to jump or run
- Limping

(continued)

✚ FIRST AID

Grade I

1. Rest the athlete from all activities causing pain.
2. Apply ice.
3. Refer the athlete to a physician if symptoms and signs worsen (occur more often, especially with daily activities) or do not subside within a few days.

Grades II and III

1. Rest the athlete from all activities.
2. Monitor and treat for shock as needed and send for emergency medical assistance if it occurs.
3. Prevent the athlete from walking on the injured foot.
4. Apply ice to the injury and send the athlete to a physician (if shock does not occur).

Playing Status

Grade I

- The athlete can return to activity if signs and symptoms subside; the toe is pain free; and the athlete has full strength, flexibility, and range of motion in the toe.
- If sent to a physician, the athlete cannot return to activity until examined and released.

Grades II and III

- The athlete cannot return to activity until examined and released by a physician; the toe is pain free; and the athlete has full strength, flexibility, and range of motion in the toe.

Prevention

- Instruct athletes to wear shoes with stiffer forefoot bend, particularly in football, soccer, baseball, and softball.

Chronic Lower Leg, Ankle, and Foot Injuries

Shin Splints

Stretch, tear, or irritation of the shin muscles, tendons, or bone covering (figure 13.20).

Causes

- Forceful contraction or stretch (tension injury) of shin muscles
- Suddenly increasing the intensity of sport or conditioning program
- Repeatedly running on an uneven or unyielding surface
- Tight calf muscles
- Tight Achilles tendon
- Weak or inflexible shin muscles
- Faulty foot mechanics that fail to absorb shock and allow shock to be transmitted up the lower leg bone
- Shoes with inadequate arch support
- Worn-out athletic shoes

Ask if Experiencing Symptoms

Grade I

- Mild pain just to the inside or outside of the tibia
- Mild pain with running and jumping activities
- Pain decreases with rest

Grades II and III

- Moderate to severe pain just to the inside or outside of the tibia
- Pain with walking

- Pain at rest
- Moderate to severe pain with running and jumping activities

Check for Signs

Grade I

- Slight point tenderness over the site of the injury

Grades II and III

- Moderate to severe point tenderness over the site of the injury
- Swelling
- Decreased ability or inability to run or jump

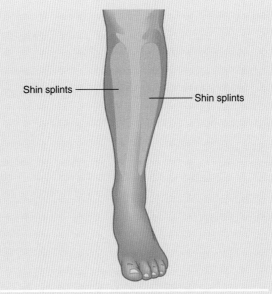

Figure 13.20 Areas of pain in shin splints.
© Breslich & Foss.

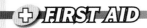

Grade I

1. Rest the athlete from all activities causing pain.
2. Apply ice.
3. Refer the athlete to a physician if symptoms and signs worsen (occur more often, especially with daily activities) or do not subside within a few days.

Grades II and III

1. Rest the athlete from all activities.
2. Monitor and treat for shock as needed and send for emergency medical assistance if it occurs.
3. Send for emergency medical assistance if any of the following are present:

a. Signs of fracture—obvious deformity, or pain at the site of the injury when compressing the tibia or fibula above, then below the site of the injury

b. Symptoms and signs of compression to nerves (tingling or numbness in foot or toes)

c. Symptoms and signs of disrupted blood supply (bluish foot or toes and are cold to the touch)

4. Prevent the athlete from walking on the injured foot.

5. Apply ice to the injury and send the athlete to a physician (if emergency medical assistance is not sent for).

Playing Status

Grade I

- The athlete can return to activity if signs and symptoms subside; the shin is pain free; and the athlete has full ankle range of motion, lower leg strength, and calf and Achilles tendon flexibility.
- If sent to a physician, the athlete cannot return to activity until examined and released.

- When returning to activity, the athlete should wear shoes with firm arch support.
- When returning to activity, the athlete should stretch the calf and Achilles tendon daily.

Grades II and III

- The athlete cannot return to activity until examined and released by a physician; the shin is pain free; and the athlete has full ankle

(continued)

range of motion, lower leg strength, and calf and Achilles tendon flexibility.

- When returning to activity, the athlete should wear shoes with firm arch support.
- When returning to activity, the athlete should stretch the calf and Achilles tendon daily.

Prevention

- Encourage athletes to do preseason exercises that strengthen the lower leg and stretch the calf and Achilles tendon.

- Instruct athletes to perform an adequate aerobic or cardiovascular warm-up before activity.
- Use appropriate increments for increasing training intensity—no greater than approximately 10 percent per week.
- Instruct athletes to wear shoes with firm arch support.

Tibial Stress Fracture

Break or crack in tibia that occurs over time.

Causes

- Suddenly increasing the intensity of sport or conditioning program (more than 10 percent per week)
- Repeatedly running or jumping on an uneven or unyielding surface
- Faulty foot mechanics that fail to absorb shock, allowing shock to be transmitted up the lower leg bone
- Shoes with inadequate arch support
- Worn-out athletic shoes
- Amenorrhea (lack of menstrual period sometimes caused by anorexia)

Ask if Experiencing Symptoms

- Pain along front of the shin
- Pain with walking
- Pain at rest
- Moderate to severe pain with running and jumping activities

Check for Signs

- Moderate to severe point tenderness over the site of the injury
- Pain at the site of the injury when tibia is pressed above or below the injury
- Swelling
- Decreased ability or inability to run or jump
- Limping

⊕ FIRST AID

1. Rest the athlete from all activities that require use of the leg.
2. Monitor and treat for shock as needed and send for emergency medical assistance if it occurs.
3. Send for emergency medical assistance if any of the following are present:
   a. Obvious deformity
   b. Symptoms and signs of compression to nerves (tingling or numbness in foot or toes)
   c. Symptoms and signs of disrupted blood supply (foot or toes appear bluish and are cold to the touch)
4. Prevent the athlete from walking on the injured leg.
5. Apply ice to the injury and send the athlete to a physician (if emergency medical assistance is not sent for).

Playing Status

- The athlete cannot return to activity until a physician has examined and released the athlete; the shin is pain free; and the athlete has full ankle range of motion, lower leg strength, and calf and Achilles tendon flexibility.
- When returning to activity, the athlete should wear shoes with firm arch support.

Prevention

- Use appropriate increments for increasing training intensity—no greater than approximately 10 percent per week.
- Instruct athletes to wear shoes with firm arch support.
- Have athletes run on shock-absorbing and even surfaces such as wood or grass.

Exertional Compartment Syndrome

Increase in pressure, typically in front of the lower leg, that constricts blood flow to the lower leg and foot.

Cause

- Unknown—possibly tight fascia (tissue) surrounding muscles, tendons, nerves, and arteries of the lower leg

Ask if Experiencing Symptoms

Mild

- Burning, aching, or cramping in front of lower leg during activity—it may subside approximately 30 minutes after activity is stopped (figure 13.21)
- Tingling in foot or toes during activity
- Feeling of fullness or tightness that may worsen as activity progresses
- Pain typically begins after starting exercise or after reaching a certain intensity level
- Pain relieved with rest and recurs upon resuming exercise

Moderate to Severe

- Pain, burning, aching, and cramping continuing into rest
- Tingling in foot or toes during activity and rest
- Toes drag when walking
- Limping

Check for Signs

Mild

- Slight swelling or tightness to touch

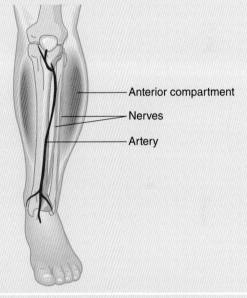

Figure 13.21 Exertional compartment syndrome.
© Breslich & Foss.

Moderate to Severe

- Muscle weakness, especially when trying to flex foot up
- Loss of sensation if swelling compresses nerve
- Bluish and cold foot or toes if swelling disrupts blood supply
- Exercise-induced swelling of lower leg

(continued)

⊕ FIRST AID

Mild

1. Rest the athlete from all activities that cause signs and symptoms.
2. Refer the athlete to a physician if symptoms and signs worsen (occur more often, especially with daily activities) or do not subside within a few days.

Moderate to Severe

1. Rest the athlete from all activities.
2. Monitor and treat for shock as needed and send for emergency medical assistance if it occurs.
3. Prevent the athlete from walking on the injured leg.
4. Instruct the athlete to elevate the leg, and send the athlete to a physician.

Playing Status

- The athlete cannot return to activity until a physician has examined and released the athlete; the leg is pain free; and the athlete has full ankle range of motion, lower leg and toe strength, and calf and Achilles tendon flexibility.

Prevention

- Unknown

➡ Playing It Safe...
With Exertional Compartment Syndrome

If an athlete complains of numbness, tingling, or weakness in the lower leg, foot, or toes, you should avoid applying a compression wrap. The added compression can worsen the condition by further restricting blood flow to the area or by compressing the nerves to the foot.

Achilles Tendinitis

Stretch, tear, or irritation to the tendon that attaches the calf muscles to the heel (figure 13.22).

Causes

- Repeated forceful contraction or stretch of the calf muscles
- Participating in repetitive, stressful activity that requires going up on the toes (gymnastics, basketball, or volleyball)

Ask if Experiencing Symptoms

Mild

- Mild pain between the heel and lower calf
- Mild pain with running and jumping
- Mild pain when pointing foot down
- Mild pain when foot is stretched up toward shin

Moderate to Severe

- Moderate to severe pain between the heel and lower calf
- Moderate to severe pain when pointing foot down
- Moderate to severe pain when foot is stretched up toward shin
- Moderate to severe pain when jumping and running

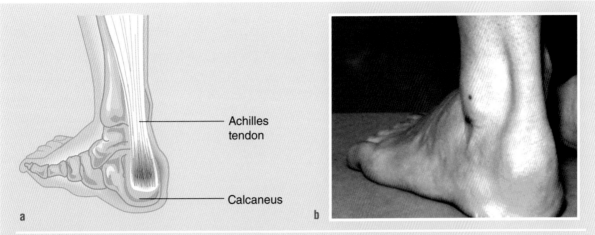

Figure 13.22 Achilles tendinitis: *(a)* irritation of the tendon and *(b)* external view.
Photo © Custom Medical Stock Photo.

Check for Signs

Mild

- Slight point tenderness

Moderate to Severe

- Moderate to severe point tenderness
- Swelling
- Thickening of the tendon
- Decreased ability or inability to point the foot down or rise up on toes
- Decreased ability or inability to jump or run
- Limping

⊕ FIRST AID

Mild

1. Rest the athlete from painful activities.
2. Apply ice.
3. Refer the athlete to a physician if symptoms and signs worsen (occur more often, especially with daily activities) or do not subside within a few days.

Moderate to Severe

1. Rest the athlete from all activities.
2. Monitor and treat for shock as needed and send for emergency medical assistance if it occurs.
3. Prevent the athlete from walking on the injured leg.
4. Apply ice to the injury and send the athlete to a physician (if shock does not occur).

Playing Status

Mild

- The athlete can return to activity if the Achilles tendon is pain free and the athlete has full range of motion in the ankle, and full strength and flexibility in the Achilles and calf.
- If sent to a physician, the athlete cannot return to activity until examined and released.
- When returning to activity, the athlete should stretch the Achilles tendon and calf daily.

Moderate to Severe

- The athlete cannot return to activity until examined and released by a physician; the Achilles tendon is pain free; and the athlete has full range of motion in the ankle, and full strength and flexibility in the Achilles and calf.
- When returning to activity, the athlete should stretch the Achilles tendon and calf daily.

Prevention

- Encourage athletes to do preseason exercises that strengthen and stretch the Achilles and calf.
- Instruct athletes to perform an adequate aerobic or cardiovascular warm-up before activity.

Plantar Fasciitis

Stretching or inflammation of the tissue that connects to the heel and toes (figure 13.23).

Causes

- Flat feet
- High arches
- Wearing shoes with inadequate arch support
- Tight calf muscles
- Increasing running intensity too fast and too soon (greater than 10 percent per week)

Ask if Experiencing Symptoms

Mild

- Mild pain along the arch or near the bottom of the heel
- Mild pain when running or jumping

Moderate to Severe

- Moderate to severe pain along the arch or near the bottom of the heel
- Feeling of muscle tightness or weakness
- Pain with walking
- Moderate to severe pain with running or jumping

Check for Signs

Mild

- Slight point tenderness

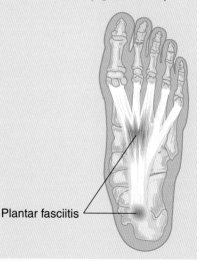

Figure 13.23　Bottom of foot: plantar fasciitis.

Moderate to Severe

- Moderate to severe point tenderness
- Arch may flatten out
- Decreased ability or inability to push off with the foot or point the foot down
- Swelling
- Limping

⊕ FIRST AID

Mild

1. Rest the athlete from painful activities.
2. Apply ice.
3. Refer the athlete to a physician if symptoms and signs worsen (occur more often, especially with daily activities) or do not subside within a few days.

Moderate to Severe

1. Rest the athlete from all activities.
2. Monitor and treat for shock as needed and send for emergency medical assistance if it occurs.
3. Prevent the athlete from walking on the injured foot.
4. Apply ice to the injury and send the athlete to a physician (if shock does not occur).

Playing Status

Mild

- The athlete can return to activity if the plantar fascia is pain free and the athlete has full calf and Achilles tendon flexibility.

- If sent to a physician, the athlete cannot return to activity until examined and released.
- When returning to activity, the athlete should stretch the calf, Achilles tendon, and plantar fascia daily.

- When returning to activity, the athlete should wear shoes with adequate heel cushions and firm arch supports.

Moderate to Severe

- The athlete cannot return to activity until examined and released by a physician; the plantar fascia is pain free; and the athlete has full calf and Achilles tendon flexibility.
- When returning to activity, the athlete should stretch the calf, Achilles tendon, and plantar fascia daily.
- When returning to activity, the athlete should wear shoes with adequate heel cushions and firm arch support.

Prevention

- Encourage athletes to do preseason exercises that stretch the calf, Achilles tendon, and plantar fascia.
- Instruct athletes to perform an adequate aerobic or cardiovascular warm-up before activity.
- Use appropriate increments for increasing training intensity—no greater than approximately 10 percent increase per week.
- Instruct athletes to wear shoes with adequate heel cushions and firm arch support.

Because of the prevalence of calf, shin, ankle, and foot injuries in sports, you'll want to be well versed in first aid techniques for the injuries presented. These common injuries and their appropriate care are summarized in appendix A on pages 295 and 296.

Chapter 13 *REPLAY*

- ☐ What are the mechanisms of an abdominal strain? (p. 187)
- ☐ What first aid techniques can be used for a side stitch? (p. 188)
- ☐ What are the signs of hip dislocation? (pp. 190-191)
- ☐ What is a hip pointer? (p. 192)
- ☐ What hip motions would cause pain if an athlete has a hip flexor strain? (p. 193)
- ☐ What are the symptoms and signs of a moderate to severe inner thigh strain? (pp. 194-195)
- ☐ What can happen if a thigh contusion is repeatedly subjected to direct blows? (p. 198)
- ☐ In a Grade II and III quadriceps strain, where might bruising (discoloration) appear? (p. 199)
- ☐ What hip and thigh motions would cause pain if an athlete has a hamstring strain? (pp. 199-200)
- ☐ What is the mechanism of injury for a knee sprain? (p. 202)
- ☐ What is the most obvious sign of a dislocated patella? (p. 204)
- ☐ What motions would cause pain if an athlete has a knee cartilage tear? (p. 205)
- ☐ What are potential causes of patellar tendinitis? (p. 205)
- ☐ What are the symptoms and signs of anterior knee pain? (p. 207)
- ☐ Where is iliotibial band pain felt? (p. 208)
- ☐ What observable signs differentiate a Grade II and III calf strain from a Grade I one? (p. 210)

☐ What are the injury mechanisms for most ankle sprains? (p. 212)

☐ What can be done to help prevent a heel contusion? (p. 215)

☐ Turf toe is actually an injury to which toe? (pp. 215-216)

☐ What are the potential causes of shin splints? (p. 216)

☐ How can you differentiate between shin splints and a tibial stress fracture? (p. 218)

☐ What are the symptoms and signs of moderate to severe exertional compartment syndrome? (p. 219)

☐ What is an observable sign of moderate to severe Achilles tendinitis? (pp. 220-221)

☐ Where does an athlete experience pain if suffering from plantar fasciitis? (p. 222)

REFERENCES

Cavanaugh, P.R., and J.R. Robinson. 1989. A biomechanical perspective on stress fractures in NBA players. A final report to the National Basketball Association. Research partially supported by and submitted to the NBA.

Comstock, R.D., C.L. Collins, and E. E. Yard. National high school sports-related injury surveillance study, 2005-06 and 2006-07 school years (Personal communication, February 1, 2008).

Hinton, R.Y., A.E. Lincoln, J.L. Almquist, W.A. Douoguih, and K.M. Sharma. 2005. Epidemiology of lacrosse injuries in high school-aged girls and boys: A 3-year prospective study. *American Journal of Sports Medicine*, 33(9): 1305-1314.

CHAPTER 1

Facial and Scalp Injuries

IN THIS CHAPTER, YOU WILL LEARN:

- ▸ How to identify serious face, eye, and mouth injuries.
- ▸ How to provide appropriate first aid care for face, eye, and mouth injuries.
- ▸ Ways to prevent face, mouth, and eye injuries.
- ▸ How to determine when a face or scalp laceration requires medical attention.

INJURIES IN THIS CHAPTER

(continued)

Sports can be tough on the face and scalp. All it takes is one quick jab of an elbow or unexpected bounce of a ball and an athlete can end up sitting in an ophthalmologist's or oral surgeon's chair. The NATA (Powell and Barber-Foss 1999) found that face and scalp injuries were most prevalent in baseball, basketball, football, and softball (table 14.1).

Because these injuries involve the vital sensory organs such as the eyes, nose, mouth, and ears as well as an athlete's appearance, great care should be taken when evaluating and providing first aid care. Also, since an extensive network of blood vessels supplies the face, these injuries tend to bleed heavily.

FACE AND SCALP LACERATIONS

Because they tend to bleed heavily, face and scalp injuries can seem intimidating. Below you will find guidelines for evaluating which injuries require medical intervention as well as how to care for such injuries.

Page 297 in appendix A summarizes first aid care for a face or scalp laceration.

Table 14.1   Face and Scalp Injuries in High School Sports

Sport	Percentage of total injuries in that sport
Baseball	8.9
Basketball	10.0 (male) 6.7 (female)
Football	2.2
Softball	8.0

Adapted, by permission, from J.W. Powell and K.D. Barber-Foss, 1999, "Injury patterns in selected high school sports: A review of the 1995-1997 seasons," *Journal of Athletic Training* 34 (3): 277-284.

Face and Scalp Laceration

Cut, usually around the eyebrow (figure 14.1), chin, forehead, nose, or scalp.

Causes

- Direct blow or contact with an object such as a ball, elbow, or racquet

Ask if Experiencing Symptoms

- Pain

Check for Signs

- Rapid bleeding (Face and scalp lacerations tend to bleed heavily because of the extensive network of blood vessels in the area. However, they often look worse than they really are.)
- Swelling
- Possible bruising

FIRST AID

If the athlete doesn't have an obvious deformity at the site of the injury or signs of brain, spine, or other serious injury, do the following:

1. Place the athlete in a seated position.
2. Cover the injury with sterile gauze and apply pressure.
3. After bleeding stops, cover the injury with sterile gauze or bandage.
4. Send the athlete to a physician if the edges of the wound gape apart (they don't touch, as in figure 14.1), if you're unable to completely clean all debris out of the wound, or if a foreign body is embedded in the wound.
5. If bleeding does not stop, athlete is experiencing breathing problems, spine or head injury, or other unstable or serious injuries:
   a. Send for emergency medical assistance
   b. Monitor breathing and provide CPR as needed
   c. Monitor and treat for shock as needed

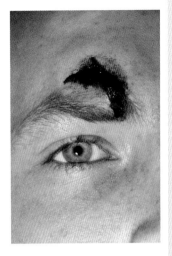

Figure 14.1 Face laceration.
© Scott Camazine/Phototake.

Playing Status

- If the edges of the wound gape open, there is concern about disfiguration, or the athlete was sent to a physician, the athlete cannot return to activity until examined and released by a physician.
- If bleeding stops, the edges of the wound are touching, and the athlete and parents are not concerned about disfiguration, the athlete can return to activity (the wound must be covered).

Prevention

- Require athletes to wear sport-appropriate protective equipment such as face masks, headgear, helmets, protective eyewear, and mouthguards.

EYE INJURIES

Sports can put the eyes at risk for devastating injuries. For instance, softball and baseball pitches have been clocked at over 90 miles per hour. Tennis, lacrosse, basketball, ice hockey, field hockey, and badminton are just as dangerous. The good news is that wearing protective eyewear or face guards can significantly reduce the risk of eye injury. In fact, the American Academy of Ophthalmology suggests that wearing protective eyewear could prevent 90 percent of eye injuries. Recommended eyewear contain polycarbonate lenses that are able to stop a sphere hurtling at 140 miles per hour or deflect an object impacting with over 1,200 pounds of force.

To fully understand eye injuries, let's look at basic eye anatomy (figure 14.2). On the outside of the eye is a tough white wall called the sclera. It's covered by a thin, moist, clear membrane, the conjunctiva, which protects and lubricates the eyeball and contains nerves and small blood vessels. The round, colored portion of the eye is the iris. It contains muscles that open and close the pupil (black dot in the center) in response to light. Light causes the muscles to contract, reducing the size of the pupil. The iris and pupil are covered by a clear membrane called the cornea that helps the eye to focus. The entire eye is housed within the orbit, a thin-walled, bony socket in the skull.

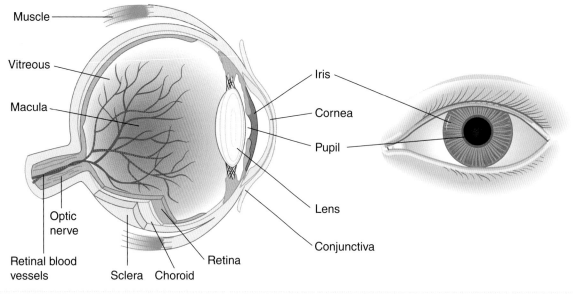

Figure 14.2 Eye anatomy.

For a summary of first aid care for serious eye injuries caused by a direct blow, see page 298 in appendix A, and page 299 summarizes first aid care for an eye abrasion.

Eye Contusion

Contusion to the structures of the eye.

Cause

- Direct blow (such as by an elbow or ball)

Ask if Experiencing Symptoms

- Blind spot
- Double vision
- Floating spots in vision
- Persistent blurred vision
- Pain
- Perception of flashing light

Check for Signs

- Blood pooling in white of eye or iris (figure 14.3)
- Restricted eye motion
- Irregularly shaped iris or pupil (figure 14.4)
- Cut to the cornea (figure 14.5)
- Dark tissue sticking out of cornea or sclera

- Pupil inequality (reaction to light, size, tracking)
- Inability to open eye
- Loss of peripheral vision
- Palpable defect of bones around the eye
- Sensitivity to light
- Pupils misaligned (one higher than other)

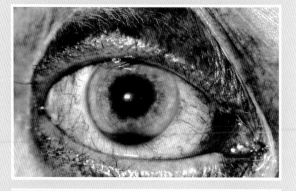

Figure 14.3 Blood pooling in eye.
© Custom Medical Stock Photo.

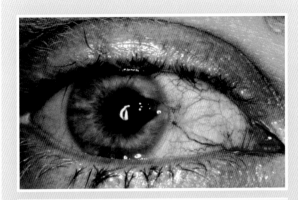

Figure 14.4 Irregular pupil.
© Bruce Coleman, Inc./Photoshot.

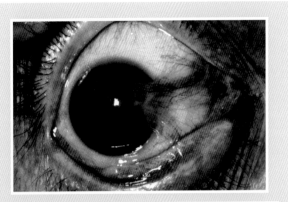

Figure 14.5 Corneal laceration.
© Custom Medical Stock Photo.

⊕ FIRST AID

1. Call for emergency medical assistance.
2. Seat the athlete in an upright or semireclining position (45 degrees).
3. If emergency assistance is delayed more than 15 minutes, loosely apply an eye patch over both eyes (to limit motion).
4. Monitor breathing and provide CPR as needed.
5. Monitor and treat for shock as needed.
6. Begin physical assessment.

Playing Status

- The athlete cannot return to activity until examined and released by a physician.

Prevention

- Encourage athletes to wear protective glasses, goggles, or face shields designed specifically for sports.

Object Embedded in Eye

Eye tissue is penetrated by a splinter or other object.

Cause

- Object punctures eye

Ask if Experiencing Symptoms

- Pain
- Burning

Check for Signs

- Blood pooling in white of eye or iris
- Irregularly shaped iris or pupil
- Cut to the cornea
- Dark tissue sticking out of cornea or sclera
- Embedded object

(continued)

⊕ FIRST AID

1. Call for emergency medical assistance.

2. Seat the athlete in an upright or semireclining position (45 degrees).

3. If emergency personnel is delayed more than 15 minutes, loosely apply a shield over the embedded object to prevent it from moving (figure 14.6).

4. Monitor breathing and provide CPR as needed.

5. Monitor and treat for shock as needed.

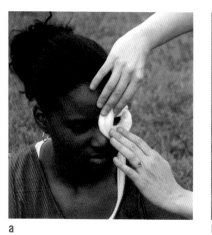
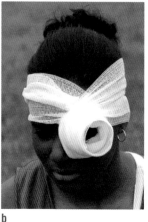

a   b

Figure 14.6   First aid care for embedded objects in eye include *(a)* loosely applying donut-shaped gauze padding around the eye and *(b)* placing paper cup securely in place with roller gauze and tape.

Playing Status

- The athlete cannot return to activity until examined and released by a physician.

Prevention

- Encourage athletes to wear protective glasses, goggles, or face shields designed specifically for sports.

Eye Abrasion

Superficial scratch to the clear part (cornea) covering the eye.

Cause

- Dirt, sand, or other foreign material in the eye

Ask if Experiencing Symptoms

- Pain
- Burning sensation
- Sensation of something in eye

Check for Signs

- Redness
- Tearing
- Possible foreign object in the eye
- Decreased vision
- Blurred vision
- Sensitivity to light
- Possible scratch on the eye

⊕ FIRST AID

Unless the object is glass, try to remove any small irritating particle such as dirt, as shown in figure 14.7. If you are unable to remove the object or decrease the athlete's pain, if the athlete experiences loss or blurring of vision, or if the object is glass, do the following:

1. Seat the athlete in a semireclining position.

2. Loosely apply an eye patch, bandage, or cup over both eyes (figure 14.8). Otherwise, movements of the uninjured eye will cause the injured eye to move.

3. Immediately send the athlete to a physician.

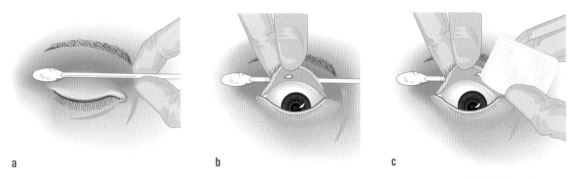

a   b   c

Figure 14.7   If the object is under the upper eyelid, *(a)* place a cotton tip applicator over the lid, *(b)* pull the lid up with your fingers, and then *(c)* remove the object with sterile gauze. (Be sure to moisten the gauze with sterile saline solution.)

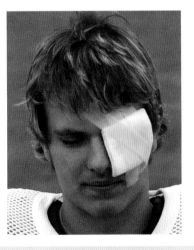

Figure 14.8   To cover the eye with a patch, loosely place sterile gauze over eye then lightly secure the gauze to the face with tape.

Playing Status

- If the athlete has persistent pain or blurred or decreased vision, the athlete cannot return to activity until examined and released by a physician.

Prevention

- Recommend wearing protective eyeglasses, goggles, or shields.

Playing It Safe...
With Eye Abrasions

If an athlete has an eye abrasion, follow these precautions:

- Do not rub the eye.
- Do not remove embedded objects.
- Do not remove glass.
- Do not remove contact lenses.
- Do not wash the eye.

Fractured Eye Socket

Break in bony socket surrounding the eye.

Cause
- Direct blow

Ask if Experiencing Symptoms
- Pain
- Altered sensation beneath the eye

Check for Signs
- Eyelid swelling
- Double vision, particularly with upward gaze
- Restricted eye motion
- Irregularly shaped iris or pupil
- Palpable defect of bones around the eye
- Pupils misaligned (one higher than other)
- Discoloration
- Possible bleeding into the white of the eye or iris
- Deformity
- Sunken eye

⊕ FIRST AID

1. Call for emergency medical assistance.
2. Seat the athlete in an upright or semireclining position (45 degrees).
3. Monitor breathing and provide CPR as needed.
4. Monitor and treat for shock as needed.

Playing Status
- The athlete cannot return to activity until examined and released by a physician.

Prevention
- Recommend wearing protective eye goggles or face shields.

NOSE, FACIAL BONE, AND JAW INJURIES

Nose, face, and jaw fractures can affect breathing passages and therefore require a quick evaluation. Also, when evaluating these injuries, you should use a light "touch" to feel for deformities.

Bloody Nose

Bleeding from the nose.

Causes
- Direct blow
- Possible head injury
- High blood pressure
- Dry nasal passages

Ask if Experiencing Symptoms
- Pain if suffered a direct blow
- Stuffiness or nasal congestion

Check for Signs
- Bleeding

⊕ FIRST AID

1. Seat the athlete with the head forward.
2. Use sterile gauze and pinch the nostrils shut for 5 to 10 minutes to apply direct pressure, as in figure 14.9.
3. Send the athlete to a physician if the bleeding doesn't stop within 15 to 20 minutes, or if it was caused by an injury.
4. Discourage the athlete from blowing nose.

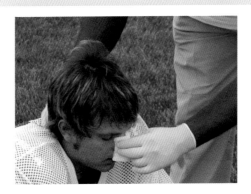

Figure 14.9   Direct pressure for bloody nose.

Playing Status

- The athlete can return to activity once the bleeding stops for five minutes.
- If the bleeding was caused by a more serious injury, the athlete must be examined and released by a physician before returning to activity.

Prevention

- Recommend wearing protective face masks and guards for football, ice hockey, and lacrosse.

Broken Nose

Break in the nose cartilage or bone.

Cause

- Direct blow

Ask if Experiencing Symptoms

- Pain
- Grating sensation

Check for Signs

- Swelling
- Discoloration
- Possible deformity
- Possible bleeding
- Inability to breathe through the nose

⊕ FIRST AID

1. Seat the athlete with the head forward to allow blood and fluid to drain from the nose.
2. Gently apply ice for 15 minutes. Gently pinch the nostrils shut with gauze if necessary to stop bleeding.
3. Send the athlete to a physician.

Playing Status

- The athlete cannot return to activity until examined and released by a physician.
- When returning to contact activity, the athlete should wear a nose protector.

Prevention

- Recommend wearing protective face masks and shields in football, lacrosse, and ice hockey.

Midface Fracture

Break of the facial bone (maxilla) above the mouth (figure 14.10).

Causes

- Direct blow

Ask if Experiencing Symptoms

- Pain
- Numbness

Check for Signs

- Inability to bring the teeth together properly
- Visual problems
- Nasal discharge (blood or other fluid)
- Bruising
- Deformity
- Tenderness when fractured area is touched

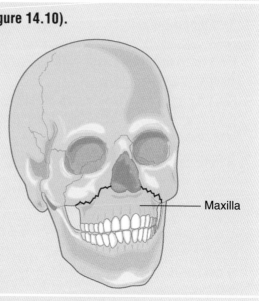

Maxilla

Figure 14.10   Midface fracture.

⊕ FIRST AID

1. If breathing is impaired or the athlete is suffering from shock, monitor breathing, administer CPR as needed, and call emergency medical personnel.

2. If the athlete is not experiencing breathing difficulties or shock, gently apply ice for 15 minutes and send the athlete to a physician.

Playing Status

- The athlete cannot return to activity until examined and released by a physician.
- When returning to activity, the athlete should wear a protective face shield.

Prevention

- Recommend wearing protective face guards for football, ice hockey, and lacrosse.

Cheekbone Fracture

Break in the cheekbone (zygomatic bone) (figure 14.11).

Causes

- Direct blow

Ask if Experiencing Symptoms

- Pain with jaw movement
- Altered sensation underneath the eye
- Pain or numbness in the face or cheeks

Check for Signs

- Flattened cheek or other deformity
- Blood in the side of the eye

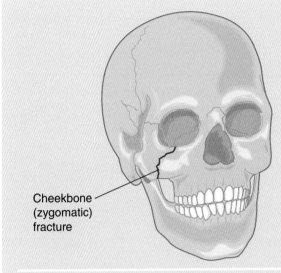

Cheekbone
(zygomatic)
fracture

Figure 14.11   Cheekbone (zygomatic) fracture.

✛ FIRST AID

1. If breathing is impaired or the athlete is suffering from shock, monitor breathing, administer CPR as needed, and call emergency medical personnel.
2. Otherwise, gently apply ice for 15 minutes and send the athlete to a physician.

Playing Status
- The athlete cannot return to activity until examined and released by physician.
- When returning to activity, the athlete should wear a protective face guard.

Prevention
- Recommend wearing protective face guards for football, ice hockey, and lacrosse.

Jaw Injury

Fracture, contusion, or dislocation of the jaw (mandible) (figure 14.12).

Causes
- Torsion injury or direct blow

Ask if Experiencing Symptoms
- Pain
- Popping sensation when opening and closing the mouth

Check for Signs
- Deformity
- Discoloration
- Swelling
- Inability to close the mouth
- Jaw may be out of place
- Occlusion—upper and lower teeth don't line up when jaw is closed

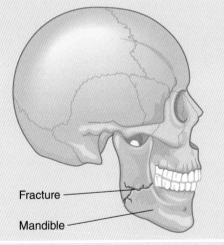

Fracture

Mandible

Figure 14.12   Jaw (mandible) fracture.

(continued)

Jaw Injury *(continued)*

✚ FIRST AID

If breathing is impaired, deformity is present, or the athlete is suffering from shock, do the following:

1. Send for emergency medical assistance.
2. Monitor breathing and administer CPR if needed.
3. If there is no suspected spine injury or shock, seat the athlete with the head forward to al-low fluid to drain from the mouth. If there is no suspected spine injury but the athlete is suffering from shock, lie the athlete on side, avoiding pressure to the jaw.

If breathing is not impaired, deformity is not present and the athlete is not suffering from shock, do the following:

1. Gently apply ice for 15 minutes and send the athlete to a physician.

Playing Status
- The athlete cannot return to activity until examined and released by a physician.

Prevention
- Recommend wearing helmets, mouth guards, and face masks when appropriate.

TOOTH INJURIES

The tooth is made up of the crown and root. The crown, the visible part, is covered by a hard outer coating (enamel). The root extends beneath the gum line and is covered by cemen-tum. Within the root, the pulp contains the blood supply for the tooth and nerve fibers that provide pain and temperature sensation. The pulp also produces the dentin. Dentin makes up most of the tooth and lies directly under the enamel. The tooth is held in a bony socket (alveolus) by a ligament and is protected by the gums (figure 14.13).

A variety of tooth injuries occur in sports, in-cluding dislocation, displacement, fracture, and chipping. Wearing custom-fitted mouth guards can prevent most of these injuries. In fact, a re-cent study of dental injuries in college basketball found that wearing custom-fitted mouth guards significantly reduced the number of dental inju-ries suffered by athletes and also the number of dental referrals for tooth injuries (Labella, Smith, and Sigurdsson 2002).

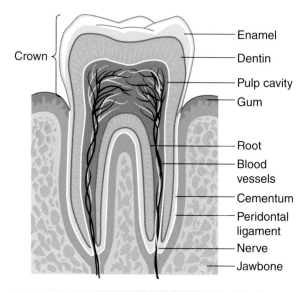

Figure 14.13 Tooth anatomy.

Dislocated Tooth

Tooth knocked out of socket.

Cause
- Direct blow

Ask if Experiencing Symptoms
- Pain

Check for Signs
- Bleeding
- Tooth totally dislodged
- Swelling of gums

➕ FIRST AID

1. Hold the tooth by the crown, not the root.
2. If the tooth is dirty, rinse (don't scrub) it with saline solution. Water can be used if saline is not available, but it can greatly decrease the chances of a successful reimplantation.
3. Place the tooth in a tooth saver container for the best chance of reimplantation. If you don't have one, placing the tooth in saline solution is the next best alternative. If saline solution isn't available, use a carton of milk.
4. Seat the athlete with the head forward to allow blood to drain from the mouth.
5. Clean bleeding wounds with saline solution or tap water.
6. Have the athlete bite down on a piece of sterile gauze to help soak up and slow bleeding.
7. Send the athlete to a dentist immediately! The best chance for successful reimplantation of the tooth is if it is done within 30 minutes of the injury.
8. If the athlete is experiencing breathing difficulties, shock, head or spine injury, compound facial fracture, or other unstable injuries:
   a. Send for emergency medical assistance
   b. Monitor breathing and provide CPR as needed
   c. Monitor and treat for shock as needed

Playing Status
- The athlete cannot return to activity until examined and released by a dentist or oral surgeon.

Prevention
- Require (if in rules) or recommend wearing mouth guards in contact sports.

Chipped Tooth

Break in a portion of tooth (figure 14.14).

Cause
- Direct blow

Ask if Experiencing Symptoms
- Pain (if broken down to the dentin or pulp)
- Sensitivity to heat, cold, or pressure if broken down to the dentin or pulp

Check for Signs
- Part of the tooth missing
- Bleeding
- Visible crack

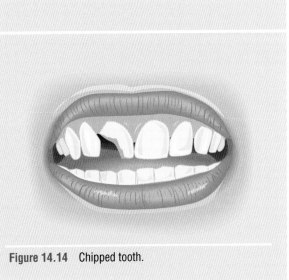

Figure 14.14 Chipped tooth.

(continued)

Chipped Tooth   *(continued)*

1. Seat the athlete with the head forward to allow blood to drain from the mouth.

2. Apply pressure with sterile gauze to areas that are bleeding.

3. Send the athlete to a dentist as quickly as possible.

Playing Status

- The athlete cannot return to activity until examined and released by a dentist.

Prevention

- Require (if in rules) or recommend wearing mouth guards in contact sports.

EAR INJURIES

The external ear is vulnerable to contusions, lacerations, and avulsions. Fortunately, these injuries are easily prevented with protective headgear and rules forbidding jewelry during practices and competitions. If an injury does occur, follow these first aid guidelines.

Ear Contusion (Cauliflower Ear)

Contusion to the ear (figure 14.15).

Causes

- Direct blow
- Repeated rubbing of the ear against a hard surface

Ask if Experiencing Symptoms

- Pain
- Burning feeling

Check for Signs

- Swelling of the outer ear
- Discoloration
- Warmth
- Redness
- Deformity

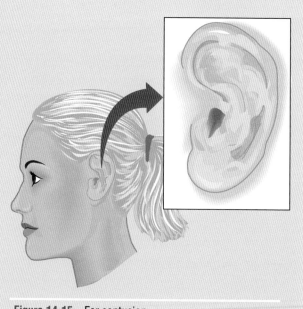

Figure 14.15   Ear contusion.

FIRST AID

1. Gently apply ice for 5 to 10 minutes.

2. Send the athlete to a physician.

Playing Status
- The athlete cannot return to activity until examined and released by a physician.

Prevention
- Recommend or require wearing protective headgear when appropriate.

Chapter 14 *REPLAY*

- ☐ Why do cuts to the face and head often bleed heavily? (p. 226)
- ☐ When should medical personnel immediately evaluate a face or scalp laceration? (p. 227)
- ☐ What can athletes do to prevent eye injuries? (p. 227)
- ☐ What are the signs and symptoms of an eye contusion (resulting from a direct blow)? (p. 228)
- ☐ Describe the first aid care for an eye with an embedded object. (p. 230)
- ☐ What part of the eye is injured in superficial abrasions? (p. 230)
- ☐ What is the first aid procedure for trying to remove a foreign object (not embedded) from the eye? (pp. 230-231)
- ☐ Describe the first aid care for a bloody nose. (p. 233)
- ☐ What are the signs and symptoms of a broken nose? (p. 233)
- ☐ What are some symptoms and signs of a facial fracture? (pp. 234-235)
- ☐ What can you do to provide the best chance to successfully reimplant a dislocated tooth? (p. 237)
- ☐ Describe the first aid care for a chipped tooth. (p. 238)
- ☐ What is a simple way to prevent ear avulsions? (p. 238)
- ☐ Describe the signs and symptoms of ear contusions. (p. 238)

REFERENCES

Labella, C.R., B.W. Smith, and A. Sigurdsson. 2002. Effect of mouth guards on dental injuries and concussions in college basketball. *Medicine and Science in Sports and Exercise* 34(1):41-44.

Powell, J.W., and K.D. Barber-Foss. 1999. Injury patterns in selected high school sports: A review of the 1995-1997 seasons. *Journal of Athletic Training* 34(3):227-284.

RESOURCES

www.aao.org (American Academy of Ophthalmology)

www.aoa.org (American Optometric Association)

www.preventblindness.org (Prevent Blindness America)

www.ada.org (American Dental Association)

www.sportsdentistry.com (Online Sports Dentistry)

CHAPTER 15

Skin Problems

IN THIS CHAPTER, YOU WILL LEARN:

- ► How to recognize and provide first aid care for common noncontagious skin conditions such as blisters and abrasions.
- ► How to recognize contagious skin conditions.
- ► When a skin condition requires a physician's evaluation.
- ► How to prevent contagious skin conditions from spreading among athletes.

Acommon characteristic of world-class athletes is the ability to concentrate or focus. Although your athletes may not be "world-class," concentration can mean the difference between winning and losing. Skin problems are a common source of distraction. And even worse, skin conditions can result in serious infections that sideline an athlete, or actually spread to other athletes.

Your first aid goal for skin problems should be to prevent your athletes from being sidelined or distracted by these seemingly minor problems. In this chapter, you'll learn how to recognize and administer first aid for skin disorders, how to determine when a skin disorder requires a physician's evaluation, and how to implement skin disorder prevention strategies. Skin disorders can be classified into two categories: noncontagious and contagious. Regardless of contagiousness, you should always wear protective gloves when handling skin conditions.

→ **Playing It Safe...**
With Skin Conditions

Always wear protective gloves when handling skin conditions, even if you think the condition is not contagious.

NONCONTAGIOUS SKIN CONDITIONS

Noncontagious skin conditions are quite common among athletes. Although they tend to be minor problems, it is important to monitor these conditions for signs of serious skin infection, such as pus, fever, and red streaks extending from the area.

See page 300 in appendix A for abrasion first aid protocol.

Blisters

Fluid-filled pockets between skin layers.

There are two types of blisters: open (figure 15.1) and closed. In closed blisters, the skin is still intact; in open blisters, the skin is torn.

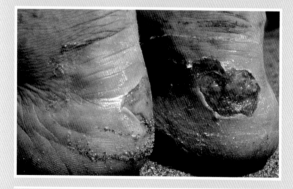

Figure 15.1 Open blister.
© Custom Medical Stock Photo.

Cause

- Friction from the skin rubbing against a surface (such as a shoe, bat, or racket handle) causes the skin layers to separate and fill with fluid

Ask if Experiencing Symptoms

- Pain
- Burning
- Warmth

Check for Signs

Closed

- Redness
- Fluid-filled bump underneath the skin

Open

- Torn skin
- Open wound or bleeding
- Redness

FIRST AID

Closed Blisters

1. Leave the blister intact (opening it may cause infection).

2. Adhere a commercial callus or corn pad (as shown in figure 15.2) over the blister to protect against further irritation and allow healing.

3. Instruct the athlete to keep the area clean.

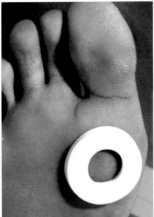

Figure 15.2 Blister donut pad.

Open Blisters

1. Clean the area with antiseptic solution or soap. Do not use iodine.

2. Dry with sterile gauze.

3. Adhere a commercial callus or corn pad (as shown in figure 15.2) over the blister to protect against further irritation and allow healing.

4. Instruct the athlete to keep the area clean.

5. Instruct the athlete to periodically check for signs of infection—redness, swelling, and warmth that progress to red streaks extending from wound, pus, and fever.

6. Immediately refer the athlete to a physician if the above signs of infection are present or if the blister doesn't heal after one to two weeks of self-care.

Playing Status

- The athlete can return to activity as long as there are no signs of serious infection.

Prevention

- Instruct athletes to file calluses to prevent excessive skin buildup.

- Instruct athletes to apply ice to "hot spots" (any skin area that is warm, red, and slightly tender, yet hasn't formed into a blister).

- Instruct athletes to apply petroleum jelly to areas of the foot that typically rub against the shoe.

- Encourage athletes to wear protective gloves in sports such as racquetball, baseball, weightlifting, and golf.

- Encourage athletes to wear appropriately fitted athletic shoes. Shoes should allow one-half of an inch between the longest toe and the end of the shoe and provide room for the widest part of the foot.

➤ Playing It Safe...
When Cleaning Wounds

When cleansing and caring for wounds, avoid using iodine. An athlete may have an iodine allergy.

Contused Nail

Blood between the nail bed and nail on a finger or toe (figure 15.3).

Cause
- Direct blow

Ask if Experiencing Symptoms
- Pain
- Feeling of pressure under nail

Check for Signs
- Blood or bruising under nail
- Swelling

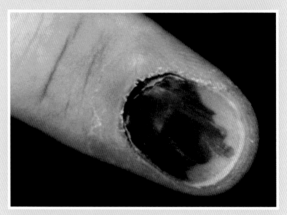

Figure 15.3 Contused nail.
© Custom Medical Stock Photo.

✛ FIRST AID

1. Apply ice immediately for 10 to 15 minutes to reduce swelling under the nail.

2. If more than 25 percent of the area of the nail bed is bruised, or if pain is severe, send the athlete to a physician.

Playing Status
- The athlete can return to activity as long as the nail is intact, the athlete is experiencing minimal pain, and there is little risk of further injury.

Prevention
- Instruct athletes to wear protective finger padding when appropriate.

Ingrown Toenail

Edge of the toenail pushes excessively into the skin (figure 15.4).

Causes
- Trimming nails at an angle—toward the sides
- Tight shoes or socks
- Toenail deformity

Ask if Experiencing Symptoms
- Pain on sides of toenail

Check for Signs
- Redness
- Warmth
- Swelling
- Pus (severe)

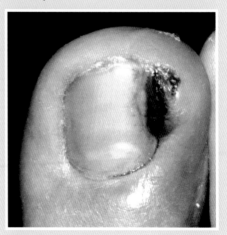

Figure 15.4 Ingrown toenail.
© Custom Medical Stock Photo.

Instruct the athlete to do the following:

1. Soak the foot in warm water.
2. Pack sterile cotton underneath the edge of the nail to reduce pressure against the skin. (Packing should be changed daily.)

3. Go to a physician if signs of infection (red streaks extending from the area, fever, pus, or warmth) appear or if the cotton packing does not help after a few days.

Playing Status

- The athlete can return to activity as long as there are no signs of serious infection—redness, swelling, and fever.

Prevention

- Instruct athletes to trim toenails straight across.
- Encourage athletes to wear properly fitted shoes.

Abrasion

Scraping injuries to the superficial skin layer that are also known as turf burns, road rash, or strawberries (figure 15.5).

Cause

- Sliding or falling against a rough or hard surface

Ask if Experiencing Symptoms

- Pain
- Tightness or pulling sensation over the abrasion
- Burning sensation

Check for Signs

- Raw, red patch of skin

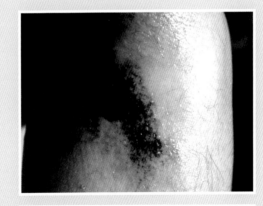

Figure 15.5 Abrasion.
© Bruce Coleman, Inc./Photoshot.

1. Rinse the area with clean running water for 5 minutes or more (use soap if necessary to remove dirt). For superficial abrasions, apply a triple antibiotic ointment or cream.
2. If the athlete is returning to activity, cover with sterile gauze.

3. To promote healing, instruct the athlete to leave the abrasion uncovered during daily activities.
4. Send the athlete to a physician if you are unable to completely clean debris from the wound, the wound edges gape open, or if it shows signs of infection.

Playing Status

- The athlete can return to activity as long as there are no signs of serious infection—pus, red streaks extending from the area, and fever.

Prevention

- Encourage athletes to wear sliding pants or to wear protective padding over the elbows, knees, and hips.

Boils

Large, infected, pus-filled bumps (figure 15.6) on the skin.

Cause

- Bacterial infection of a hair follicle

Ask if Experiencing Symptoms

- Pain
- Warmth

Check for Signs

- Red or white bump on the skin
- Localized swelling

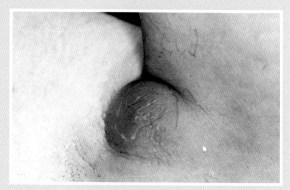

Figure 15.6　Boil.
© Welcome Trust Images/Custom Medical Stock Photo.

⊕ FIRST AID

Instruct the athlete to do the following:

1. Leave the boil intact.

2. Go to a physician.

Playing Status

- The athlete can return to activity as long as there are no signs of serious infection—redness, swelling, and fever.

Prevention

- Encourage athletes to shower after every practice and competition.

- Discourage athletes from wearing soiled, damp practice clothes.
- Encourage athletes to wear newly laundered athletic clothes for each practice and competition.

Poisonous Plant Rash

Skin reaction caused by contact with the oil from the sap of a poison ivy, poison oak, or poison sumac plant.

Causes

- Direct contact with poison ivy (figure 15.7), poison oak (figure 15.8), or poison sumac (figure 15.9) plant
- Contact with animals, clothing, tools, or sports equipment that are contaminated with the plant's oil
- Inhalation of or skin exposure to airborne oil particles of burning plants

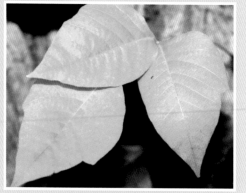

Figure 15.7　Poison ivy.
© Sally Weigand.

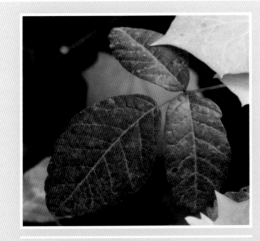

Figure 15.8 Poison oak.
© Custom Medical Stock Photo.

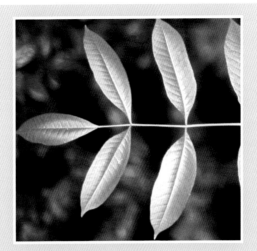

Figure 15.9 Poison sumac.
© David Liebman.

Ask if Experiencing Symptoms

Usually Within 12 to 48 Hours

- Burning
- Itching

Check for Signs

Usually Within 12 to 48 Hours

- Redness
- Rash
- Swelling
- Blisters
- High fever (if severe)
- Crusting and scaling of blisters

✛ FIRST AID

Within 5 minutes of exposure, instruct the athlete to do the following:

1. Carefully remove all contaminated clothing.
2. Flush exposed skin with cold, running water.

After rash develops, have the athlete do the following:

3. Go to a physician.
4. Avoid scratching the rash.

Playing Status

- The athlete can return to activity as long as there are no signs of serious infection—redness, swelling, and fever.

Prevention

- Learn to identify poison ivy, poison oak, and poison sumac plants.

- Clear the playing area of poison plants.
- Educate athletes about poison ivy and warn them of infested areas.
- If you suspect exposure to a poisonous plant, skin reaction may be decreased, if, within five minutes of exposure, contaminated clothing is removed and exposed skin is flushed with cool, running water.

CONTAGIOUS SKIN CONDITIONS

The following infections are considered contagious. Any athletes exhibiting signs and symptoms of these conditions should be sent to a physician for an evaluation of the condition, appropriate treatment, and release for return to participation.

Your role is to help detect such conditions and prevent infected athletes from coming into direct or indirect contact with others. You can prevent the spread of skin infections by assigning individual towels and water bottles and requiring shower shoes. It may be necessary to withhold athletes from participation until examined and released by a physician. For example, the National Federation of State High School Associations prohibits wrestlers with suspected skin infections from participating until examined and released by a physician (figure 15.10 on page 249). Regardless of contagiousness, you should always wear protective gloves when handling skin conditions. This is particularly important because of the recent increase in dangerous antibiotic-resistant bacteria that can infect damaged skin.

Community-acquired, Methicillin-resistant *Staphylococcus aureus* (CA-MRSA)

Reports of outbreaks of a potentially dangerous bacteria, methicillin-resistant *Staphylococcus aureus* (MRSA), have increased in the past few years. This bacteria can infect athletes' wounds. Staphylococcus aureus, also known as "staph," is estimated by the Center for Disease Control and Prevention (CDC) to be carried within the nose of about 30 percent of the population. The CDC also estimates that about one percent of the population carries the particularly dangerous variety that is resistant to methicillin and other related antibiotics.

Community-acquired MRSA (CA-MRSA) has been found to spread through person-to-person contact, shared towels, soaps, and improperly disinfected whirlpools and equipment. So as a coach, it's vital for you to be able to take steps to not only prevent the possible spread of infections, but also to recognize the symptoms and signs of possible CA-MRSA infections.

CA-MRSA infections typically appear as skin infections, like pimples or boils (see figure 15.11). The danger is that these infections may spread to other areas of the body and cause pneumonia and blood infections.

SAMPLE FORM
NATIONAL FEDERATION OF STATE HIGH SCHOOL ASSOCIATIONS
MEDICAL RELEASE FOR WRESTLER TO PARTICIPATE WITH SKIN LESION

Name _____

Date of exam _____ / _____ / _____

Mark location AND number of lesion(s)

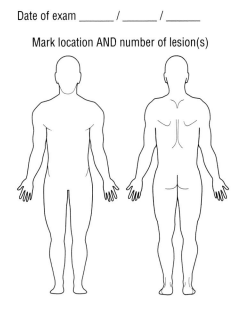

Diagnosis _____

_____

Location AND number of lesion(s) _____

_____

Medication(s) used to treat lesion(s) _____

_____

Date treatment started _____ / _____ / _____

Form expiration date: _____ / _____ / _____

Earliest date may return to participation _____ / _____ / _____

Provider signature _____

Provider name (must be legible)

_____

Office phone # _____

Office address _____

Note to appropriate health-care professionals: Noncontagious lesions do not require treatment prior to return to participation (e.g., eczema, psoriasis, etc.). Please familiarize yourself with NFHS Wrestling Rules 4-2-3, 4-2-4 and 4-2-5 which state:

ART.3: If a participant is suspected by the referee or coach of having a communicable skin disease or any other condition that makes participation appear inadvisable, the coach shall provide current written documentation, as defined by the NFHS or the state associations, from an appropriate health-care professional stating that the suspected disease or condition is not communicable and that the athlete's participation would not be harmful to any opponent. This document shall be furnished at the weigh-in for the dual meet or tournament. The only exception would be if a designated, on-site meet appropriate health-care professional is present and is able to examine the wrestler either immediately prior to or immediately after the weigh-in. Covering a communicable condition shall not be considered acceptable and does not make the wrestler eligible to participate.

ART.4: If a designated on-site meet appropriate health-care professional is present, he or she may overrule the diagnosis of the appropriate health-care professional signing the medical release form for a wrestler to participate or not participate with a particular skin condition.

ART.5: A contestant may have documentation from an appropriate health-care professional only indicating a specific condition such as a birthmark or other noncommunicable skin conditions such as psoriasis and eczema, and that documentation is valid for the duration of the season. It is valid with the understanding that a chronic condition could become secondarily infected and may require reevaluation.

Once a lesion is not considered contagious, it may be covered to allow participation.

Below are some treatment guidelines that suggest MINIMUM TREATMENT before return to wrestling:

Bacterial diseases (impetigo, boils): To be considered noncontagious, all lesions must be scabbed over with no oozing or discharge, and no new lesions should have occurred in the preceding 48 hours. Oral antibiotic for three days is considered a minimum to achieve that status. If new lesions continue to develop or drain after 72 hours, MRSA (Methicillin-Resistant Staphylococcus Aureus) should be considered.

Herpetic lesions (Simplex, fever blisters/cold sores, Zoster, Gladiatorum): To be considered noncontagious, all lesions must be scabbed over with no oozing or discharge, and no new lesions should have occurred in the preceding 48 hours. For primary (first episode of Herpes Gladiatorum), wrestlers should be treated and not allowed to compete for a minimum of 10 days. If general body signs and symptoms like fever and swollen lymph nodes are present, that minimum period of treatment should be extended to 14 days. Recurrent outbreaks require a minimum of 120 hours or five full days of oral antiviral treatment, again so long as no new lesions have developed and all lesions are scabbed over.

Tinea lesions (ringworm scalp, skin): Oral or topical treatment for 72 hours on skin and 14 days on scalp.

Scabies, head lice: 24 hours after appropriate topical management.

Conjunctivitis (pink eye): 24 hours of topical or oral medication and no discharge.

Revised/Approved by NFHS SMAC - April 2013

Figure 15.10 Sample contagious skin condition release form.

Adapted, with permission, from the National Federation of State High School Associations, 2013. [Online]. Available: www.nfhs.org [June 14, 2013].

Community-acquired, Methicillin-resistant Staphylococcus aureus (CA-MRSA)

A dangerous skin infection that can be transmitted in communal situations through personal contact or sharing toiletries or equipment.

Ask if Experiencing Symptoms

- Fever
- Localized pain at the site of the wound

Check for Signs

A wound that has

- Redness that spreads
- Swelling
- Pus
- Fluid drainage

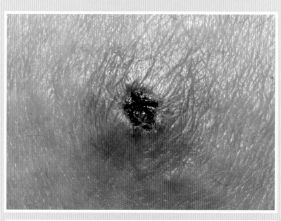

Figure 15.11 CA-MRSA infection
© Scott Camazine/PhotoTake USA.

✚ FIRST AID

1. Clean wounds with soap and water.
2. Cover wound to prevent spread.
3. Refer an athlete to a physician immediately if he or she shows symptoms or signs of a CA-MRSA infection.

Playing Status

- The athlete cannot return to activity until examined and released by a physician.

Prevention

1. Enforce strict hygiene policies:
   a. Showering immediately after activity
   b. Washing hands thoroughly and regularly with soap and water
   c. Prohibiting sharing of towels, water bottles, athletic equipment, and razors
   d. Washing athletic clothing and towels after each use
2. Regularly clean equipment, such as pads and helmets.
3. Regularly clean facilities such as mats, showers, floors, etc.
4. Cover all wounds before allowing an athlete to participate in practices or competitions.
5. Carefully watch wounds for signs of CA-MRSA infection.
6. Educate parents and athletes about proper hygiene and the signs and symptoms of CA-MRSA infections.
7. Prohibit athletes with open wounds from using shared whirlpools or tubs.

Molluscum Contagiosum

Skin growth caused by a viral infection in the top layers of the skin.

Cause

- Direct skin contact with the virus. Usually occurs at hair follicles or where the skin is broken.

Check for Signs

- Small flesh-colored or pink dome-shaped growths (figure 15.12)
- Often found in clusters on the skin of the chest, abdomen, arms, groin, or buttock and sometimes on face and eyelids
- May appear shiny
- Small indentation in the center
- May become red or inflamed

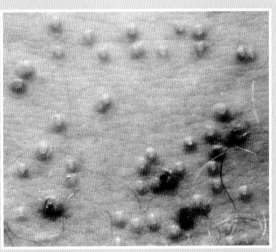

Figure 15.12 Molluscum contagiosum.
© Wellcome Image Library/Custom Medical Stock Photo.

⊕ FIRST AID

1. Send the athlete to a physician for accurate diagnosis and appropriate medication or treatment.

Playing Status

- Check your sport rules for regulations regarding participation with molluscum contagiosum.

Prevention

- Prevent direct contact of an infected athlete with other athletes.
- Prevent indirect contact with an infected athlete via shared towels, and shower and locker room floors (use shower shoes).
- Regularly clean facilities such as mats, showers, floors, etc.

Wart

Abnormal skin growth.

There are two types of warts: common (figure 15.13), found on the fingers, back of the hand, and nail beds; and plantar (figure 15.14), found on the sole of the foot.

Cause

- Direct skin contact with the human papillomavirus (HPV). Usually occurs where the skin is broken.

Ask if Experiencing Symptoms

- Pain

Check for Signs

- Localized skin growth
- "Seeds"—black dots in the wart caused by blood vessels (plantar wart)

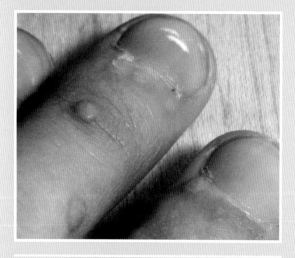

Figure 15.13 Common wart.
© Custom Medical Stock Photo.

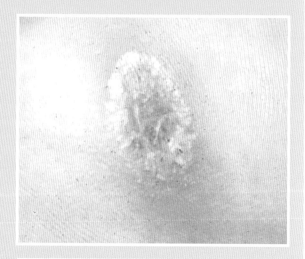

Figure 15.14 Plantar wart.
© Custom Medical Stock Photo.

⊕ FIRST AID

1. Send the athlete to a physician for accurate diagnosis and appropriate medication or treatment.

Playing Status

- The athlete can participate in activity if an exposed common wart is covered with sterile gauze.

Prevention

- Prevent direct contact of an infected athlete with other athletes.
- Prevent indirect contact with an infected athlete via shared towels, and shower and locker room floors (use shower shoes).

Herpes Simplex

Fever blister or cold sore (figure 15.15) on lips, mouth, nose, chin, or cheek.

Cause

- Contact with type 1 herpes simplex virus. Usually occurs from direct contact with an individual who carries the virus.

Ask if Experiencing Symptoms

- Itching
- Sensitive skin

Check for Signs

- Tiny, fluid-filled blisters
- Clear fluid oozing from broken blisters

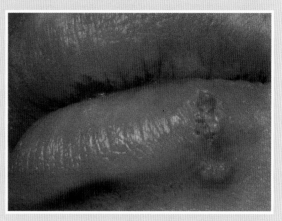

Figure 15.15 Herpes simplex (fever blister or cold sore).
© Bruce Coleman Inc./Photoshot.

⊕ FIRST AID

1. Send the athlete to a physician for accurate diagnosis and appropriate medication.

Playing Status

- Check your sport rules for regulations regarding participation with herpes simplex.

Prevention

- Prevent direct contact of an infected athlete with other athletes.
- Prevent indirect contact with an infected athlete via shared water bottles, towels, and the like.

Ringworm

Fungal infection of skin.

Cause

Direct contact with infected humans and animals, and less common, with infected soil. Of the skin disorders surveyed in the National Athletic Trainers' Association high school injury study (1997-1999), ringworm accounted for 83.8 percent of all reported skin conditions.

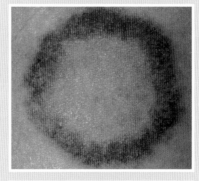

Figure 15.16 Ringworm.
© Custom Medical Stock Photo.

Ask if Experiencing Symptoms

- Pain
- Itching
- Burning

Check for Signs

- Red, scaly patches of skin
- As healing progresses from the middle of the infected area, the lesion will begin to look like a "ring" (figure 15.16)

(continued)

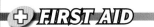 **FIRST AID**

1. Send the athlete to a physician for accurate diagnosis and appropriate treatment.

Playing Status

• Check your sport rules for regulations regarding participation with ringworm.

Prevention

• Prevent direct contact of an infected athlete with other athletes.

• Prevent indirect contact with an infected athlete via towels and clothing.

Athlete's Foot

Fungal infection affecting the feet (figure 15.17).

Cause

• Prolonged exposure of feet to a sweaty, hot, and poorly ventilated environment. (An example would be leather shoes with dirty, wet socks.)

Ask if Experiencing Symptoms

• Burning

• Itching

Check for Signs

• Red, scaly rash around the toes and other areas of the feet

• Peeling or cracking skin

• Blisters (severe cases)

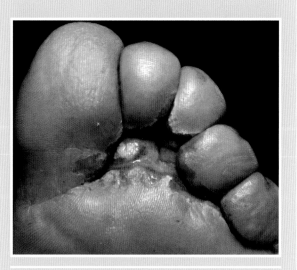

Figure 15.17 Athlete's foot.
© Custom Medical Stock Photo.

FIRST AID

Instruct the athlete to do the following:

1. Frequently change socks to keep feet dry.
2. Wash and thoroughly dry feet daily.
3. Apply antifungal cream or powder to the area.
4. Go to a physician if symptoms persist.

Playing Status

• The athlete can participate as long as the infected area is not exposed to other athletes.

Prevention

• Instruct athletes to keep feet clean and dry.

• Encourage athletes to use foot powder to absorb sweat.

• Encourage athletes to always wear clean socks.

• Require shower shoes to prevent fungus from spreading among athletes.

Jock Itch

Fungal infection affecting the genital area.

Cause

- Prolonged exposure of the skin to a sweaty, hot environment. (An example would be re-wearing soiled, damp practice clothes.)

Ask if Experiencing Symptoms

- Burning
- Itching

Check for Signs

- Red, scaly patches of skin

✚ FIRST AID

Instruct the athlete to do the following:

1. Keep the area dry by changing wet, sweaty clothing.
2. Apply cream or antifungal powder to the infected area.
3. See a physician if symptoms persist.

Playing Status

- The athlete can participate in activity as tolerated.

Prevention

- Instruct athletes to use powder to help absorb sweat.
- Encourage athletes to wear clean workout clothes daily.

Chapter 15 REPLAY

- ☐ How should you protect yourself when providing first aid care for skin conditions? (p. 242)
- ☐ What are the signs and symptoms of a serious skin infection? (p. 242)
- ☐ What can be applied to blisters to prevent further irritation? (p. 243)
- ☐ When should a nail contusion be evaluated and treated by a physician? (p. 244)
- ☐ What first aid technique may help relieve pressure from an ingrown toenail? (p. 245)
- ☐ What first aid technique helps promote healing of abrasions? (p. 245)
- ☐ What is a boil? (p. 246)
- ☐ What first aid technique can be immediately used to reduce the skin reaction caused by poisonous (ivy, oak, and sumac) plants? (p. 247)
- ☐ What substances cause contagious skin infections? (pp. 250-255)
- ☐ Describe the steps that can be taken to reduce the spread of a contagious skin condition among athletes. (pp. 250-255)
- ☐ What can athletes do to help prevent bacterial and fungal skin infections? (pp. 250-255)

REFERENCES

Center for Disease Control and Prevention. Community-Associated MRSA Information for the Public. Retrieved at www.cdc.gov/ncidod/dhqp/ar_mrsa_ca_public.html#2.

National Athletic Trainers Association. (2005). Official Statement from the National Athletic Trainers Association on Community-Acquired MRSA Infections (CA-MRSA). Retrieved at www.nata.org/statements/official/MRSA_Statement.pdf.

National Athletic Trainers' Association. High school wrestlers risk contagious skin infections. Press release. Accessed at www.nata.org/publications/otherpub/injuryinformation.htm.

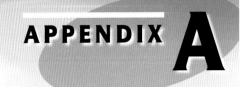

First Aid Protocols

(continued)

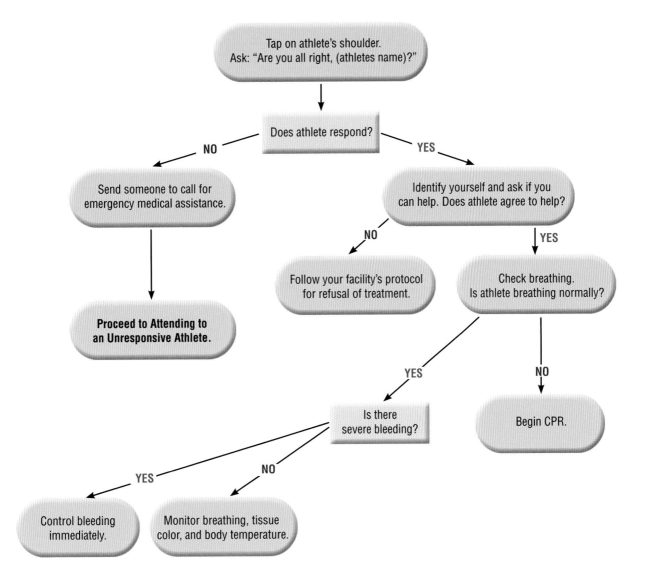

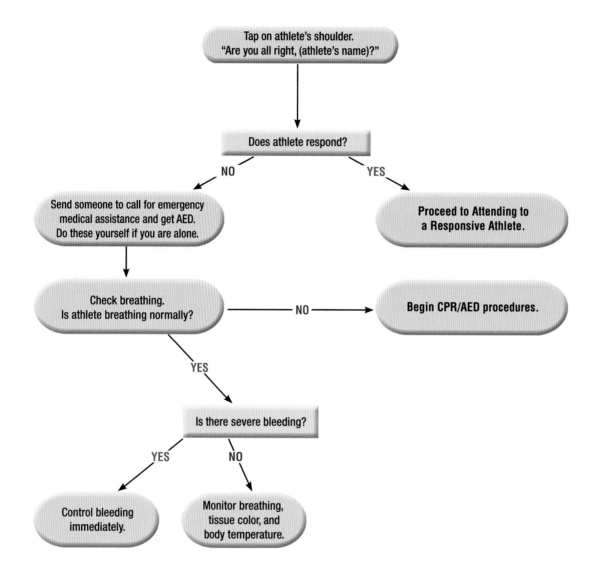

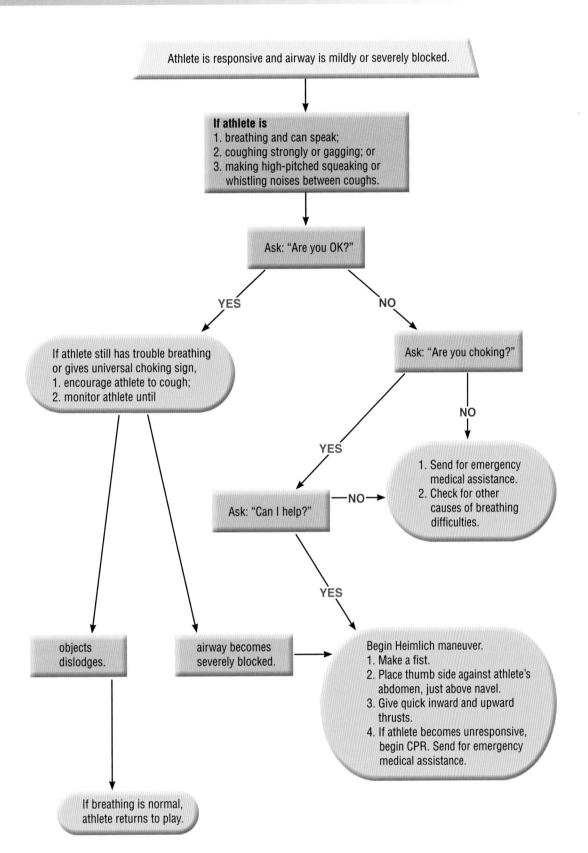

Athlete is responsive and airway is mildly or severely blocked.

If athlete is
1. breathing and can speak;
2. coughing strongly or gagging; or
3. making high-pitched squeaking or whistling noises between coughs.

Ask: "Are you OK?"

YES

NO

If athlete still has trouble breathing or gives universal choking sign,
1. encourage athlete to cough;
2. monitor athlete until

Ask: "Are you choking?"

NO

1. Send for emergency medical assistance.
2. Check for other causes of breathing difficulties.

YES

Ask: "Can I help?"

NO

YES

objects dislodges.

airway becomes severely blocked.

Begin Heimlich maneuver.
1. Make a fist.
2. Place thumb side against athlete's abdomen, just above navel.
3. Give quick inward and upward thrusts.
4. If athlete becomes unresponsive, begin CPR. Send for emergency medical assistance.

If breathing is normal, athlete returns to play.

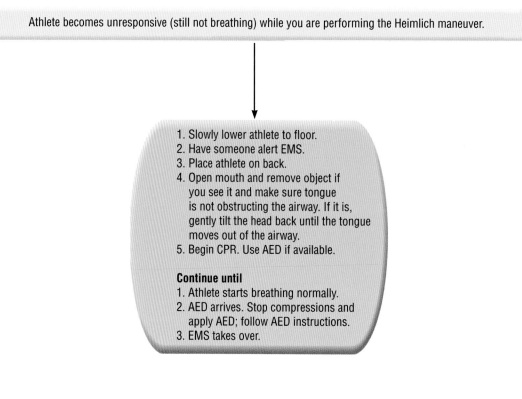

Athlete becomes unresponsive (still not breathing) while you are performing the Heimlich maneuver.

1. Slowly lower athlete to floor.
2. Have someone alert EMS.
3. Place athlete on back.
4. Open mouth and remove object if you see it and make sure tongue is not obstructing the airway. If it is, gently tilt the head back until the tongue moves out of the airway.
5. Begin CPR. Use AED if available.

Continue until
1. Athlete starts breathing normally.
2. AED arrives. Stop compressions and apply AED; follow AED instructions.
3. EMS takes over.

Note: Athlete may not return to play until he or she has been evaluated by EMS and checked by a physician.

Cardiopulmonary Resuscitation (CPR)

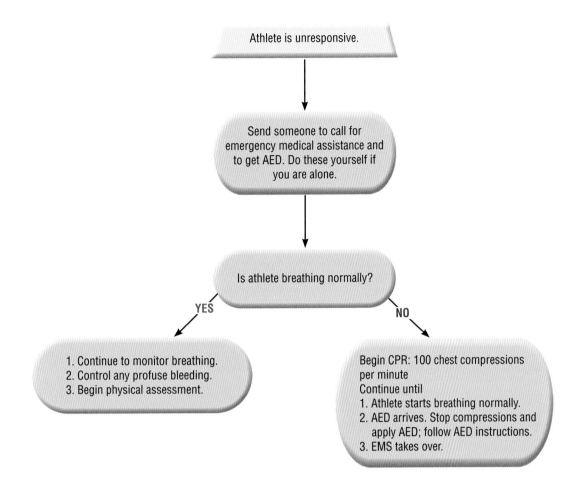

Athlete is unresponsive.

Send someone to call for emergency medical assistance and to get AED. Do these yourself if you are alone.

Is athlete breathing normally?

YES

1. Continue to monitor breathing.
2. Control any profuse bleeding.
3. Begin physical assessment.

NO

Begin CPR: 100 chest compressions per minute
Continue until
1. Athlete starts breathing normally.
2. AED arrives. Stop compressions and apply AED; follow AED instructions.
3. EMS takes over.

Using an Automated External Defibrillator (AED)

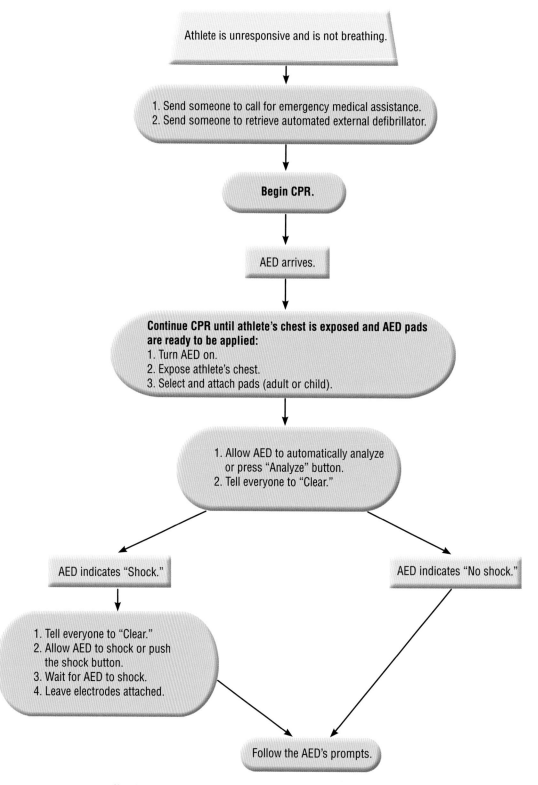

Athlete is unresponsive and is not breathing.

1. Send someone to call for emergency medical assistance.
2. Send someone to retrieve automated external defibrillator.

Begin CPR.

AED arrives.

Continue CPR until athlete's chest is exposed and AED pads are ready to be applied:
1. Turn AED on.
2. Expose athlete's chest.
3. Select and attach pads (adult or child).

1. Allow AED to automatically analyze or press "Analyze" button.
2. Tell everyone to "Clear."

AED indicates "Shock."

1. Tell everyone to "Clear."
2. Allow AED to shock or push the shock button.
3. Wait for AED to shock.
4. Leave electrodes attached.

AED indicates "No shock."

Follow the AED's prompts.

Note: If athlete becomes responsive and is breathing, monitor breathing and do physical assessment.

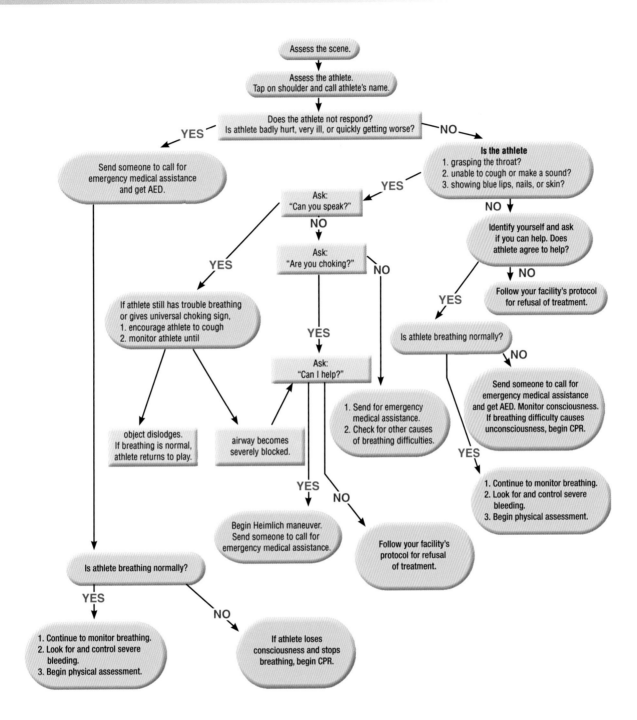

History

Determine:

injury location,
whether a reinjury,
injury mechanism, or
symptoms (e.g., headache,
pain, or numbness).

Inspection

Look for:

bleeding,
skin appearance,
pupil size and reaction,
deformities,
vomiting or coughing,
swelling,
discoloration,
ability to walk,
position of an upper
extremity, or
pulse rate.

Touch

Feel for:
point tenderness,
skin temperature,
sensation or numbness, or
deformity.

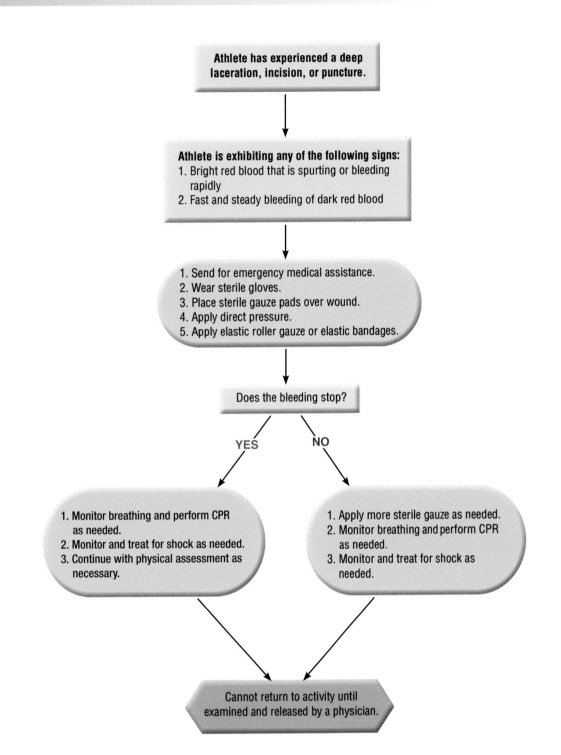

Athlete has experienced a deep laceration, incision, or puncture.

Athlete is exhibiting any of the following signs:
1. Bright red blood that is spurting or bleeding rapidly
2. Fast and steady bleeding of dark red blood

1. Send for emergency medical assistance.
2. Wear sterile gloves.
3. Place sterile gauze pads over wound.
4. Apply direct pressure.
5. Apply elastic roller gauze or elastic bandages.

Does the bleeding stop?

YES

NO

1. Monitor breathing and perform CPR as needed.
2. Monitor and treat for shock as needed.
3. Continue with physical assessment as necessary.

1. Apply more sterile gauze as needed.
2. Monitor breathing and perform CPR as needed.
3. Monitor and treat for shock as needed.

Cannot return to activity until examined and released by a physician.

Splinting Techniques for Unstable Injuries

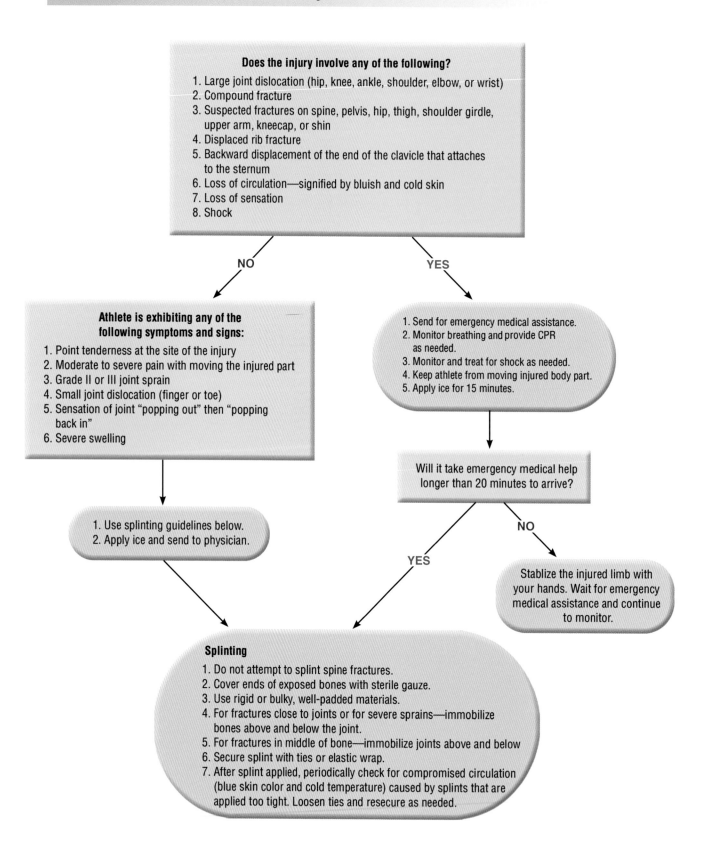

Does the injury involve any of the following?
1. Large joint dislocation (hip, knee, ankle, shoulder, elbow, or wrist)
2. Compound fracture
3. Suspected fractures on spine, pelvis, hip, thigh, shoulder girdle, upper arm, kneecap, or shin
4. Displaced rib fracture
5. Backward displacement of the end of the clavicle that attaches to the sternum
6. Loss of circulation—signified by bluish and cold skin
7. Loss of sensation
8. Shock

NO

YES

Athlete is exhibiting any of the following symptoms and signs:
1. Point tenderness at the site of the injury
2. Moderate to severe pain with moving the injured part
3. Grade II or III joint sprain
4. Small joint dislocation (finger or toe)
5. Sensation of joint "popping out" then "popping back in"
6. Severe swelling

1. Send for emergency medical assistance.
2. Monitor breathing and provide CPR as needed.
3. Monitor and treat for shock as needed.
4. Keep athlete from moving injured body part.
5. Apply ice for 15 minutes.

1. Use splinting guidelines below.
2. Apply ice and send to physician.

Will it take emergency medical help longer than 20 minutes to arrive?

YES

NO

Stablize the injured limb with your hands. Wait for emergency medical assistance and continue to monitor.

Splinting
1. Do not attempt to splint spine fractures.
2. Cover ends of exposed bones with sterile gauze.
3. Use rigid or bulky, well-padded materials.
4. For fractures close to joints or for severe sprains—immobilize bones above and below the joint.
5. For fractures in middle of bone—immobilize joints above and below
6. Secure splint with ties or elastic wrap.
7. After splint applied, periodically check for compromised circulation (blue skin color and cold temperature) caused by splints that are applied too tight. Loosen ties and resecure as needed.

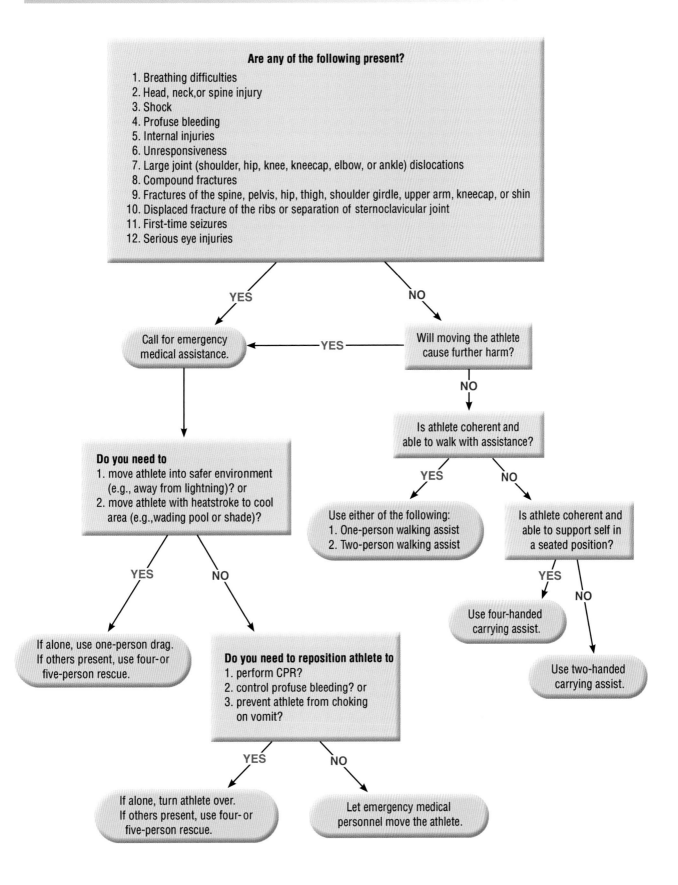

Are any of the following present?

1. Breathing difficulties
2. Head, neck, or spine injury
3. Shock
4. Profuse bleeding
5. Internal injuries
6. Unresponsiveness
7. Large joint (shoulder, hip, knee, kneecap, elbow, or ankle) dislocations
8. Compound fractures
9. Fractures of the spine, pelvis, hip, thigh, shoulder girdle, upper arm, kneecap, or shin
10. Displaced fracture of the ribs or separation of sternoclavicular joint
11. First-time seizures
12. Serious eye injuries

YES → Call for emergency medical assistance.

NO → Will moving the athlete cause further harm?

YES → Call for emergency medical assistance.

NO → Is athlete coherent and able to walk with assistance?

YES → Use either of the following:
1. One-person walking assist
2. Two-person walking assist

NO → Is athlete coherent and able to support self in a seated position?

YES → Use four-handed carrying assist.

NO → Use two-handed carrying assist.

Do you need to
1. move athlete into safer environment (e.g., away from lightning)? or
2. move athlete with heatstroke to cool area (e.g., wading pool or shade)?

YES → If alone, use one-person drag. If others present, use four- or five-person rescue.

NO → **Do you need to reposition athlete to**
1. perform CPR?
2. control profuse bleeding? or
3. prevent athlete from choking on vomit?

YES → If alone, turn athlete over. If others present, use four- or five-person rescue.

NO → Let emergency medical personnel move the athlete.

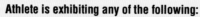

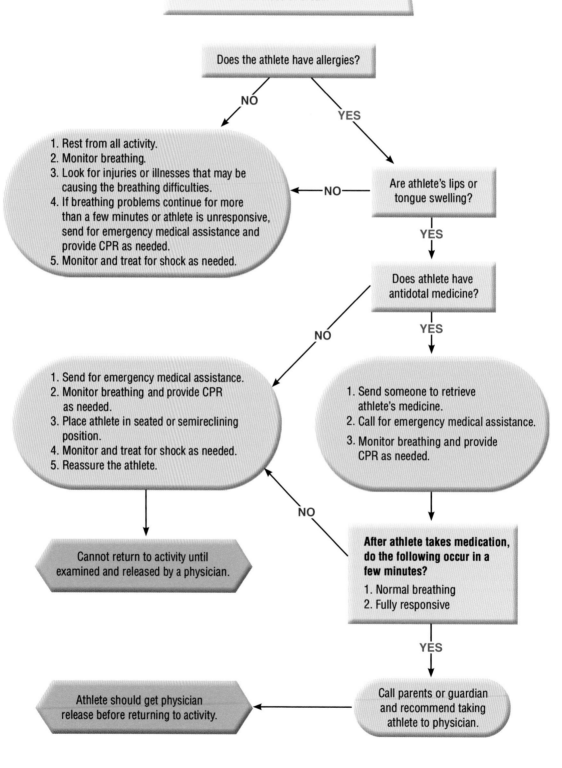

Athlete is exhibiting any of the following:
1. Wheezing
2. Coughing
3. Shortness of breath

Does the athlete have allergies?

NO   YES

1. Rest from all activity.
2. Monitor breathing.
3. Look for injuries or illnesses that may be causing the breathing difficulties.
4. If breathing problems continue for more than a few minutes or athlete is unresponsive, send for emergency medical assistance and provide CPR as needed.
5. Monitor and treat for shock as needed.

NO

Are athlete's lips or tongue swelling?

YES

Does athlete have antidotal medicine?

NO   YES

1. Send for emergency medical assistance.
2. Monitor breathing and provide CPR as needed.
3. Place athlete in seated or semireclining position.
4. Monitor and treat for shock as needed.
5. Reassure the athlete.

1. Send someone to retrieve athlete's medicine.
2. Call for emergency medical assistance.
3. Monitor breathing and provide CPR as needed.

Cannot return to activity until examined and released by a physician.

NO

After athlete takes medication, do the following occur in a few minutes?
1. Normal breathing
2. Fully responsive

YES

Athlete should get physician release before returning to activity.

Call parents or guardian and recommend taking athlete to physician.

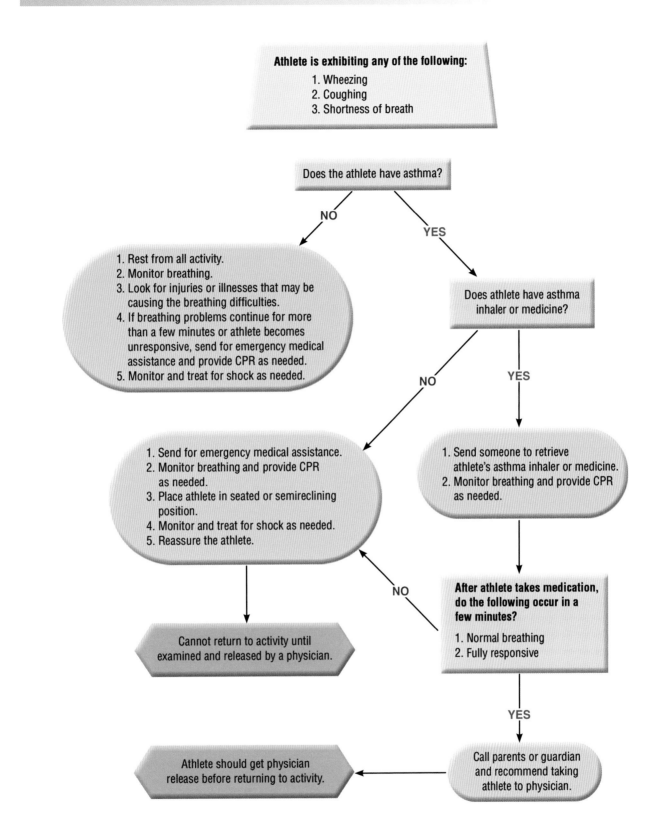

Athlete is exhibiting any of the following:
1. Wheezing
2. Coughing
3. Shortness of breath

Does the athlete have asthma?

NO

YES

1. Rest from all activity.
2. Monitor breathing.
3. Look for injuries or illnesses that may be causing the breathing difficulties.
4. If breathing problems continue for more than a few minutes or athlete becomes unresponsive, send for emergency medical assistance and provide CPR as needed.
5. Monitor and treat for shock as needed.

Does athlete have asthma inhaler or medicine?

NO

YES

1. Send for emergency medical assistance.
2. Monitor breathing and provide CPR as needed.
3. Place athlete in seated or semireclining position.
4. Monitor and treat for shock as needed.
5. Reassure the athlete.

1. Send someone to retrieve athlete's asthma inhaler or medicine.
2. Monitor breathing and provide CPR as needed.

Cannot return to activity until examined and released by a physician.

NO

After athlete takes medication, do the following occur in a few minutes?

1. Normal breathing
2. Fully responsive

YES

Athlete should get physician release before returning to activity.

Call parents or guardian and recommend taking athlete to physician.

271

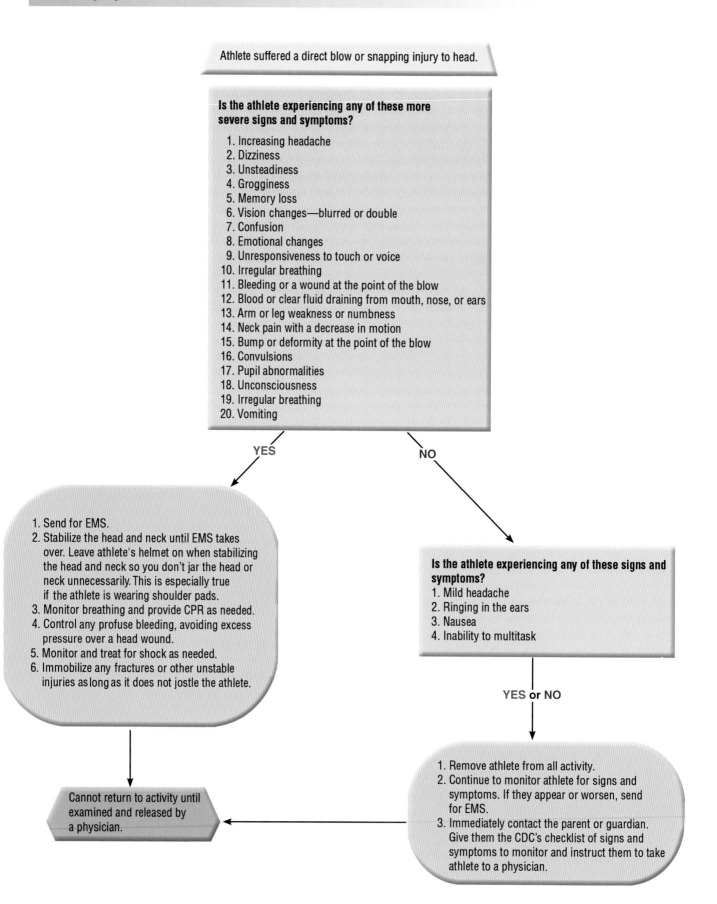

Athlete suffered a direct blow or snapping injury to head.

Is the athlete experiencing any of these more severe signs and symptoms?

1. Increasing headache
2. Dizziness
3. Unsteadiness
4. Grogginess
5. Memory loss
6. Vision changes—blurred or double
7. Confusion
8. Emotional changes
9. Unresponsiveness to touch or voice
10. Irregular breathing
11. Bleeding or a wound at the point of the blow
12. Blood or clear fluid draining from mouth, nose, or ears
13. Arm or leg weakness or numbness
14. Neck pain with a decrease in motion
15. Bump or deformity at the point of the blow
16. Convulsions
17. Pupil abnormalities
18. Unconsciousness
19. Irregular breathing
20. Vomiting

YES

NO

1. Send for EMS.
2. Stabilize the head and neck until EMS takes over. Leave athlete's helmet on when stabilizing the head and neck so you don't jar the head or neck unnecessarily. This is especially true if the athlete is wearing shoulder pads.
3. Monitor breathing and provide CPR as needed.
4. Control any profuse bleeding, avoiding excess pressure over a head wound.
5. Monitor and treat for shock as needed.
6. Immobilize any fractures or other unstable injuries as long as it does not jostle the athlete.

Is the athlete experiencing any of these signs and symptoms?
1. Mild headache
2. Ringing in the ears
3. Nausea
4. Inability to multitask

YES or NO

Cannot return to activity until examined and released by a physician.

1. Remove athlete from all activity.
2. Continue to monitor athlete for signs and symptoms. If they appear or worsen, send for EMS.
3. Immediately contact the parent or guardian. Give them the CDC's checklist of signs and symptoms to monitor and instruct them to take athlete to a physician.

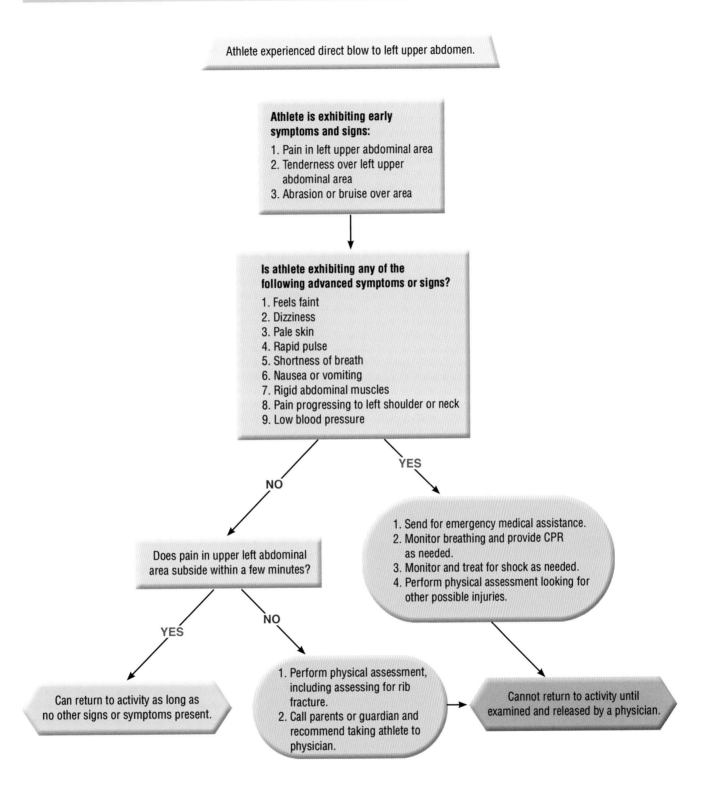

Athlete experienced direct blow to left upper abdomen.

Athlete is exhibiting early symptoms and signs:

1. Pain in left upper abdominal area
2. Tenderness over left upper abdominal area
3. Abrasion or bruise over area

Is athlete exhibiting any of the following advanced symptoms or signs?

1. Feels faint
2. Dizziness
3. Pale skin
4. Rapid pulse
5. Shortness of breath
6. Nausea or vomiting
7. Rigid abdominal muscles
8. Pain progressing to left shoulder or neck
9. Low blood pressure

NO

YES

Does pain in upper left abdominal area subside within a few minutes?

1. Send for emergency medical assistance.
2. Monitor breathing and provide CPR as needed.
3. Monitor and treat for shock as needed.
4. Perform physical assessment looking for other possible injuries.

YES

NO

Can return to activity as long as no other signs or symptoms present.

1. Perform physical assessment, including assessing for rib fracture.
2. Call parents or guardian and recommend taking athlete to physician.

Cannot return to activity until examined and released by a physician.

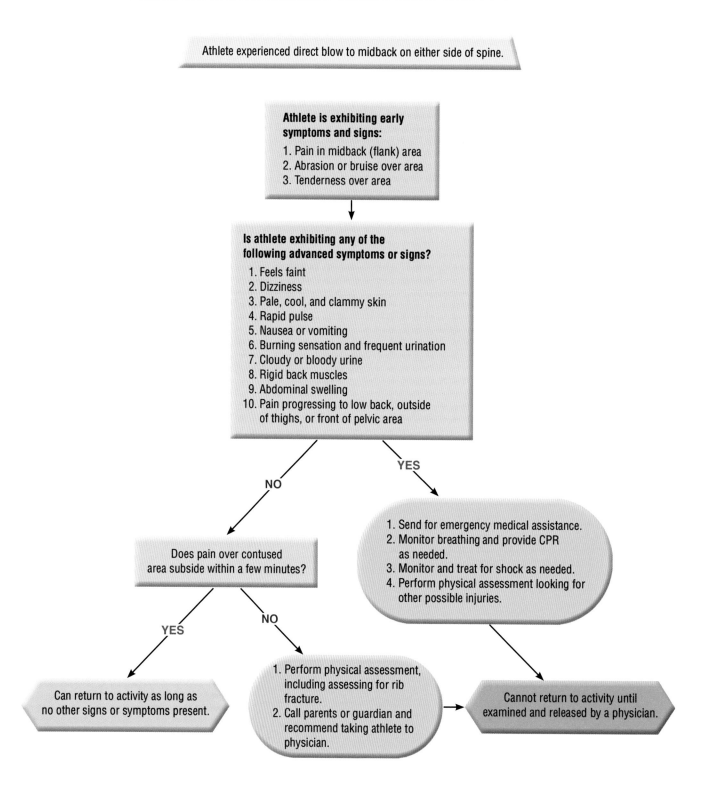

Athlete experienced direct blow to midback on either side of spine.

Athlete is exhibiting early symptoms and signs:

1. Pain in midback (flank) area
2. Abrasion or bruise over area
3. Tenderness over area

Is athlete exhibiting any of the following advanced symptoms or signs?

1. Feels faint
2. Dizziness
3. Pale, cool, and clammy skin
4. Rapid pulse
5. Nausea or vomiting
6. Burning sensation and frequent urination
7. Cloudy or bloody urine
8. Rigid back muscles
9. Abdominal swelling
10. Pain progressing to low back, outside of thighs, or front of pelvic area

NO

YES

Does pain over contused area subside within a few minutes?

1. Send for emergency medical assistance.
2. Monitor breathing and provide CPR as needed.
3. Monitor and treat for shock as needed.
4. Perform physical assessment looking for other possible injuries.

YES

NO

Can return to activity as long as no other signs or symptoms present.

1. Perform physical assessment, including assessing for rib fracture.
2. Call parents or guardian and recommend taking athlete to physician.

Cannot return to activity until examined and released by a physician.

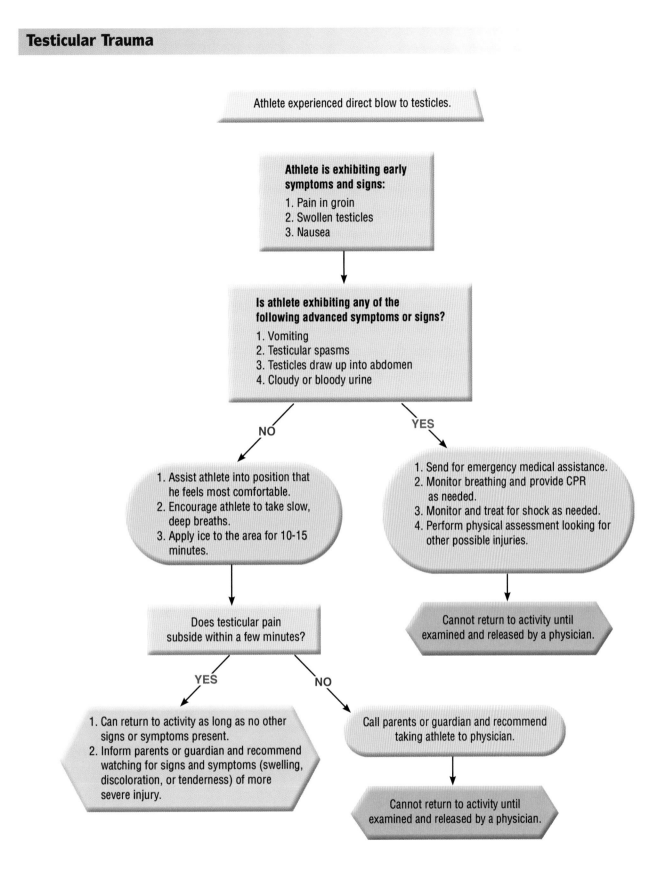

Athlete experienced direct blow to testicles.

Athlete is exhibiting early symptoms and signs:

1. Pain in groin
2. Swollen testicles
3. Nausea

Is athlete exhibiting any of the following advanced symptoms or signs?

1. Vomiting
2. Testicular spasms
3. Testicles draw up into abdomen
4. Cloudy or bloody urine

NO

1. Assist athlete into position that he feels most comfortable.
2. Encourage athlete to take slow, deep breaths.
3. Apply ice to the area for 10-15 minutes.

YES

1. Send for emergency medical assistance.
2. Monitor breathing and provide CPR as needed.
3. Monitor and treat for shock as needed.
4. Perform physical assessment looking for other possible injuries.

Does testicular pain subside within a few minutes?

Cannot return to activity until examined and released by a physician.

YES

1. Can return to activity as long as no other signs or symptoms present.
2. Inform parents or guardian and recommend watching for signs and symptoms (swelling, discoloration, or tenderness) of more severe injury.

NO

Call parents or guardian and recommend taking athlete to physician.

Cannot return to activity until examined and released by a physician.

Insulin Reaction

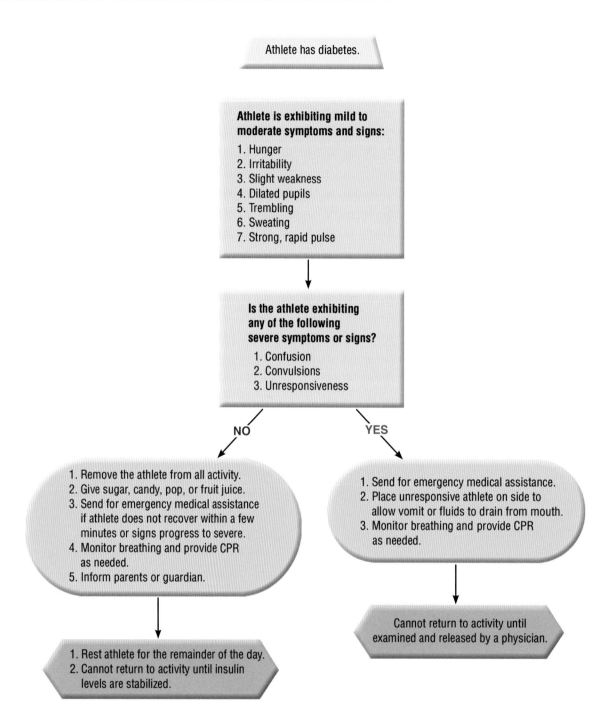

Athlete has diabetes.

Athlete is exhibiting mild to moderate symptoms and signs:

1. Hunger
2. Irritability
3. Slight weakness
4. Dilated pupils
5. Trembling
6. Sweating
7. Strong, rapid pulse

Is the athlete exhibiting any of the following severe symptoms or signs?

1. Confusion
2. Convulsions
3. Unresponsiveness

NO

1. Remove the athlete from all activity.
2. Give sugar, candy, pop, or fruit juice.
3. Send for emergency medical assistance if athlete does not recover within a few minutes or signs progress to severe.
4. Monitor breathing and provide CPR as needed.
5. Inform parents or guardian.

YES

1. Send for emergency medical assistance.
2. Place unresponsive athlete on side to allow vomit or fluids to drain from mouth.
3. Monitor breathing and provide CPR as needed.

1. Rest athlete for the remainder of the day.
2. Cannot return to activity until insulin levels are stabilized.

Cannot return to activity until examined and released by a physician.

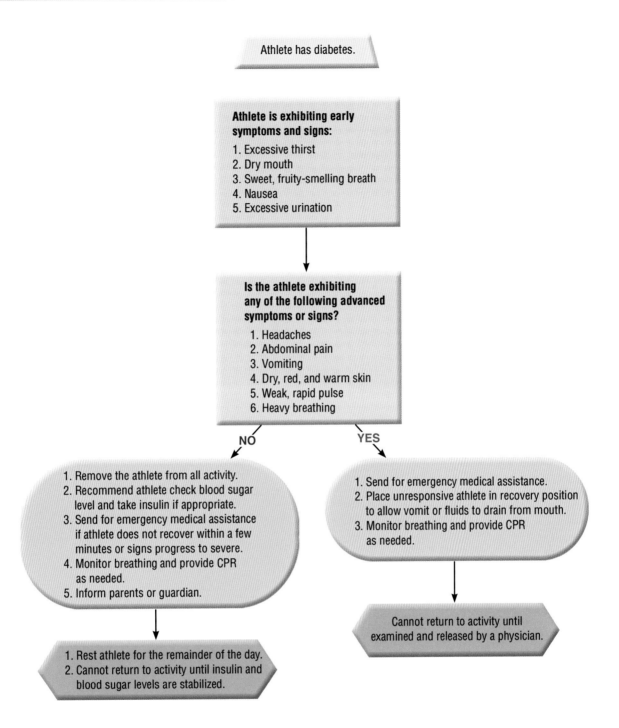

Athlete has diabetes.

Athlete is exhibiting early symptoms and signs:

1. Excessive thirst
2. Dry mouth
3. Sweet, fruity-smelling breath
4. Nausea
5. Excessive urination

Is the athlete exhibiting any of the following advanced symptoms or signs?

1. Headaches
2. Abdominal pain
3. Vomiting
4. Dry, red, and warm skin
5. Weak, rapid pulse
6. Heavy breathing

NO

1. Remove the athlete from all activity.
2. Recommend athlete check blood sugar level and take insulin if appropriate.
3. Send for emergency medical assistance if athlete does not recover within a few minutes or signs progress to severe.
4. Monitor breathing and provide CPR as needed.
5. Inform parents or guardian.

YES

1. Send for emergency medical assistance.
2. Place unresponsive athlete in recovery position to allow vomit or fluids to drain from mouth.
3. Monitor breathing and provide CPR as needed.

Cannot return to activity until examined and released by a physician.

1. Rest athlete for the remainder of the day.
2. Cannot return to activity until insulin and blood sugar levels are stabilized.

Seizure

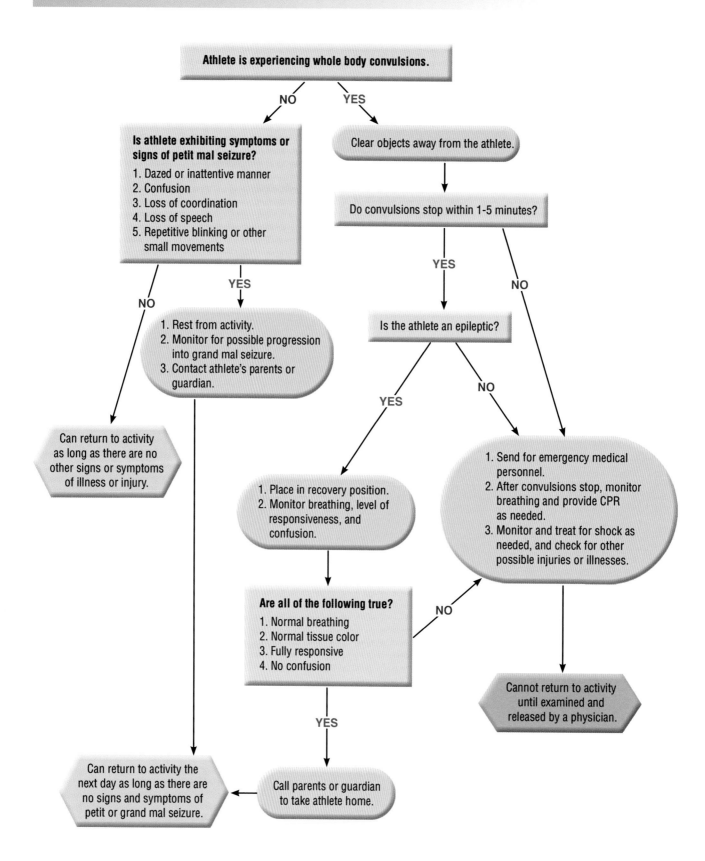

Athlete is experiencing whole body convulsions.

NO →

Is athlete exhibiting symptoms or signs of petit mal seizure?
1. Dazed or inattentive manner
2. Confusion
3. Loss of coordination
4. Loss of speech
5. Repetitive blinking or other small movements

YES →
1. Rest from activity.
2. Monitor for possible progression into grand mal seizure.
3. Contact athlete's parents or guardian.

NO → Can return to activity as long as there are no other signs or symptoms of illness or injury.

Can return to activity the next day as long as there are no signs and symptoms of petit or grand mal seizure.

YES → Clear objects away from the athlete.

Do convulsions stop within 1-5 minutes?

YES → Is the athlete an epileptic?

YES →
1. Place in recovery position.
2. Monitor breathing, level of responsiveness, and confusion.

Are all of the following true?
1. Normal breathing
2. Normal tissue color
3. Fully responsive
4. No confusion

NO → (to emergency medical personnel box)

YES → Call parents or guardian to take athlete home.

NO →
1. Send for emergency medical personnel.
2. After convulsions stop, monitor breathing and provide CPR as needed.
3. Monitor and treat for shock as needed, and check for other possible injuries or illnesses.

Cannot return to activity until examined and released by a physician.

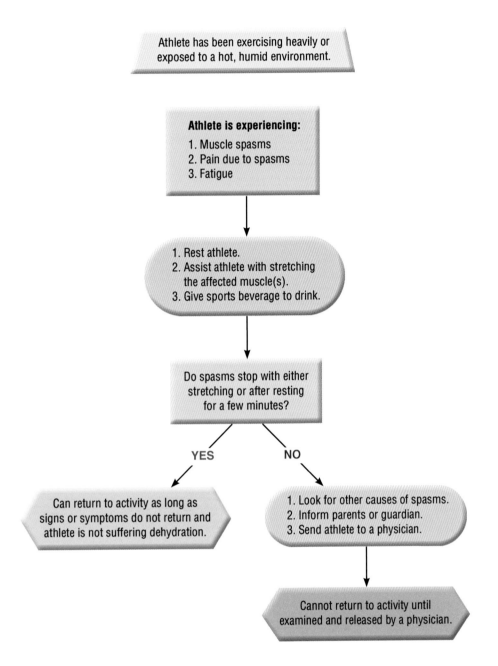

Athlete has been exercising heavily or exposed to a hot, humid environment.

Athlete is experiencing:
1. Muscle spasms
2. Pain due to spasms
3. Fatigue

1. Rest athlete.
2. Assist athlete with stretching the affected muscle(s).
3. Give sports beverage to drink.

Do spasms stop with either stretching or after resting for a few minutes?

YES

NO

Can return to activity as long as signs or symptoms do not return and athlete is not suffering dehydration.

1. Look for other causes of spasms.
2. Inform parents or guardian.
3. Send athlete to a physician.

Cannot return to activity until examined and released by a physician.

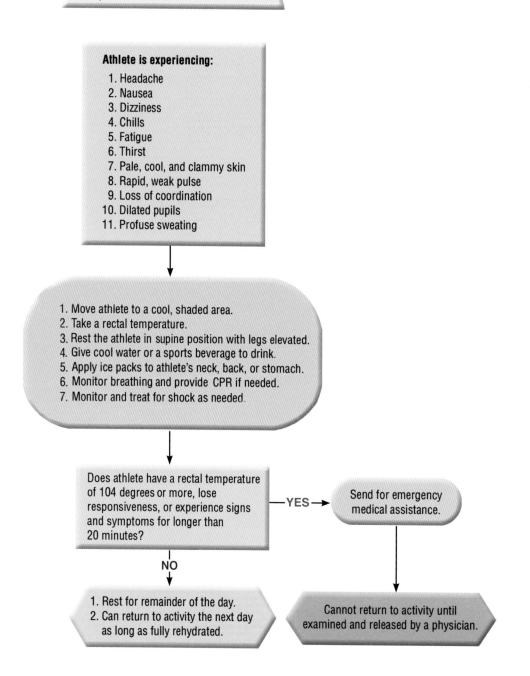

Athlete has been exercising heavily or exposed to a hot, humid environment.

Athlete is experiencing:
1. Headache
2. Nausea
3. Dizziness
4. Chills
5. Fatigue
6. Thirst
7. Pale, cool, and clammy skin
8. Rapid, weak pulse
9. Loss of coordination
10. Dilated pupils
11. Profuse sweating

1. Move athlete to a cool, shaded area.
2. Take a rectal temperature.
3. Rest the athlete in supine position with legs elevated.
4. Give cool water or a sports beverage to drink.
5. Apply ice packs to athlete's neck, back, or stomach.
6. Monitor breathing and provide CPR if needed.
7. Monitor and treat for shock as needed.

Does athlete have a rectal temperature of 104 degrees or more, lose responsiveness, or experience signs and symptoms for longer than 20 minutes?

YES → Send for emergency medical assistance.

NO

1. Rest for remainder of the day.
2. Can return to activity the next day as long as fully rehydrated.

Cannot return to activity until examined and released by a physician.

Athlete has been exercising heavily or exposed to a hot, humid environment.

Athlete is experiencing:

1. Extremely hot feelings
2. Nausea
3. Irritability
4. Fatigue
5. Hot and red skin
6. Rectal temperature of 104 degrees or more
7. Rapid breathing
8. Rapid pulse
9. Vomiting
10. Constricting pupils
11. Diarrhea
12. Confusion
13. Seizures
14. Unresponsiveness
15. Respiratory or circulatory arrest

1. Send for emergency medical assistance.
2. Move athlete to a cool, shaded area.
3. Immerse (in a semireclining position) into cold water pool or tank.
4. Remove equipment and excess clothing.
5. Monitor breathing and provide CPR if needed.
6. Monitor and treat for shock as needed.
7. If responsive and coherent, give cool water or sports beverage to drink.

Cannot return to activity until examined and released by a physician.

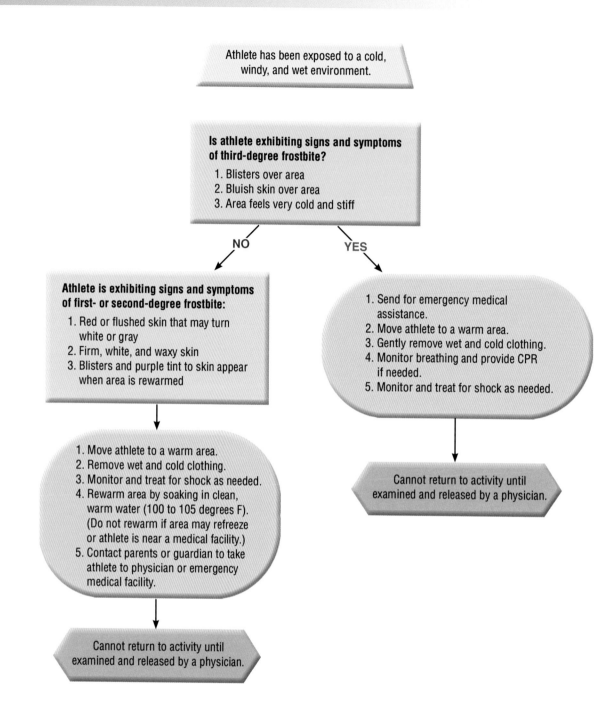

Athlete has been exposed to a cold, windy, and wet environment.

Is athlete exhibiting signs and symptoms of third-degree frostbite?

1. Blisters over area
2. Bluish skin over area
3. Area feels very cold and stiff

NO

YES

Athlete is exhibiting signs and symptoms of first- or second-degree frostbite:

1. Red or flushed skin that may turn white or gray
2. Firm, white, and waxy skin
3. Blisters and purple tint to skin appear when area is rewarmed

1. Send for emergency medical assistance.
2. Move athlete to a warm area.
3. Gently remove wet and cold clothing.
4. Monitor breathing and provide CPR if needed.
5. Monitor and treat for shock as needed.

1. Move athlete to a warm area.
2. Remove wet and cold clothing.
3. Monitor and treat for shock as needed.
4. Rewarm area by soaking in clean, warm water (100 to 105 degrees F). (Do not rewarm if area may refreeze or athlete is near a medical facility.)
5. Contact parents or guardian to take athlete to physician or emergency medical facility.

Cannot return to activity until examined and released by a physician.

Cannot return to activity until examined and released by a physician.

Athlete has been exposed to a cold, windy, and wet environment.

Is athlete exhibiting signs and symptoms of severe hypothermia?

1. Hallucinations
2. Dilated pupils
3. Slowed, erratic, or no pulse
4. Slowed breathing or respiratory arrest
5. Confusion
6. Partial responsiveness, unresponsiveness
7. No shivering
8. Muscle rigidity
9. Exposed skin is puffy and blue
10. Temperature 89 degrees or less

NO

YES

Athlete is exhibiting signs and symptoms of mild to moderate hypothermia:

1. Irritability
2. Confusion
3. Drowsiness
4. Lethargy
5. Loss of coordination
6. Loss of sensation
7. Shivering
8. Pale and hard skin
9. Numbness
10. Depression
11. Withdrawn
12. Slow, irregular pulse
13. Slowed breathing
14. Sluggish movements
15. Inability to walk
16. Difficulty speaking
17. Body temperature of 95 to 90 degrees

1. Send for emergency medical assistance.
2. Cover athlete with warm blankets.
3. Handle athlete very carefully and avoid moving as much as possible.
4. Monitor breathing and provide CPR if needed.
5. Monitor and treat for shock as needed.

Cannot return to activity until examined and released by a physician.

1. Send for emergency medical assistance.
2. Move athlete to a warm area.
3. Gently remove wet and cold clothing.
4. Wrap athlete in blankets.
5. Monitor and treat for shock as needed.

Cannot return to activity until examined and released by a physician.

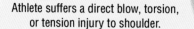

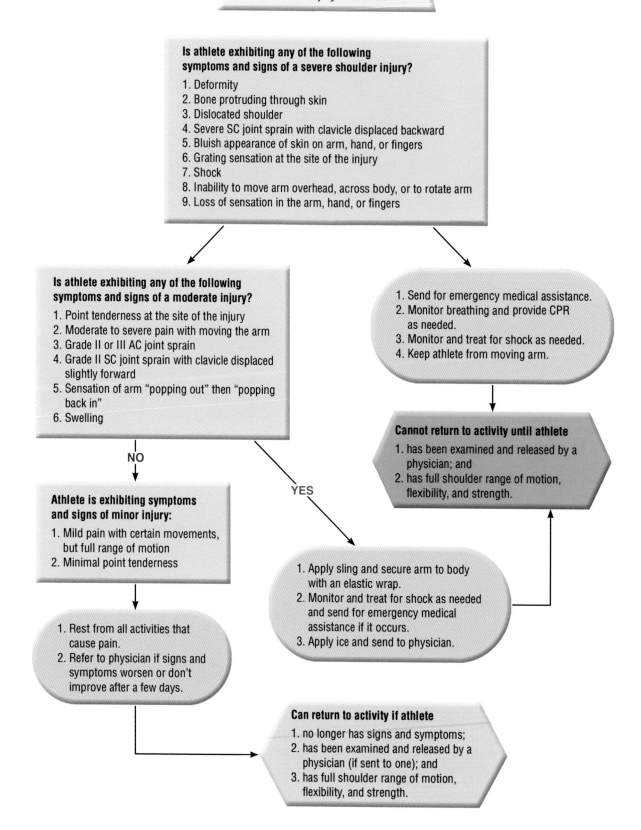

Athlete suffers a direct blow, torsion, or tension injury to shoulder.

Is athlete exhibiting any of the following symptoms and signs of a severe shoulder injury?

1. Deformity
2. Bone protruding through skin
3. Dislocated shoulder
4. Severe SC joint sprain with clavicle displaced backward
5. Bluish appearance of skin on arm, hand, or fingers
6. Grating sensation at the site of the injury
7. Shock
8. Inability to move arm overhead, across body, or to rotate arm
9. Loss of sensation in the arm, hand, or fingers

Is athlete exhibiting any of the following symptoms and signs of a moderate injury?

1. Point tenderness at the site of the injury
2. Moderate to severe pain with moving the arm
3. Grade II or III AC joint sprain
4. Grade II SC joint sprain with clavicle displaced slightly forward
5. Sensation of arm "popping out" then "popping back in"
6. Swelling

1. Send for emergency medical assistance.
2. Monitor breathing and provide CPR as needed.
3. Monitor and treat for shock as needed.
4. Keep athlete from moving arm.

Cannot return to activity until athlete

1. has been examined and released by a physician; and
2. has full shoulder range of motion, flexibility, and strength.

NO

YES

Athlete is exhibiting symptoms and signs of minor injury:

1. Mild pain with certain movements, but full range of motion
2. Minimal point tenderness

1. Apply sling and secure arm to body with an elastic wrap.
2. Monitor and treat for shock as needed and send for emergency medical assistance if it occurs.
3. Apply ice and send to physician.

1. Rest from all activities that cause pain.
2. Refer to physician if signs and symptoms worsen or don't improve after a few days.

Can return to activity if athlete

1. no longer has signs and symptoms;
2. has been examined and released by a physician (if sent to one); and
3. has full shoulder range of motion, flexibility, and strength.

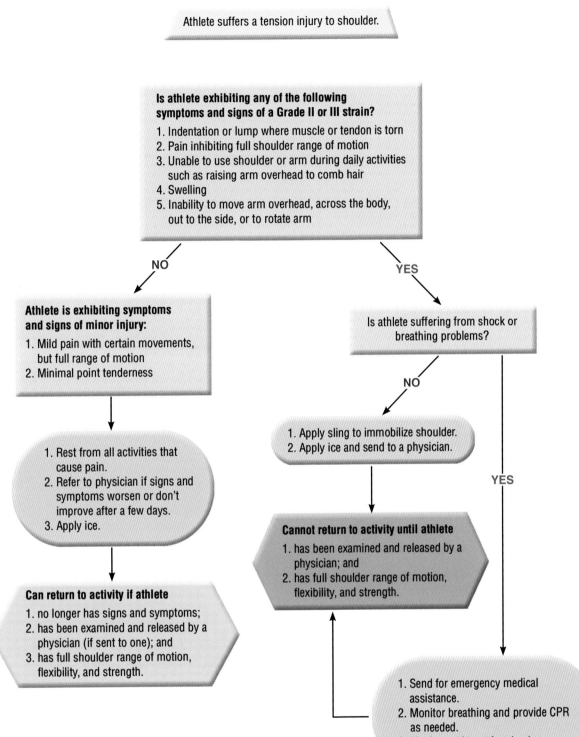

Athlete suffers a tension injury to shoulder.

Is athlete exhibiting any of the following symptoms and signs of a Grade II or III strain?

1. Indentation or lump where muscle or tendon is torn
2. Pain inhibiting full shoulder range of motion
3. Unable to use shoulder or arm during daily activities such as raising arm overhead to comb hair
4. Swelling
5. Inability to move arm overhead, across the body, out to the side, or to rotate arm

NO

YES

Athlete is exhibiting symptoms and signs of minor injury:

1. Mild pain with certain movements, but full range of motion
2. Minimal point tenderness

Is athlete suffering from shock or breathing problems?

NO

YES

1. Apply sling to immobilize shoulder.
2. Apply ice and send to a physician.

1. Rest from all activities that cause pain.
2. Refer to physician if signs and symptoms worsen or don't improve after a few days.
3. Apply ice.

Cannot return to activity until athlete

1. has been examined and released by a physician; and
2. has full shoulder range of motion, flexibility, and strength.

Can return to activity if athlete

1. no longer has signs and symptoms;
2. has been examined and released by a physician (if sent to one); and
3. has full shoulder range of motion, flexibility, and strength.

1. Send for emergency medical assistance.
2. Monitor breathing and provide CPR as needed.
3. Monitor and treat for shock.

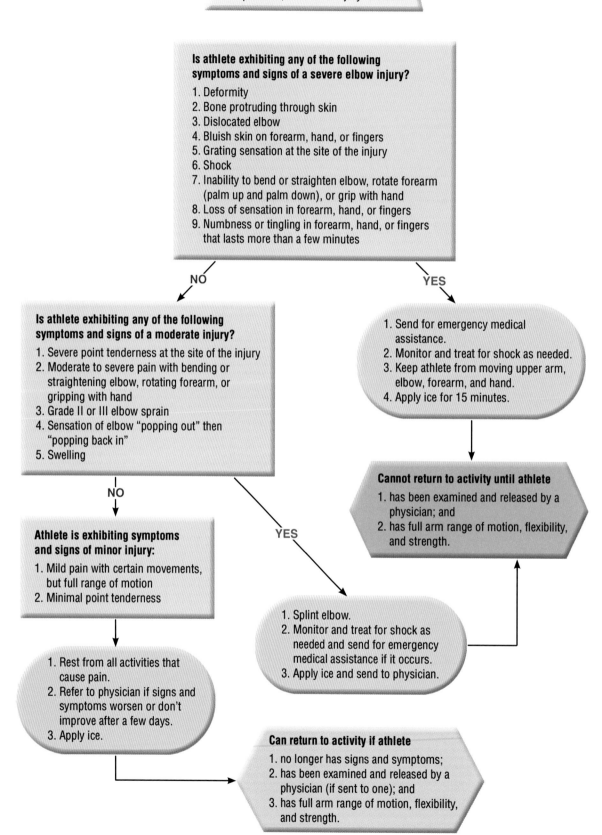

Athlete suffers a direct blow, torsion, compression, or tension injury to elbow.

Is athlete exhibiting any of the following symptoms and signs of a severe elbow injury?

1. Deformity
2. Bone protruding through skin
3. Dislocated elbow
4. Bluish skin on forearm, hand, or fingers
5. Grating sensation at the site of the injury
6. Shock
7. Inability to bend or straighten elbow, rotate forearm (palm up and palm down), or grip with hand
8. Loss of sensation in forearm, hand, or fingers
9. Numbness or tingling in forearm, hand, or fingers that lasts more than a few minutes

NO

YES

Is athlete exhibiting any of the following symptoms and signs of a moderate injury?

1. Severe point tenderness at the site of the injury
2. Moderate to severe pain with bending or straightening elbow, rotating forearm, or gripping with hand
3. Grade II or III elbow sprain
4. Sensation of elbow "popping out" then "popping back in"
5. Swelling

1. Send for emergency medical assistance.
2. Monitor and treat for shock as needed.
3. Keep athlete from moving upper arm, elbow, forearm, and hand.
4. Apply ice for 15 minutes.

NO

YES

Athlete is exhibiting symptoms and signs of minor injury:

1. Mild pain with certain movements, but full range of motion
2. Minimal point tenderness

Cannot return to activity until athlete

1. has been examined and released by a physician; and
2. has full arm range of motion, flexibility, and strength.

1. Splint elbow.
2. Monitor and treat for shock as needed and send for emergency medical assistance if it occurs.
3. Apply ice and send to physician.

1. Rest from all activities that cause pain.
2. Refer to physician if signs and symptoms worsen or don't improve after a few days.
3. Apply ice.

Can return to activity if athlete

1. no longer has signs and symptoms;
2. has been examined and released by a physician (if sent to one); and
3. has full arm range of motion, flexibility, and strength.

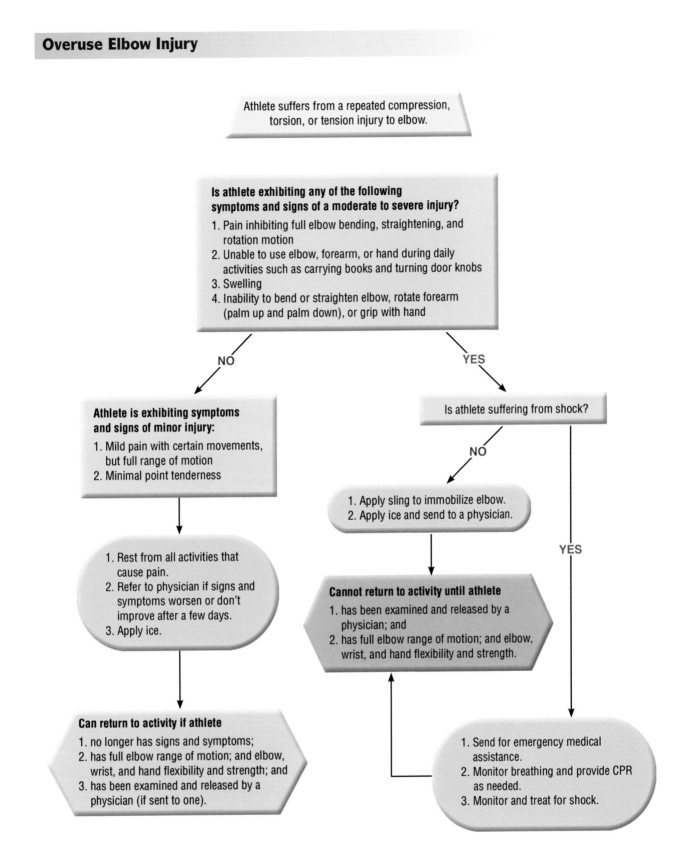

Athlete suffers from a repeated compression, torsion, or tension injury to elbow.

Is athlete exhibiting any of the following symptoms and signs of a moderate to severe injury?

1. Pain inhibiting full elbow bending, straightening, and rotation motion
2. Unable to use elbow, forearm, or hand during daily activities such as carrying books and turning door knobs
3. Swelling
4. Inability to bend or straighten elbow, rotate forearm (palm up and palm down), or grip with hand

NO

YES

Athlete is exhibiting symptoms and signs of minor injury:

1. Mild pain with certain movements, but full range of motion
2. Minimal point tenderness

Is athlete suffering from shock?

NO

1. Apply sling to immobilize elbow.
2. Apply ice and send to a physician.

1. Rest from all activities that cause pain.
2. Refer to physician if signs and symptoms worsen or don't improve after a few days.
3. Apply ice.

Cannot return to activity until athlete

1. has been examined and released by a physician; and
2. has full elbow range of motion; and elbow, wrist, and hand flexibility and strength.

YES

Can return to activity if athlete

1. no longer has signs and symptoms;
2. has full elbow range of motion; and elbow, wrist, and hand flexibility and strength; and
3. has been examined and released by a physician (if sent to one).

1. Send for emergency medical assistance.
2. Monitor breathing and provide CPR as needed.
3. Monitor and treat for shock.

Acute Forearm, Wrist, or Hand Injury

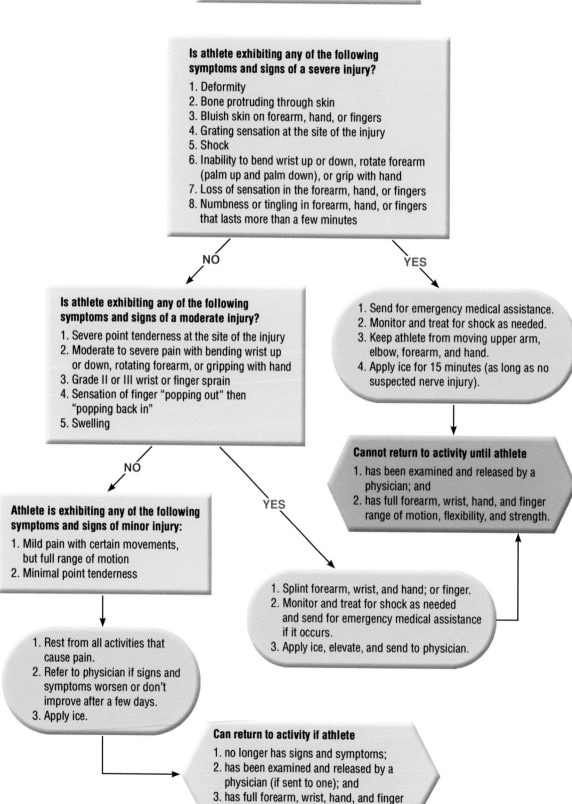

Athlete suffers a direct blow, torsion, compression, or tension injury to forearm, wrist, hand, or finger.

Is athlete exhibiting any of the following symptoms and signs of a severe injury?

1. Deformity
2. Bone protruding through skin
3. Bluish skin on forearm, hand, or fingers
4. Grating sensation at the site of the injury
5. Shock
6. Inability to bend wrist up or down, rotate forearm (palm up and palm down), or grip with hand
7. Loss of sensation in the forearm, hand, or fingers
8. Numbness or tingling in forearm, hand, or fingers that lasts more than a few minutes

NO — YES

YES:
1. Send for emergency medical assistance.
2. Monitor and treat for shock as needed.
3. Keep athlete from moving upper arm, elbow, forearm, and hand.
4. Apply ice for 15 minutes (as long as no suspected nerve injury).

Is athlete exhibiting any of the following symptoms and signs of a moderate injury?

1. Severe point tenderness at the site of the injury
2. Moderate to severe pain with bending wrist up or down, rotating forearm, or gripping with hand
3. Grade II or III wrist or finger sprain
4. Sensation of finger "popping out" then "popping back in"
5. Swelling

NO — YES

Cannot return to activity until athlete
1. has been examined and released by a physician; and
2. has full forearm, wrist, hand, and finger range of motion, flexibility, and strength.

Athlete is exhibiting any of the following symptoms and signs of minor injury:

1. Mild pain with certain movements, but full range of motion
2. Minimal point tenderness

1. Splint forearm, wrist, and hand; or finger.
2. Monitor and treat for shock as needed and send for emergency medical assistance if it occurs.
3. Apply ice, elevate, and send to physician.

1. Rest from all activities that cause pain.
2. Refer to physician if signs and symptoms worsen or don't improve after a few days.
3. Apply ice.

Can return to activity if athlete
1. no longer has signs and symptoms;
2. has been examined and released by a physician (if sent to one); and
3. has full forearm, wrist, hand, and finger range of motion, flexibility, and strength.

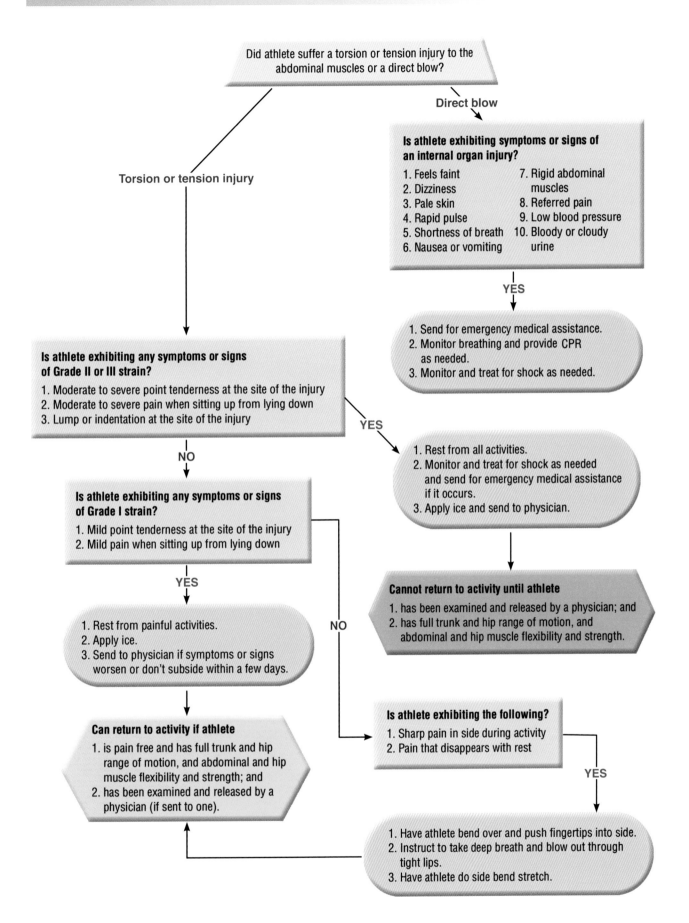

Did athlete suffer a torsion or tension injury to the abdominal muscles or a direct blow?

Direct blow

Is athlete exhibiting symptoms or signs of an internal organ injury?

1. Feels faint
2. Dizziness
3. Pale skin
4. Rapid pulse
5. Shortness of breath
6. Nausea or vomiting
7. Rigid abdominal muscles
8. Referred pain
9. Low blood pressure
10. Bloody or cloudy urine

YES

1. Send for emergency medical assistance.
2. Monitor breathing and provide CPR as needed.
3. Monitor and treat for shock as needed.

Torsion or tension injury

Is athlete exhibiting any symptoms or signs of Grade II or III strain?

1. Moderate to severe point tenderness at the site of the injury
2. Moderate to severe pain when sitting up from lying down
3. Lump or indentation at the site of the injury

YES

1. Rest from all activities.
2. Monitor and treat for shock as needed and send for emergency medical assistance if it occurs.
3. Apply ice and send to physician.

NO

Is athlete exhibiting any symptoms or signs of Grade I strain?

1. Mild point tenderness at the site of the injury
2. Mild pain when sitting up from lying down

YES

1. Rest from painful activities.
2. Apply ice.
3. Send to physician if symptoms or signs worsen or don't subside within a few days.

Cannot return to activity until athlete

1. has been examined and released by a physician; and
2. has full trunk and hip range of motion, and abdominal and hip muscle flexibility and strength.

NO

Can return to activity if athlete

1. is pain free and has full trunk and hip range of motion, and abdominal and hip muscle flexibility and strength; and
2. has been examined and released by a physician (if sent to one).

Is athlete exhibiting the following?

1. Sharp pain in side during activity
2. Pain that disappears with rest

YES

1. Have athlete bend over and push fingertips into side.
2. Instruct to take deep breath and blow out through tight lips.
3. Have athlete do side bend stretch.

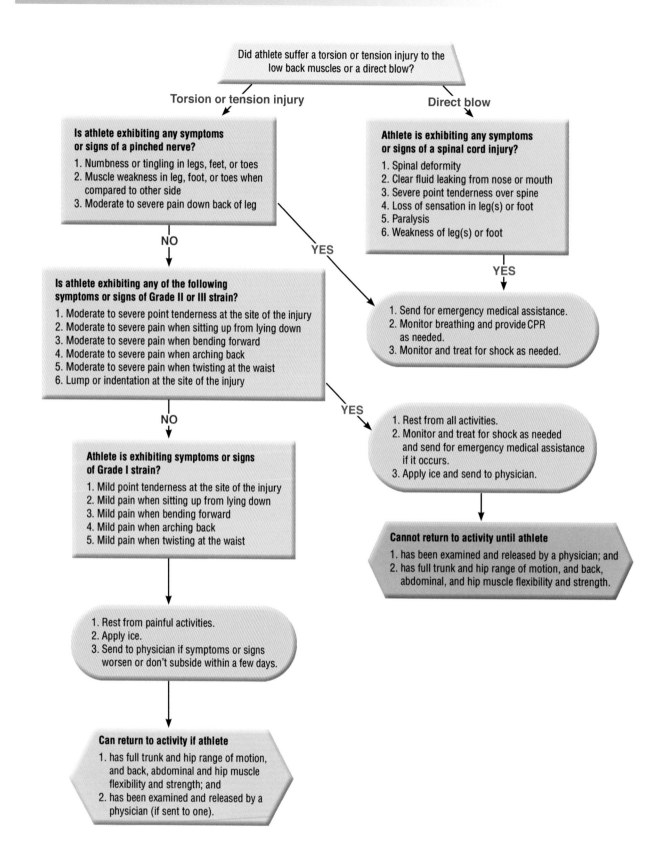

Did athlete suffer a torsion or tension injury to the low back muscles or a direct blow?

Torsion or tension injury

Is athlete exhibiting any symptoms or signs of a pinched nerve?

1. Numbness or tingling in legs, feet, or toes
2. Muscle weakness in leg, foot, or toes when compared to other side
3. Moderate to severe pain down back of leg

NO

Is athlete exhibiting any of the following symptoms or signs of Grade II or III strain?

1. Moderate to severe point tenderness at the site of the injury
2. Moderate to severe pain when sitting up from lying down
3. Moderate to severe pain when bending forward
4. Moderate to severe pain when arching back
5. Moderate to severe pain when twisting at the waist
6. Lump or indentation at the site of the injury

NO

Athlete is exhibiting symptoms or signs of Grade I strain?

1. Mild point tenderness at the site of the injury
2. Mild pain when sitting up from lying down
3. Mild pain when bending forward
4. Mild pain when arching back
5. Mild pain when twisting at the waist

1. Rest from painful activities.
2. Apply ice.
3. Send to physician if symptoms or signs worsen or don't subside within a few days.

Can return to activity if athlete

1. has full trunk and hip range of motion, and back, abdominal and hip muscle flexibility and strength; and
2. has been examined and released by a physician (if sent to one).

Direct blow

Athlete is exhibiting any symptoms or signs of a spinal cord injury?

1. Spinal deformity
2. Clear fluid leaking from nose or mouth
3. Severe point tenderness over spine
4. Loss of sensation in leg(s) or foot
5. Paralysis
6. Weakness of leg(s) or foot

YES

YES

1. Send for emergency medical assistance.
2. Monitor breathing and provide CPR as needed.
3. Monitor and treat for shock as needed.

YES

1. Rest from all activities.
2. Monitor and treat for shock as needed and send for emergency medical assistance if it occurs.
3. Apply ice and send to physician.

Cannot return to activity until athlete

1. has been examined and released by a physician; and
2. has full trunk and hip range of motion, and back, abdominal, and hip muscle flexibility and strength.

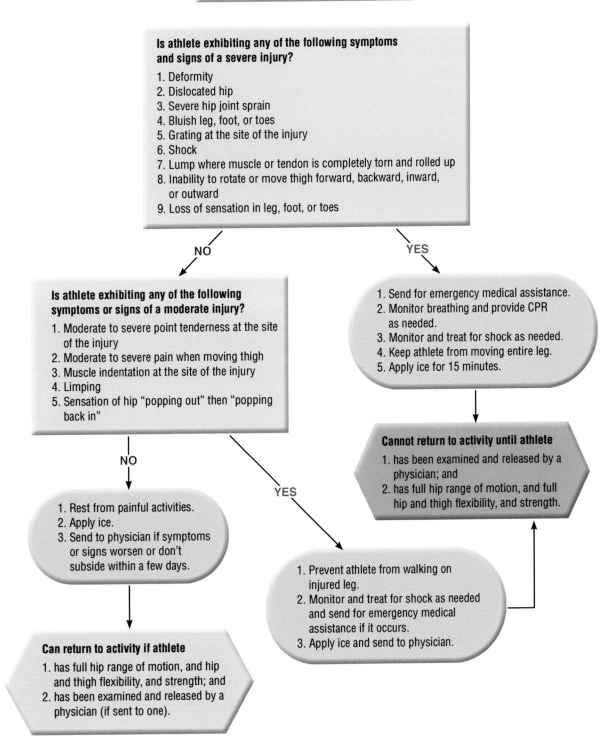

Athlete suffers a compression, torsion, or tension injury to the hip.

Is athlete exhibiting any of the following symptoms and signs of a severe injury?

1. Deformity
2. Dislocated hip
3. Severe hip joint sprain
4. Bluish leg, foot, or toes
5. Grating at the site of the injury
6. Shock
7. Lump where muscle or tendon is completely torn and rolled up
8. Inability to rotate or move thigh forward, backward, inward, or outward
9. Loss of sensation in leg, foot, or toes

NO

YES

Is athlete exhibiting any of the following symptoms or signs of a moderate injury?

1. Moderate to severe point tenderness at the site of the injury
2. Moderate to severe pain when moving thigh
3. Muscle indentation at the site of the injury
4. Limping
5. Sensation of hip "popping out" then "popping back in"

1. Send for emergency medical assistance.
2. Monitor breathing and provide CPR as needed.
3. Monitor and treat for shock as needed.
4. Keep athlete from moving entire leg.
5. Apply ice for 15 minutes.

NO

YES

1. Rest from painful activities.
2. Apply ice.
3. Send to physician if symptoms or signs worsen or don't subside within a few days.

Cannot return to activity until athlete

1. has been examined and released by a physician; and
2. has full hip range of motion, and full hip and thigh flexibility, and strength.

1. Prevent athlete from walking on injured leg.
2. Monitor and treat for shock as needed and send for emergency medical assistance if it occurs.
3. Apply ice and send to physician.

Can return to activity if athlete

1. has full hip range of motion, and hip and thigh flexibility, and strength; and
2. has been examined and released by a physician (if sent to one).

291

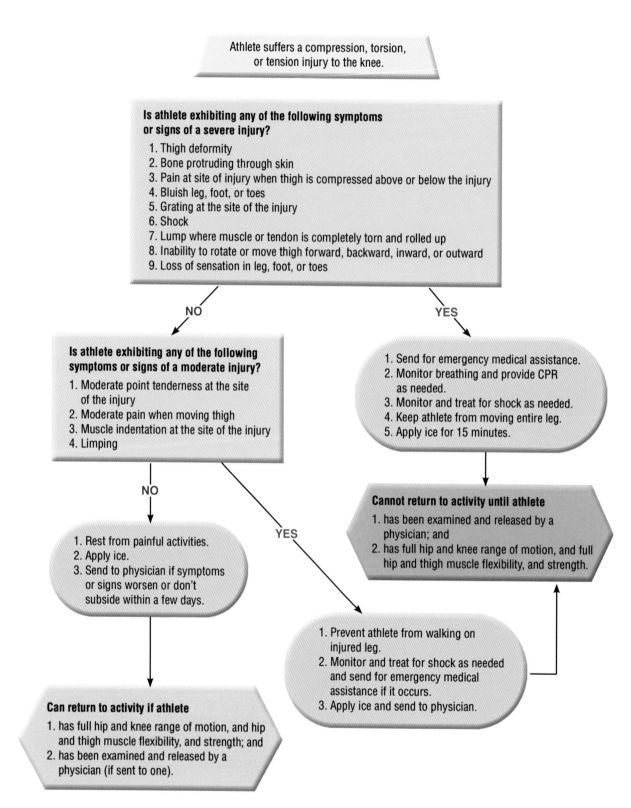

Athlete suffers a compression, torsion, or tension injury to the knee.

Is athlete exhibiting any of the following symptoms or signs of a severe injury?

1. Thigh deformity
2. Bone protruding through skin
3. Pain at site of injury when thigh is compressed above or below the injury
4. Bluish leg, foot, or toes
5. Grating at the site of the injury
6. Shock
7. Lump where muscle or tendon is completely torn and rolled up
8. Inability to rotate or move thigh forward, backward, inward, or outward
9. Loss of sensation in leg, foot, or toes

NO

YES

Is athlete exhibiting any of the following symptoms or signs of a moderate injury?

1. Moderate point tenderness at the site of the injury
2. Moderate pain when moving thigh
3. Muscle indentation at the site of the injury
4. Limping

1. Send for emergency medical assistance.
2. Monitor breathing and provide CPR as needed.
3. Monitor and treat for shock as needed.
4. Keep athlete from moving entire leg.
5. Apply ice for 15 minutes.

NO

YES

1. Rest from painful activities.
2. Apply ice.
3. Send to physician if symptoms or signs worsen or don't subside within a few days.

Cannot return to activity until athlete

1. has been examined and released by a physician; and
2. has full hip and knee range of motion, and full hip and thigh muscle flexibility, and strength.

1. Prevent athlete from walking on injured leg.
2. Monitor and treat for shock as needed and send for emergency medical assistance if it occurs.
3. Apply ice and send to physician.

Can return to activity if athlete

1. has full hip and knee range of motion, and hip and thigh muscle flexibility, and strength; and
2. has been examined and released by a physician (if sent to one).

Acute Knee Injury

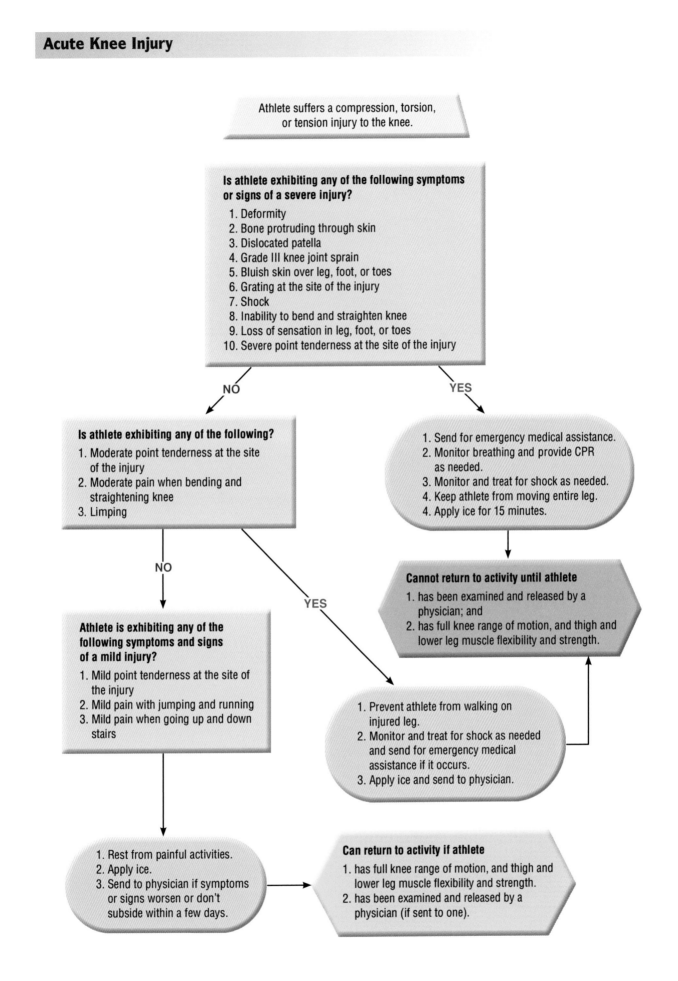

Athlete suffers a compression, torsion, or tension injury to the knee.

Is athlete exhibiting any of the following symptoms or signs of a severe injury?

1. Deformity
2. Bone protruding through skin
3. Dislocated patella
4. Grade III knee joint sprain
5. Bluish skin over leg, foot, or toes
6. Grating at the site of the injury
7. Shock
8. Inability to bend and straighten knee
9. Loss of sensation in leg, foot, or toes
10. Severe point tenderness at the site of the injury

NO

YES

Is athlete exhibiting any of the following?

1. Moderate point tenderness at the site of the injury
2. Moderate pain when bending and straightening knee
3. Limping

1. Send for emergency medical assistance.
2. Monitor breathing and provide CPR as needed.
3. Monitor and treat for shock as needed.
4. Keep athlete from moving entire leg.
4. Apply ice for 15 minutes.

NO

YES

Cannot return to activity until athlete

1. has been examined and released by a physician; and
2. has full knee range of motion, and thigh and lower leg muscle flexibility and strength.

Athlete is exhibiting any of the following symptoms and signs of a mild injury?

1. Mild point tenderness at the site of the injury
2. Mild pain with jumping and running
3. Mild pain when going up and down stairs

1. Prevent athlete from walking on injured leg.
2. Monitor and treat for shock as needed and send for emergency medical assistance if it occurs.
3. Apply ice and send to physician.

1. Rest from painful activities.
2. Apply ice.
3. Send to physician if symptoms or signs worsen or don't subside within a few days.

Can return to activity if athlete

1. has full knee range of motion, and thigh and lower leg muscle flexibility and strength.
2. has been examined and released by a physician (if sent to one).

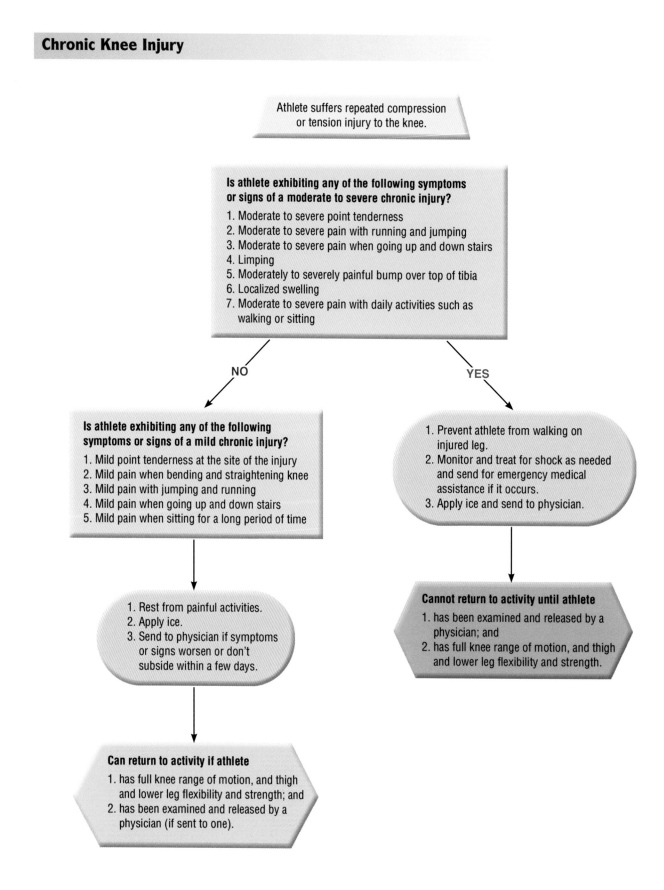

Athlete suffers repeated compression or tension injury to the knee.

Is athlete exhibiting any of the following symptoms or signs of a moderate to severe chronic injury?

1. Moderate to severe point tenderness
2. Moderate to severe pain with running and jumping
3. Moderate to severe pain when going up and down stairs
4. Limping
5. Moderately to severely painful bump over top of tibia
6. Localized swelling
7. Moderate to severe pain with daily activities such as walking or sitting

NO

YES

Is athlete exhibiting any of the following symptoms or signs of a mild chronic injury?

1. Mild point tenderness at the site of the injury
2. Mild pain when bending and straightening knee
3. Mild pain with jumping and running
4. Mild pain when going up and down stairs
5. Mild pain when sitting for a long period of time

1. Prevent athlete from walking on injured leg.
2. Monitor and treat for shock as needed and send for emergency medical assistance if it occurs.
3. Apply ice and send to physician.

1. Rest from painful activities.
2. Apply ice.
3. Send to physician if symptoms or signs worsen or don't subside within a few days.

Cannot return to activity until athlete

1. has been examined and released by a physician; and
2. has full knee range of motion, and thigh and lower leg flexibility and strength.

Can return to activity if athlete

1. has full knee range of motion, and thigh and lower leg flexibility and strength; and
2. has been examined and released by a physician (if sent to one).

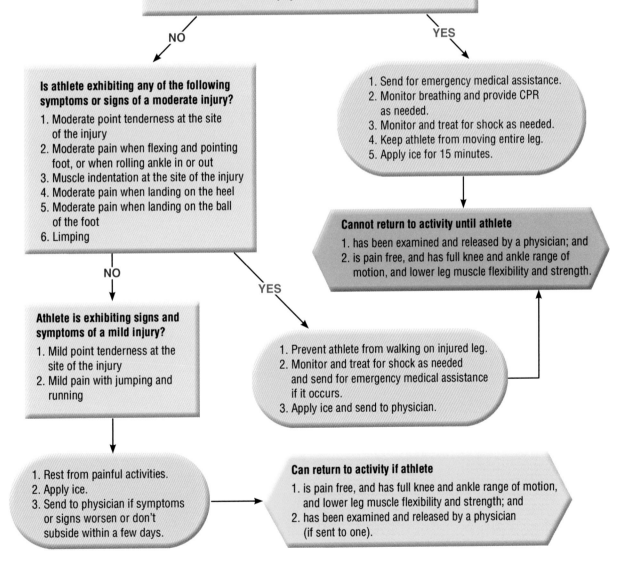

Athlete suffers a compression, torsion, or tension injury to the leg, ankle, or foot.

Is athlete exhibiting any of the following symptoms or signs of a severe injury?

1. Deformity
2. Bone protruding through skin
3. Dislocated ankle
4. Grade III ankle joint sprain
5. Lump where completely torn calf or Achilles tendon is rolled up
6. Bluish skin over leg, foot, or toes
7. Grating at the site of the injury
8. Shock
9. Inability to flex up and point foot or to roll ankle in or out
10. Loss of sensation in leg, foot, or toes
11. Severe point tenderness at the site of the injury
12. Pain at site of injury when tibia and fibula squeezed above and below the site of the injury

NO →

YES →

YES path:
1. Send for emergency medical assistance.
2. Monitor breathing and provide CPR as needed.
3. Monitor and treat for shock as needed.
4. Keep athlete from moving entire leg.
5. Apply ice for 15 minutes.

Cannot return to activity until athlete
1. has been examined and released by a physician; and
2. is pain free, and has full knee and ankle range of motion, and lower leg muscle flexibility and strength.

Is athlete exhibiting any of the following symptoms or signs of a moderate injury?

1. Moderate point tenderness at the site of the injury
2. Moderate pain when flexing and pointing foot, or when rolling ankle in or out
3. Muscle indentation at the site of the injury
4. Moderate pain when landing on the heel
5. Moderate pain when landing on the ball of the foot
6. Limping

NO →

YES →

YES path:
1. Prevent athlete from walking on injured leg.
2. Monitor and treat for shock as needed and send for emergency medical assistance if it occurs.
3. Apply ice and send to physician.

Athlete is exhibiting signs and symptoms of a mild injury?
1. Mild point tenderness at the site of the injury
2. Mild pain with jumping and running

1. Rest from painful activities.
2. Apply ice.
3. Send to physician if symptoms or signs worsen or don't subside within a few days.

Can return to activity if athlete
1. is pain free, and has full knee and ankle range of motion, and lower leg muscle flexibility and strength; and
2. has been examined and released by a physician (if sent to one).

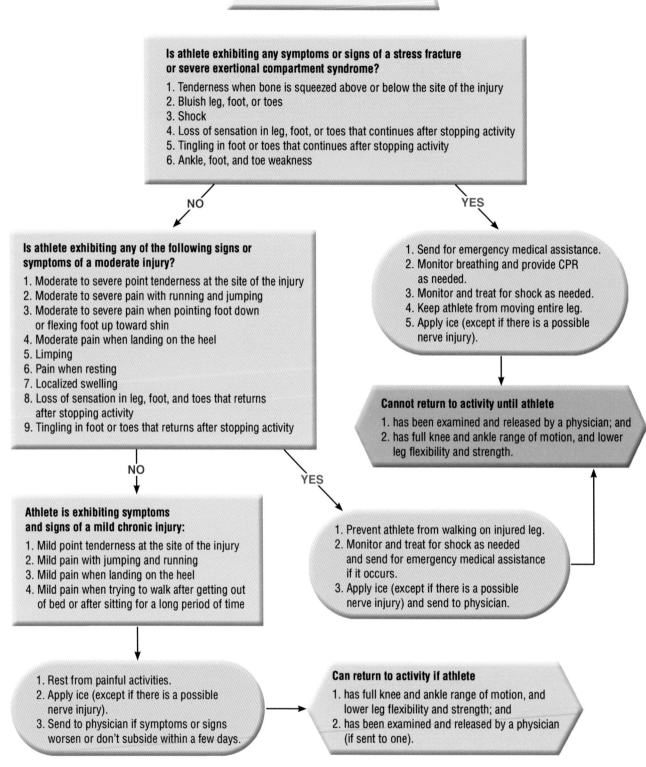

Athlete suffers from a repetitive, overuse injury to the leg, ankle, or foot.

Is athlete exhibiting any symptoms or signs of a stress fracture or severe exertional compartment syndrome?

1. Tenderness when bone is squeezed above or below the site of the injury
2. Bluish leg, foot, or toes
3. Shock
4. Loss of sensation in leg, foot, or toes that continues after stopping activity
5. Tingling in foot or toes that continues after stopping activity
6. Ankle, foot, and toe weakness

NO → / YES →

YES:
1. Send for emergency medical assistance.
2. Monitor breathing and provide CPR as needed.
3. Monitor and treat for shock as needed.
4. Keep athlete from moving entire leg.
5. Apply ice (except if there is a possible nerve injury).

Is athlete exhibiting any of the following signs or symptoms of a moderate injury?

1. Moderate to severe point tenderness at the site of the injury
2. Moderate to severe pain with running and jumping
3. Moderate to severe pain when pointing foot down or flexing foot up toward shin
4. Moderate pain when landing on the heel
5. Limping
6. Pain when resting
7. Localized swelling
8. Loss of sensation in leg, foot, and toes that returns after stopping activity
9. Tingling in foot or toes that returns after stopping activity

NO / YES

Cannot return to activity until athlete

1. has been examined and released by a physician; and
2. has full knee and ankle range of motion, and lower leg flexibility and strength.

Athlete is exhibiting symptoms and signs of a mild chronic injury:

1. Mild point tenderness at the site of the injury
2. Mild pain with jumping and running
3. Mild pain when landing on the heel
4. Mild pain when trying to walk after getting out of bed or after sitting for a long period of time

1. Prevent athlete from walking on injured leg.
2. Monitor and treat for shock as needed and send for emergency medical assistance if it occurs.
3. Apply ice (except if there is a possible nerve injury) and send to physician.

1. Rest from painful activities.
2. Apply ice (except if there is a possible nerve injury).
3. Send to physician if symptoms or signs worsen or don't subside within a few days.

Can return to activity if athlete

1. has full knee and ankle range of motion, and lower leg flexibility and strength; and
2. has been examined and released by a physician (if sent to one).

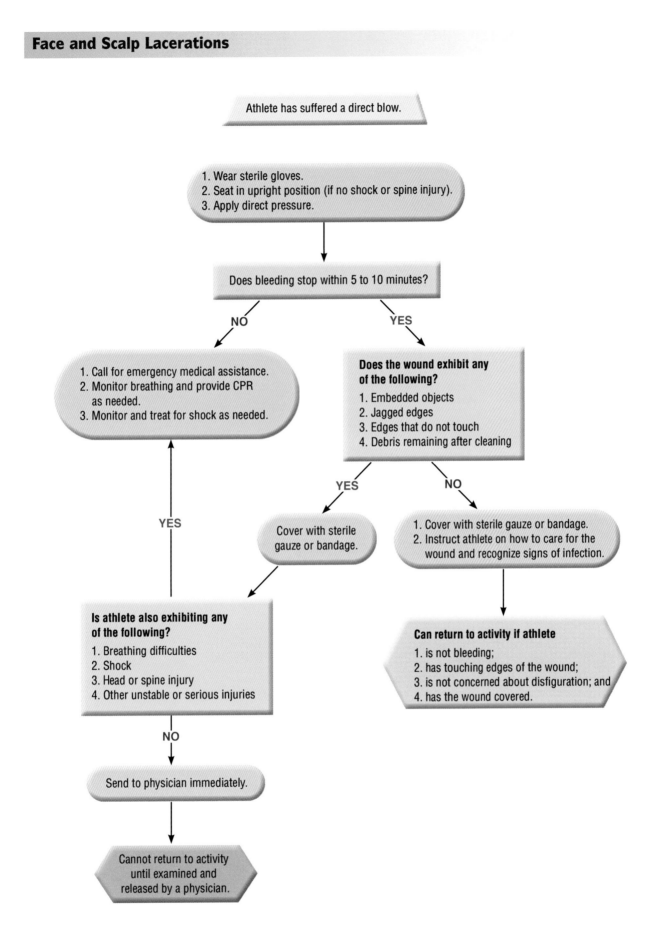

Athlete has suffered a direct blow.

1. Wear sterile gloves.
2. Seat in upright position (if no shock or spine injury).
3. Apply direct pressure.

Does bleeding stop within 5 to 10 minutes?

NO

1. Call for emergency medical assistance.
2. Monitor breathing and provide CPR as needed.
3. Monitor and treat for shock as needed.

YES

Does the wound exhibit any of the following?
1. Embedded objects
2. Jagged edges
3. Edges that do not touch
4. Debris remaining after cleaning

YES

Cover with sterile gauze or bandage.

NO

1. Cover with sterile gauze or bandage.
2. Instruct athlete on how to care for the wound and recognize signs of infection.

YES

Is athlete also exhibiting any of the following?
1. Breathing difficulties
2. Shock
3. Head or spine injury
4. Other unstable or serious injuries

NO

Send to physician immediately.

Cannot return to activity until examined and released by a physician.

Can return to activity if athlete
1. is not bleeding;
2. has touching edges of the wound;
3. is not concerned about disfiguration; and
4. has the wound covered.

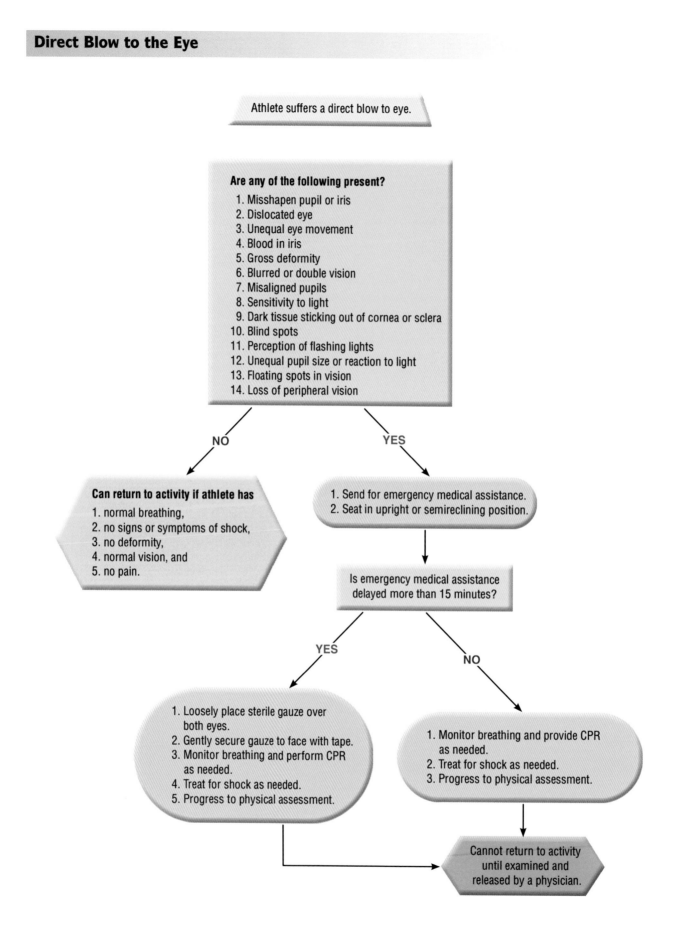

Athlete suffers a direct blow to eye.

Are any of the following present?
1. Misshapen pupil or iris
2. Dislocated eye
3. Unequal eye movement
4. Blood in iris
5. Gross deformity
6. Blurred or double vision
7. Misaligned pupils
8. Sensitivity to light
9. Dark tissue sticking out of cornea or sclera
10. Blind spots
11. Perception of flashing lights
12. Unequal pupil size or reaction to light
13. Floating spots in vision
14. Loss of peripheral vision

NO

YES

Can return to activity if athlete has
1. normal breathing,
2. no signs or symptoms of shock,
3. no deformity,
4. normal vision, and
5. no pain.

1. Send for emergency medical assistance.
2. Seat in upright or semireclining position.

Is emergency medical assistance delayed more than 15 minutes?

YES

NO

1. Loosely place sterile gauze over both eyes.
2. Gently secure gauze to face with tape.
3. Monitor breathing and perform CPR as needed.
4. Treat for shock as needed.
5. Progress to physical assessment.

1. Monitor breathing and provide CPR as needed.
2. Treat for shock as needed.
3. Progress to physical assessment.

Cannot return to activity until examined and released by a physician.

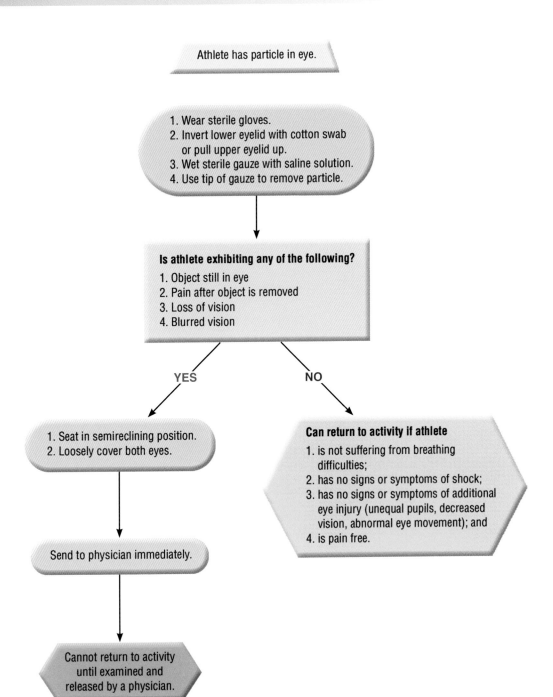

Athlete has particle in eye.

1. Wear sterile gloves.
2. Invert lower eyelid with cotton swab or pull upper eyelid up.
3. Wet sterile gauze with saline solution.
4. Use tip of gauze to remove particle.

Is athlete exhibiting any of the following?
1. Object still in eye
2. Pain after object is removed
3. Loss of vision
4. Blurred vision

YES

NO

1. Seat in semireclining position.
2. Loosely cover both eyes.

Send to physician immediately.

Cannot return to activity until examined and released by a physician.

Can return to activity if athlete
1. is not suffering from breathing difficulties;
2. has no signs or symptoms of shock;
3. has no signs or symptoms of additional eye injury (unequal pupils, decreased vision, abnormal eye movement); and
4. is pain free.

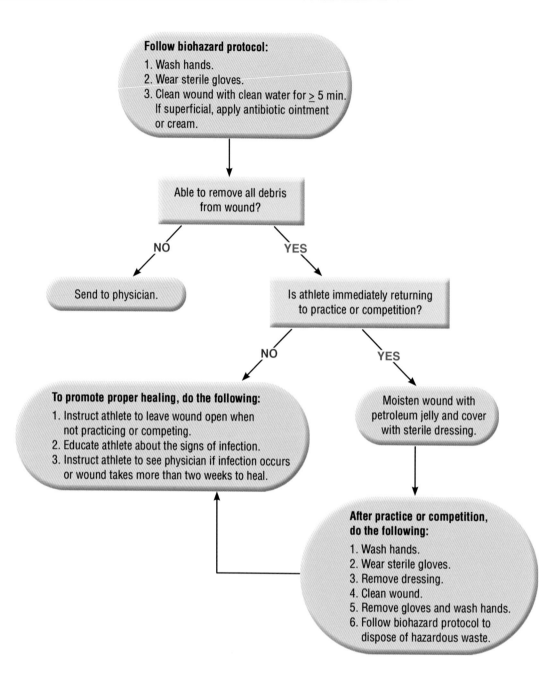

Follow biohazard protocol:
1. Wash hands.
2. Wear sterile gloves.
3. Clean wound with clean water for ≥ 5 min. If superficial, apply antibiotic ointment or cream.

Able to remove all debris from wound?

NO → Send to physician.

YES → Is athlete immediately returning to practice or competition?

NO → **To promote proper healing, do the following:**
1. Instruct athlete to leave wound open when not practicing or competing.
2. Educate athlete about the signs of infection.
3. Instruct athlete to see physician if infection occurs or wound takes more than two weeks to heal.

YES → Moisten wound with petroleum jelly and cover with sterile dressing.

After practice or competition, do the following:
1. Wash hands.
2. Wear sterile gloves.
3. Remove dressing.
4. Clean wound.
5. Remove gloves and wash hands.
6. Follow biohazard protocol to dispose of hazardous waste.

ASEP Coaches Education Programs

The question no longer is whether coaches should be trained, but *how* coaches should be trained. The American Sport Education Program (ASEP) has educated more than 1.5 million coaches since 1981 through the development and implementation of coaching education courses and resources.

ASEP PROFESSIONAL EDUCATION PROGRAM

The ASEP Professional Education Program offers coaches a three-course credentialing program known as the Bronze Level, which educates coaches across three critical disciplines. Bronze Level courses include Coaching Principles, Sport First Aid, and Coaching [Sport] Technical and Tactical Skills. To receive the Bronze Level credential, coaches must complete these three courses and also be certified in CPR. The Bronze Level is especially appropriate for coaches at the high school, college, Olympic, and serious club sport levels. In fact, 30 state high school associations, 200 colleges and universities, and 13 national governing bodies currently use, require, or recommend the Bronze Level in whole or in part to meet coaching education requirements for their organizations.

Coaching Principles provides essential education for serious coaches. *Successful Coaching, Fourth Edition,* is the text for the course. Through this course, coaches are challenged to define who they are as coaches (their coaching philosophy, objectives, and style); enhance communication and motivational skills; become more effective teachers and trainers; and improve team, relationship, risk management, and self-management skills. Coaching Principles is a study of the fundamentals of being a successful coach—before even stepping on the playing field.

Sport First Aid provides clear and up-to-date information on preventing, evaluating, and responding to more than 110 athletic injuries and illnesses. Potentially lifesaving actions covered in this course are developing a sport first aid game plan, following the emergency action steps, moving injured athletes, and following step-by-step protocols for injuries and illnesses.

The ASEP professional coaching curriculum includes the following courses and certifications:

- Coaching Principles course
- Sport First Aid course
- Bronze Level sport-specific courses (in selected sports)
- Bronze Level Certification Designation (requires CPR certification, not offered by ASEP, plus completion of Coaching Principles, Sport First Aid, and a Bronze Level sport-specific course)

Bronze Level courses are sport-specific Xs and Os courses providing coaches with practical tools for advanced-level coaching. Available courses include the following:

- Coaching Baseball Technical and Tactical Skills
- Coaching Basketball Technical and Tactical Skills
- Coaching Football Technical and Tactical Skills

- Coaching Soccer Principles
- Coaching Wrestling Principles
- Coaching Cheerleading Principles
- Coaching Softball Technical and Tactical Skills
- Coaching Swimming Principles
- Coaching Track & Field Principles
- Coaching Volleyball Principles
- Coaching Golf Principles
- Coaching Tennis Technical and Tactical Skills
- Coaching Strength and Conditioning Principles

Watch the ASEP website at www.asep.com for updates on course release dates.

Coaching Principles and Sport First Aid are offered as classroom courses taught by certified instructors and alternatively as online courses. The Coaching Principles classroom course consists of an 8-hour clinic followed by self-study of the course text and a test. The self-study and test require 32 hours to complete. The Sport First Aid classroom course follows the same format, except it is a 4-hour clinic.

Coaching Principles and Sport First Aid courses are also offered online and can be accessed via the ASEP website (www.asep.com). This approach allows coaches the flexibility to complete the course on a schedule that's right for them. After registering, each coach receives a copy of the book *Successful Coaching, Fourth Edition*, or *Sport First Aid, Fifth Edition*. In this interactive environment, coaches read sections of the book, view video, and participate in virtual exercises that simulate classroom learning and put the coach in practice- and game-day situations. These online courses provide a convenient way for coaches to learn at their own pace and save time attending in-person classroom clinics.

ASEP VOLUNTEER EDUCATION PROGRAM

For volunteer coaches, the ASEP Volunteer Education Program provides beginning and intermediate education for coaches of athletes 13 years of age and younger, plus courses and resources for parents, officials, and sport administrators working with this age group. Ideal for park and recreation departments, national youth sport organizations, YMCAs, Boys and Girls Clubs, middle schools, military and religious sport teams, and nonaffiliated local sports clubs, Coaching Youth [Sport] courses are available as online courses or through classroom instruction for baseball, basketball, football, soccer, softball, tennis, volleyball, and wrestling.

ASEP PHILOSOPHY

Built on the philosophy of "Athletes first, winning second," ASEP is committed to improving amateur sport by providing coaches with the education to put that philosophy to work. For additional information on ASEP professional and volunteer education programs, visit www.asep.com or call 800-747-5698.

Glossary

30-30 rule—Recommends suspending recreational or sporting activities and seeking shelter if thunder occurs within 30 seconds of distant lightning. Rule also promotes staying in a shelter until 30 minutes after the last lightning strike or clap of thunder.

abrasion—Scraping injury. Examples include turf burns and strawberries.

acclimatization—Period of time (approximately 7 to 10 days) used to allow the body to adjust to high heat and humidity.

Achilles tendon—Tendon attaching the calf muscles to the heel bone.

acromioclavicular (AC) joint—Area where clavicle attaches to the shoulder blade.

acute—Occurring suddenly. Examples include fractures and sprains.

airway—Passage through which air travels to the lungs. Includes the nose, mouth, and windpipe (trachea).

alveoli—Air sacs where oxygen and carbon dioxide are exchanged by the capillaries in the lungs.

anaphylactic shock—Life-threatening allergic reaction that can cause the air passages to close. Commonly happens as the result of bee stings.

anterior knee pain—Irritation between the patella and femur.

arterial bleeding—Bleeding that results from an incision, laceration, or puncture of an artery. Usually indicated by rapid bleeding or spurting of bright red blood.

artery—Large blood vessel that carries oxygen to the tissues.

asthma—Condition in which the air passages in the lungs constrict and interfere with normal breathing.

athlete's foot—Fungal infection to the foot caused by exposure to a moist, warm environment.

automated external defibrillator (AED)—Designed for use during CPR, a machine that assesses the heart's electrical rhythm, and if the rhythm is abnormal, delivers an electrical charge in attempt to restore normal rhythm.

avulsion—Forceful tearing of a structure, especially the bones or skin.

biceps muscle—Muscle along the front of the humerus, spanning from the shoulder to the elbow. Assists with raising humerus forward and bending the elbow.

blister—Fluid-filled bump between skin layers, caused by friction between layers.

boil—Large infected bump on the skin.

brachial artery—Major artery supplying oxygen-carrying blood to the arm.

bronchial tubes—Tubes through which air passes through to the lungs.

burner—Pinched nerve in the neck or shoulder.

bursa—Fluid-filled sacs located in the joints. Help to reduce friction between tendons, bones, and other joint structures.

bursitis—Inflammation of the bursa, which causes it to swell and become warm.

callus—Skin buildup over areas of friction, especially on the palm of the hands, the heels, or the feet.

capillaries—Smallest blood vessel that aids in the exchange of oxygen and carbon dioxide between blood and tissue cells.

capillary bleeding—Slow, steady oozing of blood from a damaged capillary.

cardiac arrest—Occurs when the heart stops beating.

cardiopulmonary resuscitation (CPR)—First aid for cardiac and respiratory arrest.

carotid pulse—Heartbeat felt at the carotid artery in the neck.

cartilage—Gristlelike connective tissue usually found covering ends of bones. It protects the bones from friction and shock.

cauliflower ear—Contusion to the outside ear.

cervical spine—Neck portion of the spinal column.

chronic—Prolonged or gradually occurring.

circulatory system—System that supplies blood to the body. Includes the heart, arteries, arterioles, veins, and capillaries, as well as other structures.

clavicle—Collarbone.

closed fracture—Broken bone that does not break through the skin.

compression—Application of pressure over an area to reduce bleeding or swelling.

compression injury—Injury resulting when tissue suffers a direct blow.

concussion—Temporary malfunction of the brain resulting from a direct blow to the head. Can cause memory loss, dizziness, headache, nausea, and unresponsiveness.

conduction—Method in which the body loses or gains heat by coming in contact with warmer or colder objects.

contusion—Bruising injury causing bleeding, swelling, and discoloration.

convection—Method by which heat is lost or gained to circulating air (wind) around the body.

dehydration—Low level of water in the body.

deltoid muscles—Muscles around the front, back, and side of the shoulder. Assist with flexing arm forward, extending arm backward, and raising the arm to the side.

dentist—Health professional who evaluates and treats conditions and injuries of the mouth, teeth, and jaw.

diabetes—Disorder in which the body is unable to produce or regulate the insulin needed to control blood sugar levels.

digestive system—System that breaks food down into substances that can be used as fuel by the body tissues.

direct pressure—Application of pressure over a wound to help stop bleeding.

dislocation—Condition in which a bone shifts out of position at a joint and does not relocate to its normal position.

elevation—Raising of a body part above heart level.

emergency action steps—Assess the scene and the athlete, alert, and attend to breathing.

emergency medical technicians (EMTs)—Health professionals specially trained to handle emergency medical conditions.

ephedra—Substance found in the herb, ma huang, that is taken as a supplement. Considered a stimulant like amphetamines.

epiphyseal fracture—Growth plate fracture.

evaporation—Method of heat transfer that involves cooling the body via sweat evaporation.

exertional compartment syndrome—Increase in pressure, typically in front of the lower leg, that constricts blood flow to the lower leg and foot.

extension—Straightening of a joint.

fainting—Temporary unresponsiveness; a mild form of shock.

femoral artery—Major blood vessel carrying oxygen-filled blood to the leg.

femur—Thigh bone.

flexion—Bending of a joint.

fracture—Break in a bone.

frostbite—Freezing of the superficial skin tissues and possible deeper tissues such as muscles.

gastrocnemius (calf)—Muscle located on the back of the lower leg. Helps to point the foot down and bend the knee.

gastroenteritis—Sudden infection or toxin exposure affecting the stomach and intestines. Includes conditions commonly referred to as the stomach flu or food poisoning.

glucose—Form of sugar used by the body for energy.

golfer's elbow—Inflammation where the wrist and forearm muscles attach to the inside of the lower part of the humerus.

grand mal seizure—Seizure resulting in sever muscle spasms or convulsions.

growth plate—Area on the ends of bones where growth takes place.

hamstrings—Muscles located on the back of the thigh. Help to bend the knee and extend the hip.

heat cramps—Muscle cramps caused by dehydration or loss of electrolytes through sweat.

heat exhaustion—Shocklike condition caused by dehydration. A key sign of heat exhaustion is profuse sweating. Other signs include cool and clammy skin.

heatstroke—Life-threatening illness caused by extreme dehydration. Body temperature rises to 105 degrees or higher and the skin is red, hot, and dry.

Heimlich maneuver—First aid for choking.

hernia—Protrusion of soft tissue through a muscle. Typically occurs in the abdominal or front hip muscles.

herpes simplex—Infectious fever blister or cold sore on lips, mouth, nose, chin, or cheek.

hip flexor—Muscles spanning from the front of the hip to the thigh. Assist with lifting the thigh up.

hip pointer—Contusion or bruise to the pelvic bone located on the front of the hip.

history—Information gathered to help determine the nature, extent, and mechanism of an injury.

humerus—Upper arm bone.

hyperextension—Straightening of a joint past its normal range.

hyperflexion—Bending of a joint beyond its normal bending range.

hyperglycemia—High blood sugar level, often caused by diabetes.

hyperventilation—Rapid breathing that creates a deficit of carbon dioxide in the bloodstream and upsets the oxygen and carbon dioxide balance.

hypoglycemia—Low blood sugar level, often caused by diabetes.

hypothermia—Condition in which the body temperature lowers to abnormally low levels. Caused by extreme fatigue and exposure to a cold, windy environment.

iliotibial band strain—Connective tissue along the outside of the thigh, spanning from the hip to the knee.

impingement—Injury in which tissue is pinched between two surfaces.

incision—Soft-tissue cut caused by a sharp object.

inflammation—Irritation to a body structure. Often causes swelling, scar tissue, and heat in the area.

influenza—Contagious viral infection affecting the respiratory system (nose, throat, and lungs).

inspection—Evaluation technique used to determine the nature of an injury. Inspection signs to look for include swelling, discoloration, deformity, and skin color.

insulin—Hormone or chemical that enables body tissue to use sugar or glucose as energy.

insulin reaction—Condition in which an athlete's glucose (sugar) levels drop below normal levels (hypoglycemia).

inversion—Injury in which the ankle is twisted inward.

jock itch—Fungal infection of the genital area.

joint—Junction between bones that allows the body to move. Examples include knee, elbow, shoulder, ankle, and wrist.

ketoacidosis—Condition caused by a severe or prolonged insulin deficiency that can result in a high blood glucose (sugar) level (hyperglycemia).

kidney—Organ of the urinary system used to help rid the body of energy breakdown waste products.

laceration—Soft-tissue cut caused by a blow with a blunt object.

ligament—Fibrous tissue that connects bone to bone and prevents bones from shifting over each other. Primary stabilizers of the body joints.

loss of function—Inability of a body part to carry out its function because of injury. An example is loss of function at the knee would be an inability to bend or straighten it.

lumbar spine—Portion of the spinal column located at the low back area.

lungs—Organs in which oxygen and carbon dioxide are exchanged between the air and the capillaries.

mechanism of injury—Cause of an injury that may be sudden or gradual. Examples include direct blow, twisting, or friction injuries.

molluscum contagiosum—Skin growth caused by a viral infection in the top layers of the skin

neurological system—System that controls and coordinates the functioning of all systems and tissues within the body. It is made up of the brain, spinal cord, and a network of nerves.

open fracture—Broken bone that pierces the skin.

ophthalmologist—Physician specializing in the medical and surgical care of the eyes and in the prevention of eye disease and injury.

optometrist—Health professional with specialized training and certification in diagnosing vision problems and eye disease. Also trained to prescribe eyeglasses, contact lenses, and drugs to treat eye disorders.

oral surgeon—Dentist who is trained in the surgical treatment of conditions affecting the mouth, teeth and jaw, and portions of the face.

orthopedist—Physician trained to diagnose and provide medical and surgical care for injuries to bones, muscles, and other joint tissues such as cartilage, tendons, ligaments, and nerves.

Osgood-Schlatter disease—Irritation to the junction where the kneecap tendon inserts into the lower leg bone.

osteoarthritis—Bone wear and tear that occurs over time.

overuse—Injury caused by overusing a weak or inflexible muscle, tendon, or bone. Can cause the tissue to gradually swell, become painful, and lose function.

paramedic—Health professional specially trained to handle emergency medical conditions.

paratendinitis—An inflammation or thickening of the tendon sheath (not a synovial sheath).

patella—Kneecap.

pectoral muscles—Chest muscles spanning form the sternum and clavicle to the humerus. Assist with bringing arm forward across the body.

petit mal seizure—Typically a brief (lasting seconds) seizure characterized by a dazed or inattentive manner, confusion, loss of coordination, possible speech loss, repetitive blinking, or other small movements.

physiatrist—Physician that specializes in diagnosing, treating, and prescribing rehabilitation for all forms of conditions that affect the musculoskeletal system.

physical assessment—Inspection conducted after the emergency action steps to determine the site, location, and severity of other injuries. Includes HIT, or history, inspection, and touch.

plantar fasciitis—Stretching or inflammation of the tissue that spans from the heel to the toes.

podiatrist—Doctor who specializes in handling disorders of the legs and feet.

pressure points—Areas where pressure should be applied to reduce blood flow to another area. Located in the upper arm and leg. Used as a last resort in controlling bleeding in the arms or legs.

PRICE—Protection, rest, ice, compression, and elevation.

puncture—Deep, narrow soft-tissue wound caused by being stabbed with a thin object.

quadriceps—Muscle located on the front of the thigh. It helps to straighten the knee and move the thigh forward.

radial pulse—Heartbeat felt at the wrist.

radiation—Method in which electromagnetic waves, such as from the sun, can increase the body's heat.

respiratory arrest—Occurs when breathing stops.

respiratory system—System that exchanges oxygen and carbon dioxide between the air and the blood. Includes the nose, mouth, windpipe, and lungs.

rhomboid muscle—Muscle between the shoulder blade and spine that pulls the shoulder blade toward the spine.

ringworm—Fungal infection of skin.

rotator cuff—Group of four muscles located on the shoulder blade. Used primarily in throwing and overhead shoulder motions, as well as in forehand and backhand strokes.

seizure—Episode of abnormal electrical activity within the brain. It can lead to sudden changes in an athlete's alertness, behavior, and muscle control.

shearing—Injury involving friction or rubbing between two surfaces.

shin splints—Overuse injury to the lower leg often caused by muscle weakness and inflexibility.

shock—Systemic body reaction to physical or emotional injury. The body deprives the skin, arms, legs, and other less essential tissues of oxygen and blood to ensure supplies to the brain, heart, and lungs.

side stitch—Pain in the side felt during endurance activities.

sign—Physical evidence of injury. Includes swelling, discoloration, and deformity.

solar plexus—Nervous system structure that assists in breathing. Located near the stomach.

spleen—Organ that acts as a reservoir of red blood cells.

sprain—Stretch or tear of a ligament.

standardized assessment of concussion (SAC)—Tests used to assess the extent of the symptoms and signs of a concussion.

sternoclavicular (SC) joint—Area where collarbone attaches to sternum.

sternum—Breastbone.

strain—Stretch or tear of a muscle or tendon.

stress fracture—Bone fracture caused by overuse. The fracture develops slowly while the bone is experiencing repeated stress such as in long-distance running.

subluxation—Condition in which a bone shifts out of position at a joint, then relocates to its normal position.

sweating—Mechanism through which the body cools itself. Water is transported to the skin, where it is evaporated to cool the body.

symptoms—Complaint(s) associated with injury Includes pain, numbness, tingling, and grating feelings.

synovial sheath—Covering around tendon fibers. Secretes and absorbs a fluid that helps to act as a lubricant between tendon fibers and bundles.

tendinitis—Inflammation of a tendon. Causes swelling, warmth, and scar tissue.

tendinosis—Condition in which micro tears occur in a tendon.

tendon—Fibroelastic structure that connects muscle to bone.

tennis elbow—Inflammation of the junction where the wrist and forearm muscles attach to the outside of the upper arm bone.

tenosynovitis—Inflammation of the synovial sheath that surrounds a tendon.

tension injury—An injury involving tissue that is stretched beyond its normal limits.

thoracic spine—Portion of the spinal column located at the upper and midback area.

tibia—Shinbone.

torsion—Twisting injury.

trachea (wind pipe)—Tube in the neck through which air passes from the nose and mouth to the lungs.

trapezius muscle—Muscle extending from the base of the skull to the outer tips of the shoulder and down to just above the low back. Different portions of the trapezius shrug the shoulders, extend the head backward, and squeeze the shoulder blades together.

triceps muscle—Muscle along the back of the humerus, spanning from the shoulder to the elbow. Assists with extending the humerus backward and straightening the elbow.

turf toe—Hyperextension injury of the big toe.

ulnar nerve—Runs behind the inside of the elbow joint. Sends impulses from the brain to the forearm and hand.

ureter—Tube that transports urine from the kidneys to the bladder.

urinary system—System that rids the body of the waste products resulting from energy breakdown. Consists of the kidneys, ureter, and bladder.

venous bleeding—Bleeding that results from an incision, laceration, or puncture of a vein. Usually indicated by rapid bleeding of dark red blood.

vertebrae—Bones of the spinal column.

windchill—Index used to indicate the effect of wind on cold temperatures.

Index

Note: The italicized *f* and *t* following page numbers refer to figures and tables, respectively.

About the Author

Melinda J. Flegel has 27 years of experience as a certified athletic trainer. For 13 years, she was head athletic trainer at the University of Illinois SportWell Center, where she oversaw sports medicine care and injury prevention education for the university's recreational and club sport athletes.

As coordinator of outreach services at the Great Plains Sports Medicine and Rehabilitation Center in Peoria, Illinois, Flegel provided athletic training services to athletes at more than 15 high schools and regularly consulted with their coaches about sport first aid. As the center's educational program coordinator and an American Red Cross CPR instructor, Flegel gained valuable firsthand experience in helping coaches become proficient first responders.

Flegel has taught a sports injury course at the University of Illinois. She holds master's and bachelor's degrees from the University of Illinois, is a member of the National Athletic Trainers' Association and the National Strength and Conditioning Association, and has been a Certified Strength and Conditioning Specialist since 1987.

In addition to writing *Sport First Aid*, Flegel has written several book chapters, including Injury Prevention and First Aid for the *Health on Demand* textbook.

Find more outstanding resources at

US.HumanKinetics.com
Canada.HumanKinetics.com

In the **U.S.** call 1-800-747-4457
Canada 1-800-465-7301
International 1-217-351-5076

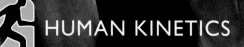
HUMAN KINETICS